MEDICAL-SURGICAL NURSING

A CONCEPT APPROACH

MEDICAL-SURGICAL NURSING

A CONCEPT APPROACH

  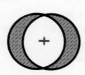 

Trish Burton

Ali Moloney

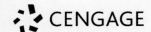

Medical-Surgical Nursing: A concept approach
1st Edition
Trish Burton
Ali Moloney

Portfolio manager: Fiona Hammond
Senior product manager: Michelle Aarons
Senior content developer: Kylie Scott / Eleanor Yeoell
Senior project editor: Nathan Katz
Text designer: Cengage Creative Studio
Cover designer: Cengage Creative Studio
Cover/concept map illustrations: Florence Chereau
Permissions/Photo researcher: Catherine Kerstjens
Editor: Sylvia Marson
Proofreader: James Anderson
Indexer: KnowledgeWorks Global Limited
Art direction: Linda Davidson / Danielle Maccarone
Typeset by KnowledgeWorks Global Limited

Any URLs contained in this publication were checked for currency during the production process. Note, however, that the publisher cannot vouch for the ongoing currency of URLs.

This first edition published in 2025

Notice to the Reader
Every effort has been made to review and confirm the accuracy of content in this publication. By following the instructions contained herein the reader willingly assumes all risks in connection with such instructions. The reader should review procedures, treatments, drug dosages or legal content. Neither the authors nor the publisher assume any liability for injury or damage to persons or property arising from any error or omission. Inclusion of proprietary names for any drugs or devices should not be interpreted as a recommendation.

Acknowledgement
Cengage acknowledges the Traditional Owners and Custodians of the lands of all First Nations Peoples of Australia. We pay respect to Elders past and present. We recognise the continuing connection of First Nations Peoples to the land, air and waters, and thank them for protecting these lands, waters and ecosystems since time immemorial. Warning – First Nations Australians are advised that this book and associated learning materials may contain images, videos or voices of deceased persons.

For product information and technology assistance,
in Australia call **1300 790 853**;
in New Zealand call **0800 449 725**

For permission to use material from this text or product, please email **aust.permissions@cengage.com**

National Library of Australia Cataloguing-in-Publication Data
ISBN: 9780170459983
A catalogue record for this book is available from the National Library of Australia.

Cengage Learning Australia
Level 5, 80 Dorcas Street
Southbank VIC 3006 Australia

For learning solutions, visit **cengage.com.au**

Printed in China by 1010 Printing International Limited.
1 2 3 4 5 6 7 28 27 26 25 24

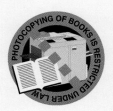

BRIEF CONTENTS

CONTENTS

PART 3

INTERPROFESSIONAL APPROACHES TO CARE   **187**

Guide to the text

As you read this text you will find a number of features in every chapter to enhance your study of Medical-Surgical Nursing and help you understand how the theory is applied in the real world.

PART-OPENING FEATURES

Refer to the part-opening **Chapter list** for an outline of the chapters in each part.

PART **03**

INTERPROFESSIONAL APPROACHES TO CARE

CHAPTER-OPENING FEATURES

Each chapter begins with a **vignette** that allows you to gain insight into how the theory and concepts covered in the chapter relate to the real world.

Identify the key concepts you will engage with through the **Learning objectives** at the start of each chapter.

Refer to the **Introduction** for a contextualised summary of the chapter.

CHAPTER **4**

CARDIOVASCULAR SYSTEM

The most common types of cardiovascular disease in Australia include coronary heart disease, atrial fibrillation, peripheral arterial disease and cardiac valve disease. Aboriginal and Torres Strait Islander peoples have a higher mortality rate than non-Aboriginal and Torres Strait Islanders from cardiovascular disease. Cardiovascular disease causes more deaths in women than any other disease. Aboriginal and Torres Strait Islander women are twice as likely to die from coronary heart disease as non-Aboriginal and Torres Strait Islander women (Australian Institute of Health and Welfare, 2019).

LEARNING OBJECTIVES
After reading this chapter, you should have an understanding of the:
1 assessment required for a person with a cardiac condition
2 prioritisation of key components in the development of plans of care for a person with the cardiac conditions of:
  – acute myocardial infarction
  – atrial fibrillation and deep vein thrombosis
  – heart valve disease – mitral regurgitation
3 prioritised and targeted nursing interventions required to promote recovery or prevent further deterioration of people presenting with the cardiac conditions of acute myocardial infarction, atrial fibrillation and deep vein thrombosis, and heart valve disease – mitral regurgitation
4 evaluation phase and how the prioritised and targeted nursing interventions inform further assessment of the person, planning of care and collaboration with the healthcare team
5 discharge planning and coordination of care required when preparing the person for discharge and subsequent continuity of care between the person and their healthcare providers.

INTRODUCTION
The cardiovascular system consists of the heart and blood vessels. The heart pumps oxygenated blood within arteries, arterioles and capillaries; deoxygenated blood is removed via the capillaries, venules and veins to be returned to the heart and the arterial system, and in turn oxygenated by the lungs. Health problems of the cardiovascular system invariably disrupt the person's activity levels and decrease their sense of wellbeing, which in turn impacts on their quality of life and lifespan. Whether the condition is newly diagnosed or is long term and considered chronic in presentation, the concepts of person-centred care are the same, with the goal of maintaining cardiovascular function so the individual can maintain a level of activities of daily living and a quality of life that represents their situation.
Common problems of the cardiovascular system can be divided into vascular disorders (hypertension, peripheral vascular disease, aneurysms, thrombus formation and shock), coronary heart disease (atherosclerosis and acute coronary syndrome), heart failure, valvular disease and dysrhythmias.

FEATURES WITHIN CHAPTERS

A **Prioritisation Planner** enables you to plan appropriate nursing care at the beginning of the shift. This aims to assist you in applying clinical decision making to nursing care. The Prioritisation Planner template appears at the end of Chapter 1 and is also available from your instructor.

NURSING PRIORITISATION PLANNER						
INTRODUCTION		Problem identification (SITUATION/BACKGROUND)	Planning	Implementation	Evaluation	Discharge planning and coordination of care
Bed/ Room No.	Name/ DOB/ Medical record number	Assessment Diagnosis (situation) Relevant medical history (Background)	Prioritise activities using the *nursing care plan, primary survey and time-sensitive indicators* Cues: ■ Primary survey – airway, breathing, circulation, disability and environment. ■ Secondary survey – head to toe assessment ■ A to G assessment for the patient/deteriorating patient ■ Time-sensitive indicators – diagnostic testing, assessment interpretation, surgical and medical treatments, medication management and interpretation to patient responses to care and potential deterioration. ■ Nursing care plan activities.	Outline the interventions (actions) for the upcoming shift. What further assessments should be initiated?		

Subjective assessment and **Objective assessment** boxes highlight key prompts for nursing assessment in each of the Part 2 clinical chapters.

Planning boxes indicate the areas that are targeted in the planning stage of assessment and nursing care for each of the common presentations explored in Part 2.

BOX 16.1 SUBJECTIVE ASSESSMENT

➤ History of illness
➤ Past health history
➤ Medications
➤ Surgery

Functional health patterns:
– Health perception and management
– Nutritional and metabolic
– Elimination
– Activity and exercise
– Sleep and rest
– Cognitive and perceptual
– Self-perception and concept
– Role relationship
– Sexuality and reproductive
– Coping and stress
– Values and beliefs
➤ Risk calculation

BOX 16.2 OBJECTIVE ASSESSMENT

➤ Inspect and palpate breasts
➤ Inspect and palpate external genitalia
➤ Diagnostic tests – hormone studies – urine and blood, cultures and smears, cytological studies, mammography, ultrasound, biopsy, and computed tomography, magnetic resonance imaging, hysteroscopy, hysterosalpingogram, colposcopy, conisation, laparoscopy, dilation and curettage
➤ Other body systems as appropriate

BOX 15.3 PLANNING CARE FOR MUSCULOSKELETAL INJURY

➤ Physical activity
➤ Medication
➤ Monitor vital signs
➤ Neurovascular observations – paraesthesia, absence of sensation
➤ Reduced or absent pulses to affected extremity
➤ Restricted function – attending to ADLs as dominant hand is right
➤ Management of cast/splint or assistive devices

BOX 6.3 PLANNING FOR AN ACUTE NEUROLOGICAL CONDITION

➤ Previous medical history
➤ Previous surgical history
➤ Nature of injury – accelerant, blunt force
➤ C-spine precautions
➤ Serum sodium levels and electrolytes
➤ Alcohol – BAL
➤ Substances of abuse screening
➤ LOC/GCS/pupillary response
➤ Medication
➤ Monitor blood pressure
➤ Thermoregulation
➤ Secondary assessment – other injuries to review

FEATURES WITHIN CHAPTERS

Concept map sequences illustrate common presentations throughout the text and are colour-coded to align with each of the steps in the nursing process. The concept maps visually demonstrate linkages between concepts, knowledge and clinical decisions for each presentation with a focus on person-centred care.

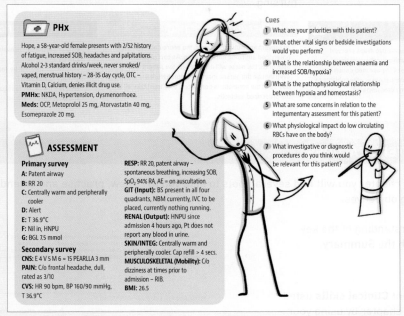

PHx

Hope, a 58-year-old female presents with 2/52 history of fatigue, increased SOB, headaches and palpitations. Alcohol 2-3 standard drinks/week, never smoked/vaped, menstrual history – 28-35 day cycle, OTC – Vitamin D, Calcium, denies illicit drug use.
PMHx: NKDA, Hypertension, dysmenorrhoea.
Meds: OCP, Metoprolol 25 mg, Atorvastatin 40 mg, Esomeprazole 20 mg.

ASSESSMENT

Primary survey
A: Patent airway
B: RR 20
C: Centrally warm and peripherally cooler
D: Alert
E: T 36.9°C
F: Nil in, HNPU
G: BGL 7.5 mmol

Secondary survey
CNS: E 4 V 5 M 6 = 15 PEARLLA 3 mm
PAIN: C/o frontal headache, dull, rated as 3/10
CVS: HR 90 bpm, BP 160/90 mmHg, T 36.9°C

RESP: RR 20, patent airway – spontaneous breathing, increasing SOB, SpO$_2$ 94% RA, AE = on auscultation.
GIT (Input): BS present in all four quadrants, NBM currently, IVC to be placed, currently nothing running.
RENAL (Output): HNPU since admission 4 hours ago, Pt does not report any blood in urine.
SKIN/INTEG: Centrally warm and peripherally cooler. Cap refill > 4 secs.
MUSCULOSKELETAL (Mobility): C/o dizziness at times prior to admission – RIB.
BMI: 26.5

Cues
1 What are your priorities with this patient?
2 What other vital signs or bedside investigations would you perform?
3 What is the relationship between anaemia and increased SOB/hypoxia?
4 What is the pathophysiological relationship between hypoxia and homeostasis?
5 What are some concerns in relation to the integumentary assessment for this patient?
6 What physiological impact do low circulating RBCs have on the body?
7 What investigative or diagnostic procedures do you think would be relevant for this patient?

CONCEPT MAP 5.1 Nursing assessment for Hope

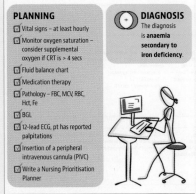

PLANNING

☑ Vital signs – at least hourly
☑ Monitor oxygen saturation – consider supplemental oxygen if CRT is > 4 secs
☑ Fluid balance chart
☑ Medication therapy
☑ Pathology – FBC, MCV, RBC, Hct, Fe
☑ BGL
☑ 12-lead ECG, pt has reported palpitations
☑ Insertion of a peripheral intravenous cannula (PIVC)
☑ Write a Nursing Prioritisation Planner

DIAGNOSIS
The diagnosis is **anaemia secondary to iron deficiency**.

CONCEPT MAP 5.2 Diagnosis and planning for Hope

INTERVENTIONS

1 Assess pain, respiratory status, and circulation frequently, as determined by ADDS.
2 ISBAR handover preparation for end-of-shift handover – what would you be handing over if your patient had an increased WOB and SOB?

What further assessments should be initiated

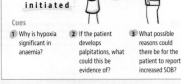

Cues
1 Why is hypoxia significant in anaemia?
2 If the patient develops palpitations, what could this be evidence of?
3 What possible reasons could there be for the patient to report increased SOB?

CONCEPT MAP 5.3 Nursing interventions for Hope

EVALUATION

The medical team have been notified of Hope's increased SOB/WOB.

Plan:
Whilst Hope was being prepared for transfer to Medical Imaging for a CXR, she has developed increased SOB and WOB associated with SpO$_2$ of 88%

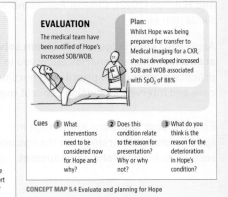

Cues
1 What interventions need to be considered now for Hope and why?
2 Does this condition relate to the reason for presentation? Why or why not?
3 What do you think is the reason for the deterioration in Hope's condition?

CONCEPT MAP 5.4 Evaluate and planning for Hope

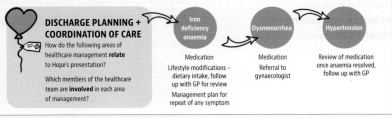

DISCHARGE PLANNING + COORDINATION OF CARE

How do the following areas of healthcare management **relate** to Hope's presentation?

Which members of the healthcare team are **involved** in each area of management?

Iron deficiency anaemia
Medication
Lifestyle modifications – dietary intake, follow up with GP for review
Management plan for repeat of any symptom

Dysmenorrhea
Medication
Referral to gynaecologist

Hypertension
Review of medication once anaemia resolved, follow up with GP

CONCEPT MAP 5.5 Discharge planning and coordination of care for Hope

At the end of the text you'll find a set of **collated concept maps**. The concept maps for each scenario have been grouped by chapter to assist with revision.

COLLATED CONCEPT MAPS

FEATURES WITHIN CHAPTERS

Identify important health and safety issues with the **Safety in nursing** boxes.

Evidence-based practice boxes link research to practice by highlighting key issues and best practices in nursing.

Reflect on your own knowledge and experience with the questions in the **Reflective practice** boxes.

SAFETY IN NURSING

For cataracts, when administering eye drops pre- and postoperatively, including health education sessions, ensure that the application tip of the eye medication does not have direct contact with the patient or other objects to ensure the tip does not become contaminated.

EVIDENCE-BASED PRACTICE

To prevent antibiotic resistance, the entire course of the prescribed antibiotic must be taken. As part of patient education, the nurse will discuss with the patient that even though the person may feel better before the entire course of the antibiotic is completed, they must take all of the prescribed antibiotic.

REFLECTIVE PRACTICE

1 Why is it important to evaluate planned strategies quickly with Sally?
2 Why would GAD not be recognised in presentations to primary health care?
3 Why is it important to regularly monitor observations and physical health?

END-OF-CHAPTER FEATURES

At the end of each chapter you will find several tools to help you to review, practise and extend your knowledge of the key learning objectives.

Review your understanding of the key chapter topics with the **Summary**.

SUMMARY

Pain is one of the most common causes for presentation to health care – be it primary or acute healthcare settings in Australia. Pain is deeply personal and reliant on many factors – physical, psychological and social.

The impact of pain, be it acute or chronic or a combination, is different for every patient. Ensuring you assess the patient and their subjective data, bearing in mind that pain is whatever the person says it is, will enable holistic person-centred care to be given.

Explore the relevant **Clinical skills** listed at the end of each chapter by using your Clinical Skills resources, such as Tollefson and Hillman (2022), *Clinical Psychomotor Skills* (8th ed.).

CLINICAL SKILLS IN PAIN MANAGEMENT

Pain management is focused on a clinical assessment to determine as much supporting or objective data as possible. The following clinical skills are required when managing a person with pain; consult your Clinical Skills resources, such as Tollefson and Hillman (2022), *Clinical Psychomotor Skills* (8th ed.).
- Pain assessment
- Physical assessment
- Mental status assessment

- Temperature, pulse and respiration measurement
- Blood pressure measurement
- Monitoring pulse oximetry
- Focused musculoskeletal health history and physical assessment and range of motion exercises (This would vary between each patient and be dependent upon the mechanism of injury or nature of the person's pain.)

Apply your knowledge with **Problem solving scenarios**. These scenarios allow you to practise planning and prioritising nursing care and interventions using concept maps.

PROBLEM-SOLVING SCENARIO

James Mansfield presents to his GP with increasing back pain. He initially injured his back two years ago at work and has ongoing chronic pain for this condition. He was doing some gardening and lifting fertiliser and has strained his lower back. He is rating his pain as 7/10 and describes it as sharp, stabbing and 'gripping' at times.

His GP is concerned about adding more medications to provide analgesia. James currently takes the following medications:
- Pregabalin 100 mg nocte
- Targin 20/10 bd
- Paracetamol 1 gm QID

Enhance your skills and knowledge in specific areas of nursing with the tips and resources for **Portfolio development**.

PORTFOLIO DEVELOPMENT

Wherever you practise nursing you will need ongoing continuing professional development to ensure that you are delivering current evidence-based nursing care that provides the best possible outcomes for the patient. The useful

websites below will assist in meeting continuing professional development activities to meet the NMBA yearly registration requirements for a Registered Nurse.

Extend your understanding with the suggested **Useful websites** and extensive **References and further reading** relevant to each chapter.

USEFUL WEBSITES

Registered Nurse Standards for Practice
The Registered Nurse Standards for Practice consist of seven crucial standards that all nurses must follow. Download and review the standards at the following link. https://www.nursingmidwiferyboard.gov.au/codes-guidelines-statements/professional-standards/registered-nurse-standards-for-practice.aspx

Australian Commission on Safety and Quality in Health Care
The clinical care standards related to acute pain assessment. There is also supporting information for pain assessment and tools to use across various patient populations.
https://www.safetyandquality.gov.au/standards/clinical-care-standards/opioid-analgesic-stewardship-acute-pain-clinical-care-standard/quality-statements/quality-statement-2-acute-

REFERENCES AND FURTHER READING

Australian Institute of Health and Welfare (AIHW). (2020). *Chronic pain in Australia*. https://www.aihw.gov.au/reports/chronic-disease/chronic-pain-in-australia/summary

Brown, D., Edwards, H., Buckley, T., Aitken, R. L., Lewis, S. L., Bucher, L., McLean Heitkemper, M., Harding, M. M., Kwong, *Fundamentals of nursing* (3rd ed.). Cengage Learning Australia.

Department of Health, Australian Government. (2021). *National strategic action plan for pain management*. https://www.health.gov.au/sites/default/files/documents/2021/05/the-national-strategic-action-plan-for-pain-

iasp-news/iasp-announces-revised-definition-of-pain

Malviya, S., Voepel-Lewis, T., Burke, C., Merkel, S., & Tait, A. R. (2006). The revised FLACC observational pain tool: improved reliability and validity for pain assessment in children with cognitive impairment. *Pediatr Anesthesia, 16*(3), 258–65.

Guide to the online resources

FOR THE INSTRUCTOR

Cengage is pleased to provide you with a selection of resources
that will help you to prepare your lectures and assessments
when you choose this textbook for your course.
Log in or request an account to access instructor resources at
au.cengage.com/instructor/account for Australia or
nz.cengage.com/instructor/account for New Zealand.

MINDTAP

Premium online teaching and learning tools are available on the MindTap platform – the personalised eLearning solution.

MindTap is a flexible and easy-to-use platform that helps build student confidence and gives you a clear picture of their progress. We partner with you to ease the transition to digital – we're with you every step of the way.

MindTap for *Medical-Surgical Nursing: A concept approach* is full of innovative resources to support critical thinking, and help your students move from memorisation to mastery! Includes:

- Burton/Moloney *Medical-Surgical Nursing: A concept approach* ebook
- Prioritisation planner template
- Concept check quizzes
- Interactive concept map sequences
  ...and more!

MindTap is a premium purchasable eLearning tool. Contact your Cengage learning consultant to find out how *MindTap* can transform your course.

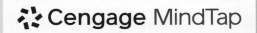

INSTRUCTOR'S MANUAL

The **Instructor's Manual** includes:

- Learning objectives
- Tips for using the Prioritisation Planner and concept map approach
- Suggested solutions to critical thinking questions/problem-solving scenarios
- Alignment with NBMA Registered nurse standards for practice, NSHQS Standards and ACQSC Aged Care Quality Standards.

COGNERO® TEST BANK

A bank of questions has been developed in conjunction with the text for creating quizzes, tests and exams for your students. Create multiple test versions in an instant and deliver tests from your LMS, your classroom, or wherever you want using Cognero. Cognero test generator is a flexible online system that allows you to import, edit and manipulate content from the text's test bank or elsewhere, including your own favourite test questions.

POWERPOINT™ PRESENTATIONS

Use the chapter-by-chapter **PowerPoint slides** to enhance your lecture presentations and handouts by reinforcing the key principles of your subject.

ARTWORK FROM THE TEXT

Add the digital files of concept maps, graphs, pictures and flow charts into your course management system, use them in student handouts, or copy them into your lecture presentations.

FOR THE STUDENT

MINDTAP

MindTap is the next-level online learning tool that helps you get better grades!

MindTap gives you the resources you need to study – all in one place and available when you need them. In the *MindTap Reader* you can make notes, highlight text and even find a definition directly from the page.

If your instructor has chosen *MindTap* for your subject this semester, log in to *MindTap* to:
- Get better grades
- Save time and get organised
- Connect with your instructor and peers
- Study when and where you want, online and mobile
- Complete assessment tasks as set by your instructor.

When your instructor creates a course using *MindTap*, they will let you know your course key so you can access the content. Please purchase *MindTap* only when directed by your instructor. Course length is set by your instructor.

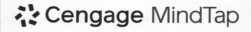

PREFACE

When undertaking their clinical placements, nursing students are required to apply theoretical foundations in the planning of their delivery of care to their patients for each of their shifts. This text aims to guide student planning in a unique way. While students often use a form of planner at the beginning of every shift to document when and what nursing care should be delivered to a patient, the structure of this text demonstrates a logical way to ensure that timely nursing assessments, interventions and evaluations can be made. Embedded in this planning is the rationale as to why students have chosen particular nursing interventions for their patients.

Concept mapping is a pedagogical method for students to apply clinical decision making in their assessment, planning, implementation and evaluation of nursing care. Concept mapping in a diagrammatical form enables students to make linkages between concepts, knowledge and clinical decisions while practising person-centred nursing care. The visual organisation, representation and linkage of knowledge in this way provides a method for students to demonstrate their articulation of clinical decision making when planning person-centred care.

The authors have designed *Medical-Surgical Nursing* for students, preceptors, clinical facilitators, nurse educators and nurse academics following this approach. Concept maps have been included for the more common acute care patient presentations. The presentation of the concept maps aims to promote student deep learning in patient-centred care, and provide the student with interactive tutorial, nursing laboratory and clinical placement experiences whilst being mentored and guided by nurses. The text also enables the student to plan the appropriate nursing care at the beginning of the shift by means of a prioritisation planner. This aims to assist the student to become less dependent on the nurse in applying clinical decision making to nursing care.

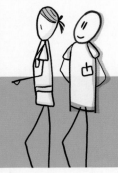

ABOUT THE AUTHORS

Trish Burton is a Senior Lecturer in Nursing and Deputy Director, Centre for Nursing and Midwifery Research (Cairns Campus) in the College of Healthcare Sciences, James Cook University, Australia. Trish has extensive experience teaching all aspects of undergraduate nursing and postgraduate studies and enjoys employing blended learning methods as central to curriculum development.

Trish has been widely published in reference books, has sat on numerous nurse education committees, developed curricula, and has participated in professional consultancies in relation to curriculum development and conducting research. Trish is a Fellow, Australian College of Nursing and Member, Australian Collaborative Education Network.

Ali Moloney has extensive experience in rural and remote health care delivery, emergency and critical care nursing, with over 27 years working as a clinical/registered nurse and in-patient care delivery. Ali has over 15 years' experience in nursing and health education. She is currently working in both the vocational and higher education sectors in nursing, with a strong passion for patient safety and student preparedness. Ali is also a Project Officer with the World Health Organization Collaborating Centre at the University of Technology Sydney in the Western Pacific Regional Office, currently focusing on curriculum development for Nursing and Community Health Workers in Papua New Guinea. Ali has a research focus on Cultural Safety and is completing a higher degree by research through the University of the Sunshine Coast.

Ali has contributed to other textbooks in the Community Services sector, including *Delivering Person Centred Care: Case Management* and is a co-author of *Holistic Mental Health Support*, and in the aged care sector with *The Australian Carer*. Ali has received two Educational Publishers Awards for co-authoring textbooks 'Holistic Mental Health Support' (2023) and the 'Clinical Placement Manual' (2021), which are both student-orientated/focused texts, and were winners of their tertiary categories. Ali continues to ensure student outcomes are supported through her teaching and through the development of textbooks to further support the learning journey of students, and also continues to promote safe and person-centred care in the health care sector.

Contributing authors

Cengage Learning and the authors would like to thank the following contributors:

- **Jason Moloney** (Assessment and diagnostic tests, Musculoskeletal system, Primary health care, Male reproductive system). Jason is a Nurse Practitioner with over 20 years of experience in healthcare. He has worked extensively in Primary Health and Emergency.
- **Dr. Josefina Talavera** (Perioperative care). Josefina is an experienced Clinical Nurse Specialist. She is currently a Sessional Lecturer in the discipline of Nursing and Midwifery, and Unit Coordinator in the Master of Nursing at Victoria University.
- **Natalie Conley** (Mental health, substance use and dependency). Natalie is an experienced Registered Nurse with a background in legal and forensic psychiatry and intellectual disability. She is currently a Lecturer at James Cook University teaching mental health and addictions nursing and culturally safe healthcare for Australia's First Peoples to undergraduate nursing students.
- **Dr Vanessa Sparke** (Integumentary systems). Vanessa is a Senior Lecturer in the discipline of Nursing and Midwifery and Course Coordinator of the Graduate Certificate of Infection Control at James Cook University.

ACKNOWLEDGEMENTS

Trish: I would like to thank Douglas and Hamish for their never-ending support in my academic ventures. A special little thankyou to Lucy, our 16-year-old Jack Russell Terrier who can always wag her tail when encouragement is required. I would like to devote this book to all of the nurses I have encountered in the past, present and will encounter in the future. Nurses make up a very special community of healthcare professionals and, as such, the nursing community always strives for making all of our lives better.

A big thank you to the Cengage publishing team and to Ali – textbook writing is an adventure and a challenge, and you have made this adventure and challenge an enriching one.

Ali: Thank you to my beautiful family for enabling me to bash the keys some more for a textbook. You will all see your names littered throughout the case studies as each of you were constantly on my mind when writing, I love you all – Mags, Haydos, Beebs, Dilemma, CJCJ and Mum. So many others have influenced and contributed to my experience as a nurse, educator and person, and I thank you all for your patience with me over the years – from fellow nurses, to students and of course my friends.

I would also like to thank Michelle Aarons for the concept behind this text and for pairing me with Trish to write. It has been wonderful to work with and learn from you both. I would like to acknowledge the entire team at Cengage; working with you is always a positive experience from start to finish. Thank you, Kylie, for your wordnerding.

Cengage Learning and the authors would also like to thank the following reviewers for their incisive and helpful feedback:

- Dr Leanne Jack, Central Queensland University
- Mariam H. Atib, Victoria University
- Ange Schafer, TAFE Queensland Gold Coast
- Bernie Kushner, Massey University (Albany)
- Melissa Arnold-Chamney, University of Adelaide
- Linda Ng, University of Southern Queensland
- Courtney Hayes, University of Canberra
- Elyse Coffey, Deakin University
- Kiriaki Stewart, University of South Australia
- Debbie Hetherington, Western Sydney University
- Darlene Archer, University of South Australia
- Nina Sivertson, Flinders University
- Mark Lock, Cultural Safety Editing Service.

INTRODUCTION

CHAPTER 1

CLINICAL DECISION MAKING AND CONCEPT MAPS

Research suggests that undergraduate nursing students, although faced with the complexity of identifying the appropriate cues within each stage of the nursing process, find that the nursing process assists them in providing person-centred care. The nursing process includes stages of conducting a health assessment, the identification of a person's healthcare needs, planning care using research evidence, implementing nursing care and evaluating outcomes against benchmarks for responses to care. The complexities of identifying cues requires a strategy that promotes meaningful learning. Concept maps are an effective strategy for meaningful learning as they promote critical thinking. Critical thinking translates to clinical decision making where person-centred care leads to safe and effective nursing practice. Effective nursing practice enables the delivery of care that promotes optimal health outcomes for the person within the healthcare team environment.

LEARNING OBJECTIVES
After reading this chapter, you should be able to:
1 explain the meaning of person-centred care
2 understand concept map methodology and its application to the Registered nurse standards for practice (NMBA, 2016)
3 describe the steps in the nursing process
4 explain the linkage between critical thinking, clinical judgement and clinical decision making and how these are employed in the nursing process
5 discuss the difference between best practice and evidence-based practice that underpins clinical decision making
6 understand the nursing prioritisation of care by applying concept map methodology
7 understand the linkage of the nursing process, primary survey and time-sensitive indicators in the prioritisation of person-centred nursing care in the concept map.

INTRODUCTION

The practice of nursing requires nurses to employ the **nursing process**, and the nursing process framework requires clinical decision making that can be presented in a concept map format. The focus of this learning resource is the clinical decision making and concept map development that is required for nurses to deliver person-centred care.

This chapter introduces the reader to person-centred care and how the nursing process can be operationalised by concept maps that are based on evidence-based nursing activities. In the planning of care delivery, the format of a Nursing Prioritisation Planner enables students to identify and prioritise activities that are person-centred and delivered in a timely manner to promote optimal healthcare outcomes. The primary survey, time-sensitive indicators, secondary survey and, where appropriate, A to G assessment for deteriorating patients and general assessment patients, are additional resources that complement the nursing process. They identify patient problems and specific care activities in the planning stage to enable effective nursing care prioritisation.

The care activities are then implemented and the patient's response to those are evaluated. As discharge planning and the coordination of care are integral components of person-centred care, they are the fifth and final component area of the concept map sequence and follow the evaluation phase of the nursing process. The Nursing Prioritisation Planner contributes to the documentation of person-centred care and is a written artefact that can contribute to the validation of a student's clinical practice.

For the body system chapters in this resource, the chapters are presented in the primary and secondary survey sequence, with the selection of common patient presentations within the acute care hospital environment. Preceding these scenarios are the subjective and objective assessment data components that are applicable to the body system that is the focus of the chapter. The patient's presentation will indicate which assessment data should be collected. These scenarios focus on the healthcare journey of these patients which is diagrammatically represented via concept maps. The concept maps are central in stimulating critical thinking around the provision of person-centred care. In the body system and common presentations and interprofessional approaches to care chapters, patient scenarios are presented as the basis for integrating concept maps using the nursing process framework, which enables the identification and prioritisation of nursing care which includes a Nursing Prioritisation Planner as a core feature.

1.1 PERSON-CENTRED CARE

Nursing care is based on discipline-specific knowledge, scientific theory, health promotion, health education, cultural competence, spirituality and evidence-based practice. The basic tenet of nursing care is person-centred care, where age-appropriate care is underpinned by ethical and legal principles, and is negotiated with the person and their significant others in equal partnership with the nurse. This resource presents concept maps for the more common acute care patient presentations using a *body systems approach*. Concept maps require critical thinking for student nurses to engage in person-centred care, by introducing new knowledge to established knowledge, which enables understanding of the complexities of a patient's clinical presentation. A concept map is considered an educational strategy for meaningful learning, where critical thinking, analysis of information, clinical decision making and organisational skills are promoted, and provides a method for linking theory to practice in the clinical setting for student nurses (Daley et al., 2016; Dorttepe & Arikan, 2019). This linkage between signs and symptoms, pathophysiology, identified problem/medical diagnosis/nursing diagnosis and associated treatment provides the foundation of developing a person-centred care plan. This linkage of knowledge increases student understanding by immersing the student as an active participant in their learning (Cook et al., 2012).

1.2 THE CONCEPT MAP

Concept maps enable student nurses to meet the NMBA (2016) Registered nurse standards for practice and Decision-making framework for nursing and midwifery (NMBA, 2020) in planning the clinical care for the person seeking health care. In each chapter the NMBA (2016) Registered nurse standards for practice, National Safety and Quality Health Service Standards (2021) and Aged Care Quality Standards (2019) are aligned to the components of the concept maps, as these national-based healthcare standards are key drivers for nurses to deliver safe person-centred care.

Concept maps provide a graphic presentation for the visualisation of information and the relationship between the patient history, current health status, identified problem/medical diagnosis/nursing diagnosis, and the nursing care plan for students to develop a person-centred care *nursing prioritisation planner* (see **Figure 1.1**). The nursing prioritisation planner is a schematic representation of the nursing process that is embedded in the concept map. The student develops their nursing prioritisation planner in response to the established nursing care plan and, in consultation with the registered nurse, reviews the prioritisation of identified problems and subsequent nursing care using the primary survey and time-sensitive indicators. The documentation within the nursing prioritisation planner enables the student to identify, prioritise and plan nursing interventions.

NURSING PRIORITISATION PLANNER					
INTRODUCTION	Problem identification (SITUATION/BACKGROUND)	Planning	Implementation	Evaluation	Discharge planning and coordination of care
Bed/ Room No.	Name/ DOB/ Medical record number	Assessment Diagnosis (situation) Relevant medical history (Background)	Prioritise activities using the *nursing care plan, primary survey* and *time-sensitive indicators* Cues: • Primary survey – airway, breathing, circulation, disability and environment. • Secondary survey – head to toe assessment • A to G assessment for the patient/deteriorating patient • Time-sensitive indicators – diagnostic testing, assessment interpretation, surgical and medical treatments, medication management and interpretation to patient responses to care and potential deterioration. • Nursing care plan activities.	Outline the interventions (actions) for the upcoming shift. What further assessments should be initiated?		

FIGURE 1.1 An example of the nursing prioritisation planner. A full template for this planner can be found at the end of Chapter 1.

The planning of interventions promotes time management and appropriate use of resources, which in turn establishes an environment of safety to deliver quality patient care. In the process of care delivery, patient responses to care are evaluated and the ongoing process of discharge planning and coordination of care is continually reviewed. There are significant skill sets required to make safe clinical decisions and asking questions is part of the critical thinker's cognitive tool box. This resource promotes the skill sets for student nurses to plan person-centred care at the beginning of each professional experience placement (PEP) episode (also known as the shift) and deliver nursing care to more than one patient, which in turn fosters student development as a healthcare team member while applying clinical decision making for person-centred care. This development in student nurse skills sets leads to effective time management and patient safety. Each chapter will guide how to plan care for people with common medical-surgical conditions, while highlighting the requirements of a comprehensive nursing prioritisation planner, which promotes effective time management and safe patient care.

1.3 NURSING PROCESS FOR CLINICAL DECISION MAKING

The *nursing process* is a systematic problem-solving tool that provides a consistent decision-making framework for collecting, validating and documenting information for person-centred care (see **Figure 1.2**). The nursing process has five phases:

1 the *assessment* of the individual seeking health care
2 the *diagnosis* which is problem identification from the assessment data
3 the *planning* of person-centred care in response to problem identification
4 the *implementation* of prioritised and targeted nursing care interventions

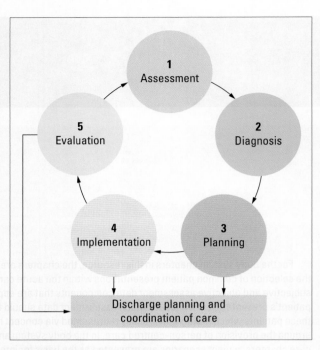

FIGURE 1.2 Stages in the nursing process

5 the *evaluation* of individual responses to the targeted interventions for improving health outcomes for the individual.

The steps of the nursing process are not linear in practice but are dynamic and overlap in response to person-centred care (McHugh Schuster, 2020) that is safe, effective and efficient. *Discharge planning* is normally embedded in the planning, implementation and evaluation phases, and is an important factor in person-centred care as patients are acutely ill, and yet are discharged home in an early stage of recovery. In this resource, to promote a continuum of care for the individual from the hospital environment to the home, *discharge planning and coordination of care* will have its own section in the concept map sequences. The aspect of the continuum of care is to reduce the fragmentation of healthcare delivery, especially when individuals with healthcare needs will be accessing various healthcare providers such as hospitals, outpatient departments, hospital in the home and community-based nursing services. When fragmentation of healthcare services occurs, missed care results, incorrect care is delivered, and person-centred needs are not addressed, which leads to reduced patient outcomes.

1.4 CRITICAL THINKING

Critical thinking has been discussed in the literature over many decades, and a contemporary definition describes critical thinking as a cognitive process of analysing information to facilitate clinical judgement and clinical decision making. Clinical judgement is used to draw conclusions for specific actions to be implemented (Phillips et al., 2021). **Clinical decision making** is a 'contextual, continuous, and evolving process, where data are gathered, interpreted, and evaluated in order to select an evidence-based choice of action' (Tiffen et al., 2014, p. 399). The collection of cues is an integral process and requires use of the critical thinking to make clinical decisions to provide patient care. Questioning which produces cues identifies issues, examines reasoning, defines the problem, and challenges assumptions to produce a reasoned conclusion. The foundational subject areas of nursing, health assessment, clinical skills, anatomy and physiology, pathophysiology and pharmacology will be embedded in the concept maps, so their relationship with nursing care can be linked to promote an increased understanding of what nursing interventions are required for safe and effective nursing care. This assists students to make sound clinical judgements with current knowledge, which in turn demonstrates effective clinical decision making.

As the level of clinical decision making increases in complexity, in tandem critical thinking ability is enhanced, which is linked to increased patient outcomes and safety (Jacob et al., 2017). **Figure 1.3** presents the three years of the Bachelor of Nursing, where fundamental concepts and their development, enhancement and consolidation are highlighted in multiple subjects to culminate in nursing knowledge that supports person-

centred care. The chapters in this resource reflect the scaffolding of knowledge in the nursing course and have concept map exemplars that draw from subject specific information. The chapters in conducting health assessments for individuals, providing culturally sensitive care, caring for persons with specific health alterations using a body systems approach, and responding to the deteriorating patient span across Years 1 and 2 of the Bachelor of Nursing. These chapters highlight the foundational elements of providing nursing care, and the time critical requirements of responding to acute illness. Mental health and substance use, complex care, pain management and perioperative care are exemplars that require specific nursing knowledge, which is presented in concept maps to stimulate critical thinking and reflect the scaffolding of nursing knowledge in Years 2 and 3. The final chapters of cancer, chronic disease management, primary health care and rural and remote health care highlight the complexity of illness as it progresses, and how to maintain health in challenging environments. These chapters denote the consolidation of nursing knowledge in Years 2 and 3. It is acknowledged that some subjects in a Bachelor of Nursing may not be sequenced as in **Figure 1.3**, but wherever the subjects are located the concepts of critical thinking, clinical judgement and clinical decision making are required for person-centred care. The use of concept maps assists in targeting appropriate planning and delivery of nursing care.

BACHELOR OF NURSING	YEAR 1 FOUNDATIONS OF HEALTH	YEAR 2 COMPLEXITY OF ILLNESS	YEAR 3 CONSOLIDATION OF NURSING KNOWLEDGE
Subjects	Nursing	Nursing – medical and surgical/acute care, mental health	Nursing – complex care, chronic disease management
	Health assessment	Health assessment – systems approach for medical and surgical presentations	Health assessment – consolidation of techniques for complex care
	Clinical skills	Clinical skills – medical and surgical, mental health	Clinical skills – complex care, chronic disease management
	Professional experience placements	Professional experience placements – medical and surgical, mental health	Professional experience placements – complex care, chronic disease management, consolidation
	Anatomy and physiology	Pathophysiology – signs and symptoms linkage, and diagnosis	
	Pharmacology	Pharmacology	Pharmacology
	Evidence-based practice	Evidence-based practice – review and apply	Evidence-based practice – critical evaluation and application
	Professional issues	Professional issues – critical thinking and reflective practice	Professional issues – evaluating practice; transitions to practice

FIGURE 1.3 Subject areas mapped across the three years of the Bachelor of Nursing course

1.5 BEST PRACTICE AND EVIDENCE-BASED PRACTICE

It is through critical thinking, and the underpinning of best practice and evidence-based practice (EBP), that appropriate and safe nursing care is documented

in the nursing care plan. The outcome of appropriate and safe nursing care is improved patient outcomes that promote health and wellbeing. Best practice in nursing is the level of agreement that strategies such as interventions or programs assist in the continuum of care, and these strategies are informed by EBP research findings in providing nursing care. In the development of a nursing care plan, best practice and EBP is employed in partnership with nursing knowledge, the individual's and significant others' preferences and providing person-centred care. The outcome of person-centred care is quality of care outcomes and appropriate utilisation of healthcare resources (Jacob et al., 2017). The provision of optimal patient outcomes using critical thinking generates interactive learning, which in turn enables authentic learning to occur and stimulates an environment for the student to feel work ready within the clinical environment. Concept mapping, with the addition of the nursing prioritisation planner, provide the framework for enabling critical thinking to be applied to the nursing process, and in turn enable the student to plan, document and provide comprehensive and person-centred care.

EVIDENCE-BASED PRACTICE

Nurses are instrumental in the prevention of the transmission of infection. A key component in preventing the transmission of infection is to implement infection-control best practices, which have been validated by research findings (evidence-based practice). Best practice includes keeping the healthcare environment clean, wearing personal protective equipment, using barrier precautions and practising the 5 moments of hygiene.

1.6 NURSING PRIORITISATION

The concept map methodology demonstrates in action how to develop a comprehensive nursing prioritisation planner for common medical-surgical conditions, with the focus of person-centred care. The outcomes of this planning are effective time management (for the student's course level) and safe patient care.

Concept maps require critical thinking. Critical thinking occurs when a patient situation is analysed and made sense of. This in turn enables the formulation of clinical decisions for person-centred care, which can often be complex decisions. Part of critical thinking is the evaluation of evidence, linking cues and asking further questions. To be a critical thinker requires employing the problem-solving method and making decisions. The *problem-solving method* requires the definition of the problem, collecting and analysing the data, identifying the cause of the problem, and creating a solution to the problem. In each of the problem-solving steps, sound clinical decision making is required. **Problem solving** in nursing is represented by the nursing process. The nursing process requires critical thinking to make complex decisions for safe and optimal patient outcomes (Sinatra-Wilhelm, 2012).

The nursing process provides a framework for the provision of nursing care, but this framework also requires additional resources to establish priorities in care. The two most influential and effective resources are the *Primary survey* and *Time-sensitive indicators*. The primary survey is an algorithm to identify and manage actual and impending health threats in patients. The secondary survey commences after the primary survey is completed and a head-to-toe assessment is conducted. The A to G assessment of patients occurs predominantly for the deteriorating patient but can also be applied to the assessment of a patient. Time-sensitive indicators are where nursing activities are prioritised in relation to the importance of the activity to be delivered in a timely manner. When a student commences their PEP episode there is the expectation that they determine how to proceed with their shift, and competently respond to the requirements of health assessments and diagnostic testing, multidisciplinary team communication, nursing procedures (e.g. administration of medications, wound dressings and healthcare teaching), and communicating with the person and their family and evaluating the person's response to care.

The primary survey and time-sensitive indicators not only prioritise nursing care for each patient, but also prioritise nursing care episodes between patients. The primary survey components of airway, breathing, circulation, disability and environment are established indicators that accurately indicate a patient's condition and where the priority of care lays to prevent the patient deteriorating. The primary survey not only prioritises the care delivered for the individual, but also between patients. For example, if there is a patient that has an exacerbation of asthma with audible wheezing and a patient with central

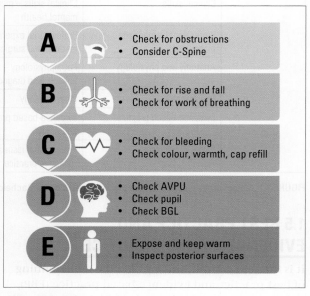

FIGURE 1.4 Components of the primary survey

chest pain with a pain scale rating of 7 out of 10, the patient with audible wheezing requires attention first, as the priority is to have a patent airway. The patient with central chest pain indicates a problem with circulation and requires attention immediately after the first patient. The central chest pain is an indicator for coronary artery disease and the evolution of a myocardial infarction.

The time-sensitive indicators such as diagnostic testing, assessment interpretation, surgical and medical treatments, medication management and interpretation to patient responses to care and potential deterioration (Jessee, 2019) direct the nurse in planning the sequence of care requirements. For example, a patient is scheduled for transfer to the operating room at 0800 hours. After receiving the morning handover at 0700 hours, the student undertakes the morning assessment of the patient, then prepares the patient for transfer to the operating room and uses the preoperative checklist as the guide for the preparation of the patient. If ordered, premedication is administered to the patient, and recorded. The patient's documentation is gathered for transfer for the patient. If the student was caring for two patients, ensuring that the second patient is stable, the nurse commences the preparation for the patient that is scheduled for surgery as the preparation is time critical for a transfer to the operating room of 0800 hours.

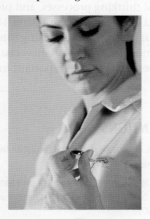

FIGURE 1.5 Time-sensitive indicators direct the nurse in planning the sequence of care requirements

SOURCE: STOCK.ADOBE.COM/MONKEY BUSINESS

The *secondary survey* commences at the completion of the primary survey and the patient's condition is stable for a health history and head-to-toe examination. The secondary survey is frequently conducted in the emergency department. The acronym AMPLE assists in gathering information about allergies, medication, past medical history including immunisation, last meal and events that have led to seeking health care. The head-to-toe examination includes head and face, neck, chest, abdomen, limbs, back, buttocks and perineum

and genitalia. During this examination phase, injuries, wounds and fractures are attended to. If the patient starts to deteriorate during this assessment, then the primary survey or the A to G assessment for the deteriorating patient is conducted. The *A to G assessment for the deteriorating patient* draws from the components of the primary and secondary survey. The A to G assessment components for the deteriorating patient are airway, breathing, circulation, disability, exposure, fluids and glucose. The A to G assessment is conducted in the areas of healthcare organisations where patients require patient care, whether episodic or long term.

The components of the concept map

The concept maps in this resource have, as their basis, the nursing process. The patient presentation and past history (PHx) are outlined. As problem identification has occurred, each concept map for person-centred care focuses on the assessment, planning, implementation and evaluation phases, and discharge planning and coordination of care. In relation to the prioritisation of nursing care interventions, the primary survey and time-sensitive indicators are used as essential resources in the concept map (please refer to the Nursing Prioritisation Planner at the end of this chapter). Where appropriate, the secondary survey is presented, and the A to G assessment for the deteriorating patient is acknowledged.

Assessment

The assessment phase involves the collection of objective and subjective data and the subsequent validation of the data to ensure accuracy (see **Figure 1.6**). The categorisation of data requires critical thinking for the identification of patterns, which leads to interpretations and accurate recording and reporting.

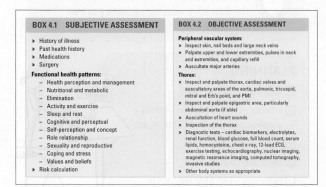

FIGURE 1.6 Examples of the subjective and objective assessment boxes used in the scenarios in Part 2 of this resource

In the assessment part of the concept map, patient history (PHx) is recorded, then assessment findings are presented and there are associated questions that are cues to stimulate critical thinking (see **Figure 1.7**).

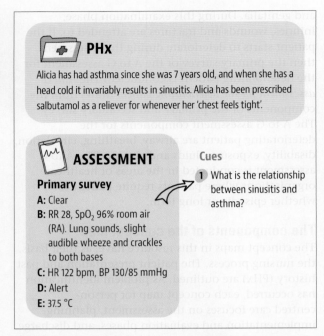

PHx

Alicia has had asthma since she was 7 years old, and when she has a head cold it invariably results in sinusitis. Alicia has been prescribed salbutamol as a reliever for whenever her 'chest feels tight'.

ASSESSMENT

Primary survey

A: Clear

B: RR 28, SpO$_2$ 96% room air (RA). Lung sounds, slight audible wheeze and crackles to both bases

C: HR 122 bpm, BP 130/85 mmHg

D: Alert

E: 37.5 °C

Cues

1 What is the relationship between sinusitis and asthma?

FIGURE 1.7 An example of an assessment concept map

The scenarios throughout the resource will be based within the hospital environment. If the patient is in the emergency department, then the primary survey and secondary survey will be recorded. The A to G assessment can also be conducted for the deteriorating and non-deteriorating patient within the hospital. If the patient is established in the ward environment, then functional health patterns may be included in the nursing care plan. Cue questions will be part of the assessment information to stimulate linkage of assessment findings.

Diagnosis and planning

From the assessment findings, problem identification is embedded in the second concept map for the medical-surgical condition (along with planning), and includes an identified problem/medical diagnosis and, if required, a nursing diagnosis.

Planning for person-centred care involves the person and their significant others and the nurse. The planning of nursing interventions is determined by the person's healthcare needs in relation to the medical diagnosis, a general plan for therapy and the individual specific nursing care plan, which includes nursing interventions for actual and potential problems and risk factors that inhibit patient recovery. The planning phase is based on effective critical thinking. The Nursing Prioritisation Planner enables the student to document the nursing care plan for the person. The student is able to include the primary survey findings and time-sensitive indicators in validating their plan of person-centred nursing activities during the shift.

Implementation (nursing interventions)

In the implementation phase, the student delivers person-centred care that encompasses skills-based nursing activities and monitors patient status and responses. Cue questions will be asked in relation to the changes in patient status and what further assessment and nursing interventions are required, which will develop critical thinking processes, and promote clinical judgement and clinical decision making. Documentation of the individual's response to nursing interventions, patient outcomes and if there are new changes to the individual's presentation, are important in this phase.

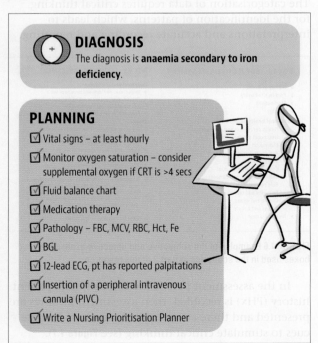

DIAGNOSIS

The diagnosis is **anaemia secondary to iron deficiency**.

PLANNING

☑ Vital signs – at least hourly

☑ Monitor oxygen saturation – consider supplemental oxygen if CRT is >4 secs

☑ Fluid balance chart

☑ Medication therapy

☑ Pathology – FBC, MCV, RBC, Hct, Fe

☑ BGL

☑ 12-lead ECG, pt has reported palpitations

☑ Insertion of a peripheral intravenous cannula (PIVC)

☑ Write a Nursing Prioritisation Planner

FIGURE 1.8 An example of a diagnosis and planning concept map

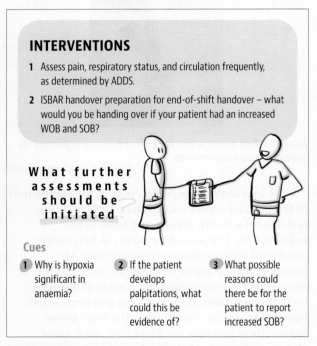

INTERVENTIONS

1 Assess pain, respiratory status, and circulation frequently, as determined by ADDS.

2 ISBAR handover preparation for end-of-shift handover – what would you be handing over if your patient had an increased WOB and SOB?

What further assessments should be initiated

Cues

1 Why is hypoxia significant in anaemia?

2 If the patient develops palpitations, what could this be evidence of?

3 What possible reasons could there be for the patient to report increased SOB?

FIGURE 1.9 An example of an implementation concept map, highlighting nursing interventions

Evaluation

The evaluation phase highlights the degree that patient goals have been met, and the communication to the healthcare team in relation to patient response to interventions and new changes to the patient's presentation. In response to lack of or unexpected progress in meeting patient goals and new changes in the patient's presentation, a plan for further assessment is documented, which in turn requires re-identification of patient problems, reviewed planning for goals and interventions. Targeted cue questions will be highlighted in promoting further reflective thinking for effective person-centred care.

Discharge planning and coordination of care

The critical thinking that occurs in the assessment, planning, intervention and evaluation phases informs discharge planning and the coordination of care, where person-centred interventions and the appropriate referrals are provided for effective home care with the person and their significant other. Cue questions will be part of the home care process, so as potential barriers and enablers to home care are further explored, and to ensure the person's home care addresses health needs and does not result in areas of missed home care that potentially leads to the person being re-admitted to the hospital.

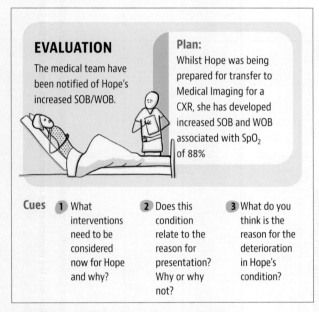

FIGURE 1.10 An example of an evaluation concept map

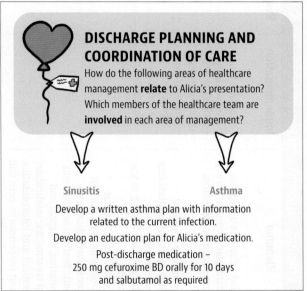

FIGURE 1.11 An example of a discharge planning and coordination of care concept map

SUMMARY

This chapter introduces the reader to the learning strategy of concept mapping and its application to the nursing process in identifying how best to provide person-centred care in the healthcare environment. The identification of an individual's healthcare needs is dependent on critical thinking processes and the subsequent application of evidence-based practice in producing a nursing care plan. The nursing care plan should be both person-centred and enable optimal health outcomes in a safe environment. A Nursing Prioritisation Planner (**Figure 1.12** at the end of this chapter) is provided to assist the student in documenting the requirements of patient care for one or more individuals and enables the student to prioritise care activities for a patient and in between patients.

CRITICAL THINKING QUESTIONS

1   Why do patient assessments that are undertaken in the emergency department not include functional health patterns?

2   How is the A to G assessment for the deteriorating patient similar to the primary and secondary survey?

NURSING PRIORITISATION PLANNER

INTRODUCTION	Problem identification (SITUATION/BACKGROUND)	Planning	Implementation	Evaluation	Discharge planning and coordination of care
Bed/ Room No.	Name/ DOB/ Medical record number	Assessment Diagnosis (situation) Relevant medical history (Background)	Prioritise activities using the *nursing care plan, primary survey and time-sensitive indicators* Cues: ■ Primary survey – airway, breathing, circulation, disability and environment. ■ Secondary survey – head to toe assessment ■ A to G assessment for the patient/deteriorating patient ■ Time-sensitive indicators – diagnostic testing, assessment interpretation, surgical and medical treatments, medication management and interpretation to patient responses to care and potential deterioration. ■ Nursing care plan activities.	Outline the interventions (actions) for the upcoming shift. What further assessments should be initiated?		

FIGURE 1.12 Nursing Prioritisation Planner. This template should be used in conjunction with key elements of the concept maps to allow nurses to prioritise and plan patient care during a shift. Ask your instructor for a digital version of this template.

PORTFOLIO DEVELOPMENT

In the nursing literature, missed care in the provision of nursing care is highlighted as a contributor to adverse patient events, decreased patient satisfaction and decreased quality of care (Jones et al., 2015). What activities may nurses undertake to equip them with skill sets that prevent incidents of missed care?

USEFUL WEBSITES

Nursing and Midwifery Board of Australia

Decision-making framework for nursing and midwifery (2020)
https://www.nursingmidwiferyboard.gov.au/codes-guidelines-statements/frameworks.aspx

Registered nurse standards for practice (2016)
https://www.nursingmidwiferyboard.gov.au/codes-guidelines-statements/professional-standards/registered-nurse-standards-for-practice.aspx

REFERENCES AND FURTHER READING

Alfaro-LeFevre, R. (2016). *Critical thinking and clinical judgement: A practical approach* (6th ed.). Saunders.

Atay, S., & Karabacak, U. (2012). Care plans using concept maps and their effects on the critical thinking dispositions of nursing students. *International Journal of Nursing Practice, 18*, 233–239. DOI: 10.1111/j.1440-172X.2012.02034.x

Cook, L. K., Dover, C., Dickson, M., & Colton, D. L. (2012). From care plan to concept map: A paradigm shift. *Teaching and Learning in Nursing, 7*, 88–92. DOI: 10.1016/j.teln.2011.11.005

Daley, B. J., Morgan, S., & Black, S. B. (2016). Concept maps in nursing education: A historical literature review and research directions. *Journal of Nursing Education, 55*(111), 631–639. DOI:10.3928/01484834-20161011-05

Dorttepe, Z. U., & Arikan, B. (2019). Use of concept maps in nursing education. *Journal of Education and Research in Nursing, 16*(2), 1–9. DOI: 10.5222/HEAD.2019.160

Garwood, J. K., Ahmed, A. H., & McComb, S. A. (2018). The effect of concept maps on undergraduate nursing students' critical thinking. *Nursing Education Perspectives, 39*(4), 208–214.

Harrison, S., & Gibbons, C. (2013). Nursing student perceptions of concept maps: From theory to practice. *Nursing Education Perspectives, 34*(6), 395–399. DOI: 10.5480/10-465

Jacob, E., Duffield, C., & Jacob, D. (2017). A protocol for the development of a critical thinking assessment tool for nurses using a Delphi technique. *Journal of Advanced Nursing, 73*, 1982–1988. DOI:10.1111/jan.13306

Jessee, M. A. (2019). Teaching prioritization: 'Who, what & why?'. *Journal of Nursing Education, 58*(5), 302–305. DOI:10.3928/01484834-20190422-10

Jones, T. L., Hamilton, P., & Murry, N. (2015). Unfinished nursing care, missed care, and implicitly rationed care: State of the science review. *International Journal of Nursing Studies, 52*(6), 1121–1137. https://doi.org/10.1016/j.ijnurstu.2015.02.012

McHugh Schuster, P. (2020). *Concept mapping: A critical thinking approach to care planning* (5th ed.). F. A. Davis.

Nibbelink, C. W., & Brewer, B. B. (2018). Decision-making in nursing practice: An integrative literature review. *Journal of Clinical Nursing, 27*, 917–928. DOI: 10.1111/jocn.14151

Nursing and Midwifery Board of Australia. (2016). *Registered nurse standards for practice*. https://www.nursingmidwifery-board.gov.au/codes-guidelines-statements/professional-standards/registered-nurse-standards-for-practice.aspx

Phillips, B. C., Morin, K., & Valiga, T.M. (2021). Clinical decision making in undergraduate nursing students: A mixed methods multisite study. *Nurse Education Today, 97*, 1–6. DOI: 10.1016/j.nedt.2020.104676

Sinatra-Wilhelm, T. (2012). Nursing care plans versus concept maps in the enhancement of critical thinking skills in nursing students enrolled in a Baccalaureate nursing program. *Creative Nursing, 18*(2), 78–84.

Tiffen J., Corbridge, S. J., & Slimmer, L. (2014). Enhancing clinical decision making: Development of a contiguous definition and conceptual framework. *Journal of Professional Nursing, 30*(5), 399–405.

CHAPTER **2**

ASSESSMENT AND DIAGNOSTIC TESTS

Nursing assessment aligns with the acronym ADPIE:

Assessment
Diagnosis
Planning
Implementation
Evaluation.

Through this process, the patient is assessed using progressive steps that are also cyclical, just like the nursing process. The nursing process, using ADPIE, ensures that the patient's needs are addressed, and the plan of care is related and formed specifically for that person.

LEARNING OBJECTIVES

After reading this chapter, you should be able to:
1 explain the difference between subjective and objective data
2 understand assessment and diagnostic testing in nursing
3 explain the stages of assessment, diagnosis, planning, implementation and evaluation (ADPIE).

INTRODUCTION

Knowing how to carry out an accurate health assessment – from taking the health history through to performing a physical examination – will help you uncover significant problems and assist in planning your care appropriately.

The acronym ADPIE represents a systematic approach to nursing care that stands for Assessment, Diagnosis, Planning, Implementation and Evaluation. It provides a framework for nurses to deliver holistic and individualised care to their patients. Let's discuss each step of the ADPIE process in detail.

Assessment

Assessment is the first step of the nursing process, where the nurse gathers comprehensive and accurate data about the patient's health status.

The nurse collects subjective data through patient interviews and obtains objective data through physical examinations, observations and reviewing medical records.

Assessment involves assessing the patient's physical, emotional, psychological, and social wellbeing, as well as their developmental, cultural and environmental factors.

The nurse uses various assessment tools and techniques to gather relevant information, such as health history questionnaires, vital signs measurements and specific assessment scales.

Diagnosis

Diagnosis involves analysing the data collected during the assessment phase to identify the patient's health problems or needs.

Nursing diagnoses are different from medical diagnoses and focus on the patient's response to the actual or potential health problems.

The nurse uses critical thinking skills and knowledge of nursing science to formulate nursing diagnoses based on the assessment data.

Planning

Planning involves developing a comprehensive care plan in collaboration with the patient, their family and other healthcare professionals.

The nurse establishes goals and outcomes that are specific, measurable, achievable, relevant, and time-bound (SMART goals).

The care plan includes nursing interventions that are evidence-based and tailored to meet the patient's individual needs.

The nurse considers the patient's preferences, cultural beliefs and available resources when developing the care plan.

Implementation

Implementation is the phase where the nurse executes the planned interventions and delivers the care outlined in the care plan.

The nurse provides direct patient care, administers medications, performs treatments, educates the patient and their family, and coordinates referrals to other healthcare professionals.

Implementation involves effective communication, therapeutic interventions, and utilising nursing knowledge and skills.

The nurse documents the interventions provided and evaluates the patient's response to the interventions.

Evaluation

Evaluation is the final step of the nursing process, where the nurse assesses the effectiveness of the care provided and the patient's progress towards achieving the established goals and outcomes.

The nurse compares the patient's actual responses to the expected outcomes and determines if the interventions were successful.

If the desired outcomes are achieved, the nurse continues with the current plan or modifies it as necessary.

If the outcomes are not met, the nurse reevaluates the care plan, identifies any barriers or issues, and modifies the interventions accordingly.

The diagnosis and planning stages of the nursing process are represented together in one section of the concept map sequences used in Part 2 of this text. As discussed in Chapter 1, discharge planning and coordination of care is generally embedded in the planning, implementation and evaluation phases of the nursing process. In this resource, to promote a continuum of care for the individual from the hospital environment to the home, discharge planning and coordination of care will have its own section in the concept map sequences presented in Part 2 of this text.

The ADPIE process is cyclic, and each phase informs the next. It is a dynamic process that promotes individualised, evidence-based and person-centred care. The systematic approach of ADPIE allows nurses to provide comprehensive care, prioritise interventions and continuously improve the patient's health outcomes.

Advances in technology also ensure the earlier availability of diagnostic tests, which provide data and give direction to history taking and physical assessment. Nurses have traditionally been responsible for patient observations and documentation. However, the interpretation of their observations has been contingent on their ability to integrate the other components of a complete health assessment (Brown et al., 2019).

2.1 DATA COLLECTION

Assessment involves collecting two kinds of data – objective and subjective.

Subjective data is the process in which information relating to the patient's problem is elicited from the patient; however, in the situation of a patient with altered level of consciousness this information can be obtained from family or friends. In the process, the nurse seeks information on psychosocial issues, past health and surgical history, family history, medications including patterns of drug use/smoking/alcohol and complementary or over-the-counter medications and allergies. A review of symptoms, including vital signs, will help with the planning process and care plan forming a baseline for the patient.

Objective data is obtained through physical assessment and interpretations of laboratory values and diagnostic tests. Objective data cannot be persuaded by the patient. That means that the data is what it is – you cannot alter the findings (Gray et al., 2019).

Objective data is obtained through observation and is verifiable – for instance, if we document a patient is febrile, we have a temperature recorded on observation charts that correlates with this and thus verifies the information. Subjective data is provided by the patient and is based on what they say – for instance, there is no way to confirm or deny that the patient has a headache, we merely act upon what our patients tell us (Brown et al., 2019; Crisp & Taylor, 2021).

All data should be recorded at the time it is gathered and not left until the end of the shift. Any variation may need to be reported immediately to senior staff for immediate intervention. Alternatively, it may be as simple as just recording the variance on a variance sheet. Any abnormal values in observation or diagnostics should be recorded in the patient's notes and verbally reported during handover.

Care plans need to be current and reflect the need requirements of the patient at that specific time; therefore, it is essential that data is collected and recorded each shift to ensure the care plan is adequate. It will become habitual to review and update care plans throughout your shift, contemporaneously (DeLaune et al., 2024; Gray et al., 2019; Joustra & Moloney, 2019; Tollefson et al., 2022).

In developing an individual database, we need to draw on a range of sources – these include objective and subjective data sources. Most subjective data is obtained by taking a health history, while objective data is gathered during physical assessment. For example, the patient complains of feeling breathless (subjective data) and on examination you note cyanosis, rapid respirations and breath sounds consistent with bronchospasm (objective data) (Joustra & Moloney, 2019).

2.2 ASSESSMENT

Physical assessment is an organised systematic process of collecting objective data based upon a health history and a head-to-toe or general systems examination. A physical assessment should be adjusted to the patient, based on their specific needs. A comprehensive patient assessment can be:
- a complete physical assessment
- an assessment of a singular body system
- an assessment of a body part.

A detailed physical assessment provides the nurse with the foundation for their nursing care plan – your observations and findings from the physical assessment play an integral part in the assessment, intervention and evaluation phases of your care, which in turn informs the discharge planning and establishment of outpatient or comprehensive care in the community. Furthermore, data collected from a thorough and thoughtful history and examination contributes to both the nursing and medical decisions for all therapeutic interventions (Brown et al., 2019; Crisp & Taylor, 2021).

During physical assessment, it is essential that the nurse:
- remain professional and show concern
- maintain dignity and privacy at all times
- maintain modesty – visualise one body system at a time
- explain to the patient what you are doing
- communicate with the patient during the assessment when appropriate.

Generally, for a physical assessment, a nurse will need the following equipment:
- thermometer
- stethoscope
- sphygmomanometer
- penlight or flashlight
- pulse oximeter (if patient not monitored)
- scales.

All nurses develop their 'own' way of performing a physical assessment. Commonly, nurses start at the head and work down to the toes. A thorough physical assessment can take up to an hour, so ensure that your time can be adequately managed (Brown et al., 2019; Crisp & Taylor, 2021; DeLaune et al., 2024; Joustra & Moloney, 2019).

The principles of health assessment for any body system follow four methods – inspection, palpation, auscultation and percussion. These four methods are applied to each body system to complete a comprehensive assessment (see Evidence-based practice box).

Inspection is used to assess colour, rashes, scars, body shape, facial expression and body structures and is an active process rather than a passive one. When conducting a respiratory assessment, for example, you will need to examine:

- the nares for flaring
- how the client is breathing – open mouthed or through the nose
- skin colour (cyanosis)
- clubbing of fingers
- chest symmetry
- intercostal recession
- tracheal tug
- use of accessory muscles, such as the abdominal muscles and diaphragm.

Auscultation is perhaps the most important and effective clinical technique you will ever learn for evaluation of a patient's respiratory function. Before you begin, bear in mind the following:

- It is important that you try to maintain a quiet environment as much as possible.
- The patient should be in proper position for auscultation – sitting up in bed if possible.
- Your stethoscope should be touching the patient's bare skin wherever possible, or you may hear rubbing noises from clothing or monitoring leads.
- Always ensure patient comfort and explain the procedure to the client before beginning to ensure cooperation. You can also warm the diaphragm of your stethoscope with your hand before you begin.

The major function of the respiratory system is to supply the body with oxygen and remove carbon dioxide. When the respiratory rate is measured, we are observing the act of ventilation. One respiration consists of one inspiration and one expiration (breathing in and breathing out). Perhaps one of the most important assessments of your client will be the respiratory rate. When assessing the respiratory rate, you need to know a normal/expected normal rate for the person's age group, and a baseline reading if available. In healthy people, the relationship between pulse and respiration is constant – being a ratio of one respiration to every four or five heartbeats. However, a normal respiratory rate is 12–20 breaths per minute.

On assessment of respirations, you should be observing the difficulty, sound, depth and pattern of breathing. Respirations are normally effortless, and you should therefore observe if the patient is dyspnoeic. Dyspnoeic patients tend to mouth breathe as there is less resistance to airflow through the mouth than the nose, and they generally prefer to sit up.

Past medical history is an excellent tool in guiding our physical assessment. It makes assessment easier and more structured if we know, for example, that the patient has hypertension or chronic obstructive pulmonary disease. It's also important to establish if there are any treatments or interventions currently being undertaken by the patient. With this information, our findings may make a 'little more sense'. However, it is not always possible to interview patients and determine past medical history due to the nature of illness and accidents. Patients can be unconscious, with no known next of kin or contact person. If the patient has just moved to the area, then there may be the added difficulty in tracking down previous GPs or treating physicians.

A health history is used to gather subjective data about the patient and to explore past and present problems. First, ask the patient about their general physical and emotional health, and then move onto specific body systems. The accuracy and amount of information you obtain from your interviewing will depend largely on your skill as an interviewer. In obtaining a health history, medical diagnosis including all disease processes, medications, laboratory values, allergies, vital signs and physical examination data are required from your patient.

Armed with this information you will be able to establish a nursing care plan tailored to your patient. The benefit of this is that person-focused care plans and assessment tools are based on needs analysis and holistic health assessment. These care plans should be developed in conjunction with family members, allied health professionals and, most importantly, the patient. Nursing assessment is the foundation for all our care provision, so it must be effective.

Holistic nursing assessment is what drives our nursing interventions, so if we do not ask relevant and open-ended questions, we are not going to have much to work with. Essentially, we need to cover all the person's day-to-day activities in our assessment – sexual function and drive, driving, going out for dinner, meals – not just all the body systems. Being unhealthy or unwell can affect a person in many ways, so having all the information is beneficial in planning and evaluating your patient's care.

Pathophysiology

Pathophysiology is the term used to describe changes in normal functioning within the body; that is, the presence of disease or illness (Brown et al., 2019; Craft & Gordon, 2019). Pathophysiology looks at the specific mechanisms that cause disease and illness in the different body systems. There are millions of diseases and types of illness, so they can't all be listed here. Familiar disease processes might be things such as:

- asthma
- pneumonia
- hypertension

- Crohn's disease
- Paget's disease
- AIDS
- hepatitis C
- cancer
- COVID-19.

As you can see, the list is endless! What will make the impact on your patient care will be using the physical assessment you perform – armed with diagnostic tests and imaging – to plan, implement and evaluate the holistic care of the patient.

EVIDENCE-BASED PRACTICE

Nursing assessment
Assessment is a key aspect of nursing practice and is aligned into the Nursing and Midwifery Board of Australia (NMBA) in the national competency standards – namely Standards 1 & 4 (NMBA, 2016). Within nursing there are many types of assessments we perform, including:

- primary assessment – airway, breathing, circulation, disability and environment/exposure (ABCDE) – often performed at bedside handover, or on initial interaction with the patient
- admission assessment – thorough assessment including history, general appearance, physical examination (including vital signs) completed on admission
- focused assessment – detailed or in-depth assessment of specific body system/s. For example, if your patient presents with shortness of breath, initially you might focus on the respiratory system.

In each assessment the structure is underpinned by:
- inspection – observe and inspect the area, look for colour, integrity, movement, etc.
- auscultation – listen with stethoscope
- palpation – skin temperature, presence of oedema, diaphoresis
- percussion – assists with locating borders of organs.

Each of these skills will be continually developed over the duration of your nursing career, and you will take with you previous assessment findings to really give you a 'database' of abnormal findings for comparison (DeLaune et al., 2024).

2.3 DIAGNOSTIC TESTING

There are many different types of diagnostic testing, and some will be considered 'routine' for patients when they present to a hospital or are having a procedure performed – including surgery. The sheer number of pathology tests can be overwhelming and

almost akin to learning another language! There are many acronyms that you will become familiar with in your direct patient care. The most common pathology tests are:

- **FBC** – Full Blood Count – includes leucocyte count/white cell count (WBC/WCC), eosinophils, erythrocyte count/red cell count (RCC, RBC), haemoglobin (Hgb, Hb) haematocrit (Hct/Packed cell volume [PCV]), mean cell volume (MCV), platelet count (Plt)
- **UEC** – Urea and Electrolytes – includes sodium (Na), potassium (K), chloride (Cl), bicarbonate (HCO_3), creatinine and urea. This test also calculates the anion gap, the urea/creatinine ratio and eGFR (estimated glomerular filtration rate).

It will be determined through local policy and procedures if it is within your role as the registered nurse (RN) to perform pathology testing – many hospitals have the provision of phlebotomists during certain hours, and after hours it is clinical staff responsibility. In rural and remote areas this changes again, dependent upon the availability of staff and pathology equipment.

Pathology testing can be undertaken through point of care (POC) diagnostics – where a basic profile can be obtained within minutes. POC testing is often used in regional facilities, primary healthcare centres and rural regions within Australia.

Any pathology test will have all information available from the test provider, including what coloured sample tubes are required. There are often flipcharts or online tools to assist you at the bedside in ensuring you have selected the correct vial/container and have undertaken the correct procedure (e.g. if it is for blood cultures, you will need to follow specific guidelines).

Radiology
Radiology is also referred to as medical imaging. For the most part, it includes x-rays (CXR = chest x-ray), ultrasound (USS), computed tomography (CT) scan, magnetic resonance imaging (MRI), angiography, mammography, interventional radiology (guided injections, insertion of vascular devices) and fluoroscopy. Radiology/medical imaging is offered in public hospitals and also through private providers in suburban areas. The availability of radiology and medical imaging is varied across areas of Australia. In rural and remote areas, there is significantly limited access to specialised imaging, so the patient may be referred to a tertiary hospital for further investigation.

As the RN, it is not within your scope of practice to assess and diagnose from a chest x-ray, for example. What is a component of the nursing role is the safe transfer of the patient to the radiology department, or the safe x-ray of the patient at the bedside. Your role will be to work collaboratively with the radiology staff, and ensure patient safety is maintained during the procedure.

X-rays are the most common of all radiological interventions, as they are used to assess the placement of invasive devices, assess organs (lungs, heart, etc.) and assess and diagnose fractures.

Within x-rays, there are densities, with the most common being white (bone) and black (air). The other densities are:

- dark grey – fat
- grey – soft tissue/water
- bright white – man-made (pacemaker, any foreign object).

Unless you have performed further training in radiology, it will not be a component of your role to perform x-rays or other interventional diagnostic procedures.

Bedside care

There are several POC or bedside care/investigations that you may be involved in. They include POC pathology, the use of glucometers (for ketones and blood glucose levels) and ward urinalysis. From these interventions, you may request 'formal' blood tests (i.e. sending a sample to the pathology lab) or further escalation of care (e.g. if there are ketones present).

Continually assessing and evaluating your patient and their response to treatment will enable you to safely report findings, and escalate care as required when your patient is not responding or their condition is deteriorating.

SAFETY IN NURSING

RISK MANAGEMENT

Blood or fluids exposure is an ongoing risk as a nurse. To mitigate this risk there are several safety practices in place to manage the disposal of sharps, and the availability of sharps disposal equipment at the bedsides of patients.

The use of sharps exposes nursing staff to the risk of many bloodborne infectious agents such as hepatitis B, hepatitis C, and human immunodeficiency virus (HIV) (National Health and Medical Research Council (NHMRC), 2019).

Within the Australian Guidelines for the Prevention and Control of Infection in Healthcare (p. 9), there are guidelines

around the use and management of sharps, including medication vials. Good practice is outlined as:

- not passing sharps directly from one hand to the other
- keeping handling of sharps to a minimum
- not recapping, bending or breaking needles after use
- disposing of single-use sharps immediately into an approved sharps container at the point of use/care.

There will be local guidelines surrounding the management of sharps containers and the steps required for any exposure to fluids – be it through needlestick injury or exposure of fluids through other membranes.

SUMMARY

In this chapter, we discussed the importance of using the assessment you perform, along with the results of any diagnostic tests and imaging, to plan, implement and evaluate the holistic care of the patient.

Assessment and diagnostic testing vary depending on the patient's needs and reason for presentation. Age is also a factor in the type or kind of testing undertaken. In some facilities there is nurse-initiated pathology and radiology, but this is reliant upon the facility and their local guidelines.

Patient safety is paramount, as are dignity, respect and collaboration with other healthcare professionals. The list of diagnostic tests and procedures is extensive and ever changing; your role will be to work collaboratively with the patient and allied health to complete the interventions.

CLINICAL SKILLS IN ASSESSMENT

The following clinical skills are required for a holistic patient assessment; consult your Clinical Skills resources, such as Tollefson and Hillman (2022), *Clinical Psychomotor Skills* (8th ed.).

- Vital signs
- Past medical/surgical history – questioning around this
- Collection of subjective and objective data to form an assessment (patient reports pain in left lower abdomen – on auscultation … on palpation …)

- POC testing – urinalysis, blood glucose level, ketones (if relevant clinically)
- Inspection – observing the patient for any abnormalities, can be related to a specific body system
- Auscultation – listening through a stethoscope for breath sounds, abdominal sounds or heart sounds.
- Palpation – assessing for warmth, oedema, skin integrity

- Percussion – not always used in nursing, but a tool for identifying organ borders (liver is a good example if you have someone with hepatitis or alcoholic liver disease)
- Documentation and escalation of care
- Re-evaluation and re-assessment

Your assessment skills will grow and improve with exposure and experience. They are one of the biggest factors in detecting patient condition changes and knowing when to escalate patient care. For a comprehensive and holistic exploration of patient assessment, refer to *Estes Health Assessment and Physical Examination* by Calleja et al. (2024).

CRITICAL THINKING QUESTIONS

1   What are the two different types of data, and why are they both important to nursing assessment?

2   Explain how physical assessment is undertaken for a patient. What are you documenting?

PORTFOLIO DEVELOPMENT

There are many continuing professional development providers that have a focus on patient assessment and phsyical assessment. Most healthcare facilities will also have

pathways in place for nursing staff to improve and increase their clinical physical assessment skills.

USEFUL WEBSITES

Registered Nurse Standards for Practice (Nursing and Midwifery Board)
The Registered Nurse Standards for Practice consist of seven crucial standards that all nurses must follow. Download and review the standards at the following link. https://www.nursingmidwiferyboard.gov.au/Codes-Guidelines-Statements/Professional-standards/registered-nurse-standards-for-practice.aspx

QLD Health Guideline: Management of occupational exposure to blood and body fluids (2017)
Guidelines from Queensland Health regarding the management of exposure to blood and body fluids. https://www.health.qld.gov.au/system-governance/policies-standards/guidelines

Managing Exposures to Blood and Body Fluids or Substances (Department of Health, Victoria)
Guidelines from Victorian Department of Health regarding the management of exposure. https://www.health.vic.gov.au/infectious-diseases/managing-exposures-to-blood-and-body-fluids-or-substances

Australian Guidelines for the Prevention and Control of Infection in Healthcare (2019)
Guidelines from the National Health and Medical Research Council that outline all requirements for healthcare facilities in infection control, including sharps management. https://www.nhmrc.gov.au/sites/default/files/documents/infection-control-guidelines-feb2020.pdf

REFERENCES AND FURTHER READING

Brown, D., Edwards, H., Buckley, T., Aitken, R., Lewis, S., Bucher, L., McLean Heitkemper, M., Harding, M., Kwong, J., & Roberts, D. (2019). *Lewis's medical-surgical nursing ANZ* (5th ed.). Elsevier.

Calleja, P., Theobald, K., & Harvey, T. (2024). *Estes Health assessment and physical examination* (3rd ed.). Cengage Learning Australia.

Craft, J., & Gordon, C. (2019). *Understanding pathophysiology* (3rd ed.). Elsevier Australia.

Crisp, J., & Taylor, C. (2021). *Potter and Perry's Fundamentals of nursing* (4th ed.). Elsevier.

DeLaune, S. C., Ladner, P. K., McTier, L., Tollefson, J., & Lawrence, J. (2024). *Australian and New Zealand fundamentals of nursing* (3rd ANZ ed.). Cengage Learning Australia.

Gray, S., Ferris, L., White, L. E., Duncan, G., & Baumle, W. (2019). *Foundations of nursing: Enrolled nurses* (2nd ANZ ed.). Cengage Learning Australia.

Joustra, C., & Moloney, A. (2019). *Clinical placement manual.* Cengage Learning Australia.

National Health and Medical Research Council (NHMRC). (2019). *Australian*

guidelines for the prevention and control of infection in healthcare. National Health and Medical Research Council.

Nursing and Midwifery Board (NMBA). (2016). *Registered nurse standards for practice.* https://www.nursingmidwiferyboard.gov.au/Codes-Guidelines-Statements/Professional-standards/registered-nurse-standards-for-practice.aspx

Tollefson, J., Watson, G., Jelly, E., & Tambree, K. (2022). *Essential clinical skills: Enrolled nurses* (5th ANZ ed.). Cengage Learning Australia.

PART **02**

BODY SYSTEMS AND COMMON PRESENTATIONS

Part 2 introduces the body systems and works through examples of common presentations for each system using the concept map approach.

CHAPTER 3

RESPIRATORY SYSTEM

Approximately 11 per cent of the Australian population have asthma. Up to 14 years of age, boys are more likely than girls to have asthma, though female adults (over the age of 25 to end of lifespan) are more likely than males of the same age group to experience asthma. Asthma is 1.6 times more prevalent in Aboriginal and Torres Strait Islander peoples than in non-Aboriginal and Torres Strait Islanders, and the presentation of asthma is more marked in older adults. People with asthma are more likely to describe their quality of life as poor, and this description is associated with people who have poorly controlled asthma (Australian Institute of Health and Welfare, 2023).

LEARNING OBJECTIVES
After reading this chapter, you should have an understanding of the:
1. assessment required for a person with a respiratory condition
2. prioritisation of key components in the development of plans of care for a person with the respiratory conditions of:
   – asthma and sinusitis
   – pneumonia
   – pneumothorax
3. prioritised and targeted nursing interventions required to promote recovery or prevent further deterioration of people presenting with the respiratory conditions of asthma and sinusitis, pneumonia and pneumothorax
4. evaluation phase and how the prioritised and targeted nursing interventions inform further assessment of the person, planning of care and collaboration with the healthcare team
5. discharge planning and coordination of care required when preparing the person for discharge and subsequent continuity of care between the person and their healthcare providers.

INTRODUCTION

The respiratory system extends from the nose through to the alveoli within the lungs. The respiratory system is divided into the upper and lower tracts. The upper respiratory tract comprises the nose, pharynx, larynx and the upper trachea. The lower respiratory tract is from the lower trachea to the lungs (Calleja et al., 2024).

People with disorders of the respiratory system experience disruption in interacting with their environment and, importantly, with other people. Whether the condition is newly diagnosed or is long term and considered chronic in presentation, the concepts of person-centred care are the same, with the goal of maintaining oxygenation so the individual can interact at the best level possible with their environment and others.

This chapter focuses on disorders of the respiratory system. Both upper and lower airway infections are presented. A non-traumatic pneumothorax is presented to highlight the issues of air collection in the pleural cavity.

3.1 ASSESSMENT OF RESPIRATORY PROBLEMS

In the collection of subjective data, previous and current person-reported information is important in the determination of respiratory symptoms. See **Box 3.1** for the health assessment data collection areas.

BOX 3.1 SUBJECTIVE ASSESSMENT

- ➤ History of illness
- ➤ Past health history
- ➤ Medications
- ➤ Surgery

Functional health patterns
- – Health perception and management
- – Nutritional and metabolic
- – Elimination
- – Activity and exercise
- – Sleep and rest
- – Cognitive and perceptual
- – Self-perception and concept
- – Role relationship
- – Sexuality and reproductive
- – Coping and stress
- – Values and beliefs
- ➤ Risk calculation

The collection of objective data is informed by the subjective data and the physical assessment and diagnostic studies focus on the respiratory system and associated body responses to oxygen-carbon dioxide exchange (see **Box 3.2**). As the physical assessment is guided by the health history, other body systems will be assessed as deemed appropriate.

BOX 3.2 OBJECTIVE ASSESSMENT

- ➤ Inspect nose and nasal cavity
- ➤ Palpate frontal and maxillary sinuses
- ➤ Respiratory rate
- ➤ Inspection of the thorax
- ➤ Palpation of the thorax
- ➤ Percussion of the thorax
- ➤ Auscultation of the lungs
- ➤ Diagnostic tests – pulse oximetry, peak flow, spirometry, sputum, arterial blood gases, chest x-ray, computed tomography, magnetic resonance imaging, pulmonary ventilation-perfusion scan, bronchoscopy, thoracentesis
- ➤ Other body systems as appropriate

3.2 ASSESSMENT FOR ASTHMA

Asthma is airflow obstruction that is characterised by episodes of wheezing, coughing, breathlessness and chest tightness. As part of a focused health assessment, please refer to **Box 3.1** and **Box 3.2**.

Presentation

Alicia Jones is an 18-year-old university student who has been admitted to the emergency department with breathlessness for the last two hours which is not responding to her salbutamol puffer. Alicia has an audible wheeze and she can only speak in short sentences. She has had a cold for the last five days, and it is now affecting her sinuses.

See **Concept map 3.1** to further explore Alicia's initial care in the emergency department.

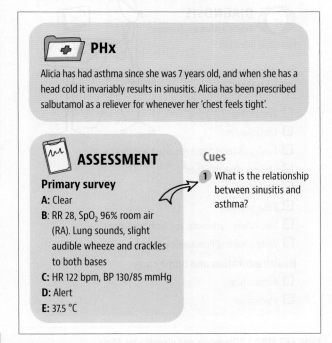

PHx

Alicia has had asthma since she was 7 years old, and when she has a head cold it invariably results in sinusitis. Alicia has been prescribed salbutamol as a reliever for whenever her 'chest feels tight'.

ASSESSMENT

Primary survey

A: Clear
B: RR 28, SpO$_2$ 96% room air (RA). Lung sounds, slight audible wheeze and crackles to both bases
C: HR 122 bpm, BP 130/85 mmHg
D: Alert
E: 37.5 °C

Cues

1 What is the relationship between sinusitis and asthma?

CONCEPT MAP 3.1 Nursing assessment for Alicia

3.3 PLANNING CARE FOR ASTHMA

Planning for the nursing care for acute asthma has the goals of:
- oxygenation
- medication management
- patient education.

Alicia, in partnership with the nurse, constructs a care plan and participates in the management of her asthma and sinusitis and ongoing asthma management at home. **Box 3.3** indicates the areas that are targeted in the planning stage of acute asthma management.

See **Concept map 3.2** to explore the initial diagnosis and planning for Alicia's care.

BOX 3.3   PLANNING FOR ACUTE ASTHMA MANAGEMENT

- ➤ Oxygenation
- ➤ Tests
- ➤ Self-care
- ➤ Medication

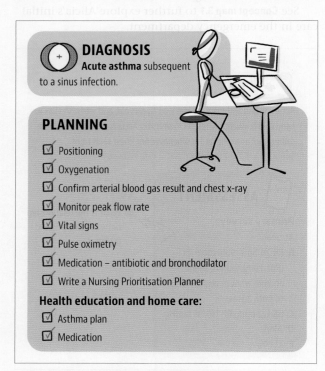

⊕ DIAGNOSIS

Acute asthma subsequent to a sinus infection.

PLANNING

- ☑ Positioning
- ☑ Oxygenation
- ☑ Confirm arterial blood gas result and chest x-ray
- ☑ Monitor peak flow rate
- ☑ Vital signs
- ☑ Pulse oximetry
- ☑ Medication – antibiotic and bronchodilator
- ☑ Write a Nursing Prioritisation Planner

Health education and home care:

- ☑ Asthma plan
- ☑ Medication

CONCEPT MAP 3.2 Diagnosis and planning for Alicia

3.4 NURSING INTERVENTIONS TO SUPPORT HEALTH CARE FOR ASTHMA

Nursing interventions are implemented as part of person-centred care, and the aim of asthma management is to reduce or reverse signs and symptoms and the associated pathophysiology of asthma.

Concept map 3.3 explores Alicia's journey in the emergency department, before discharge to home.

INTERVENTIONS

1 Position upright
2 Oxygen 10 L/min
3 Vital signs and pulse oximetry, frequency as determined by ADDS
4 Salbutamol 5 mg via nebuliser
5 Peak expiratory flow
6 Confirm arterial blood gas result and chest x-ray
7 Patient health education

Health education and home care:

- Asthma plan including peak flow
- Medication – antibiotic and bronchodilator

What further assessments should be initiated?

Cues   **1** What other assessments should we undertake for Alicia?

CONCEPT MAP 3.3 Nursing interventions for Alicia

3.5 EVALUATION OF CARE FOR ASTHMA

As part of the further assessment of Alicia's presentation, **Concept map 3.4** asks further questions in relation to Alicia's management.

EVALUATION

Alicia is responding to the treatment protocol for asthma in the emergency department. Respiratory rate and heart rate have returned to be within normal range. No audible wheeze, but crackles remain in both bases of the lungs.

Plan:
Alicia's mother will take her home after Alicia has responded to the asthma treatment protocol plan.

Cues

1 Why is it important that Alicia continues to administer salbutamol?

2 Alicia has been prescribed an antibiotic for her sinusitis. Why is it important that the sinusitis is treated?

CONCEPT MAP 3.4 Evaluation and planning for Alicia

EVIDENCE-BASED PRACTICE 🔍

To prevent antibiotic resistance, ensure that all of the antibiotic medication is taken in the prescribed time frame.

3.6 DISCHARGE PLANNING AND COORDINATION OF CARE FOR ASTHMA

Alicia's asthma and sinusitis requires discharge planning and further management at home in the form of an asthma management plan. **Concept map 3.5** explores this further.

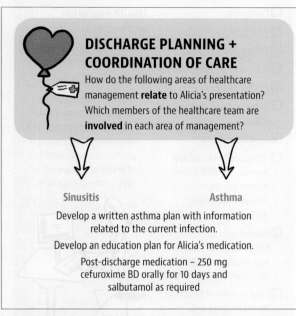

DISCHARGE PLANNING + COORDINATION OF CARE

How do the following areas of healthcare management **relate** to Alicia's presentation? Which members of the healthcare team are **involved** in each area of management?

Sinusitis   Asthma

Develop a written asthma plan with information related to the current infection.

Develop an education plan for Alicia's medication.

Post-discharge medication – 250 mg cefuroxime BD orally for 10 days and salbutamol as required

CONCEPT MAP 3.5 Discharge planning and coordination of care for Alicia

3.7 ASSESSMENT FOR PNEUMONIA

The pathophysiology of pneumonia depends on the infecting organism, with organisms triggering inflammatory responses which are exhibited by vascular permeability and fluid filled alveoli, and this leads to hypoxia. Also, there is increased mucus production that impacts air flow and in turn reduces gas exchange. The person presents with a cough, fever, chills, tachypnoea, limited breath sounds for the infected lung and pleuritic chest pain. Dyspnoea is common when larger areas of lung are infected. See **Box 3.1** and **Box 3.2** to guide the data collection for Patrice's health assessment.

Presentation

Patrice Bell is a 62-year-old widow who was brought into the emergency department by her daughter. Patrice had an appointment with her general practitioner (GP) this morning as she felt she had the flu, and when her daughter arrived at the family home to take her mother to the GP she noticed her mother was being vague. While in the car Patrice appeared to have trouble concentrating so her daughter drove her to the emergency department. Patrice's daughter stated to the triage nurse that she thought Patrice is having a stroke, with Patrice stating 'it's the flu and not a stroke, as I'm aching all over with a roaring headache'.

See **Concept map 3.6** to further explore Patrice's initial care in the emergency department.

 PHx

Patrice has **enjoyed good health,** which she attributes to being a keen gardener. She had her **annual influenza injection** so cannot understand why she has the flu this year.

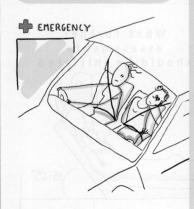
➕ EMERGENCY

 ASSESSMENT

Primary survey
A: Clear
B: RR 24, pulse oximetry 96% on room air, lung sounds reveal bilateral lower lobe fine crackles
C: Pulse 122 bpm, BP 140/80 mmHg, skin flushed, cap refill >2 seconds
D: Alert and orientated. Headache predominantly in sinuses but radiates into forehead, pain scale 5/10. Equal limb strength
E: 38.3 °C

Secondary survey
CNS: Alert and orientated, with patient stating that she has to concentrate to respond to questions. Still has a frontal headache, 5/10 pain scale unchanged
CVS: BP 135/90 mmHg, HR 118 bpm, T 38.6 °C, well perfused with cap refill <2 seconds, peripherally perfused
Resp: Sinuses tender on palpation, occasional dry cough, bilateral lower lobe fine crackles in lungs. RR 26, SaO₂ 96%.
GIT: Bowel sounds present with a non-tender abdomen. Poor appetite for the last 3 days, so eating chicken soup and drinking lemon tea.

Renal: Urine concentrated but no abnormalities detected.
Metabolic: BGL 5.7 mmol/L
Integumentary: Warm dry skin.
Musculoskeletal: Equal limb strength with muscle pain in the thighs and lower back and joint pain in hands and knees.
White blood cell count: 15.9 (3.5–11 nL)
Neutrophils: 10.6 (1.5–7.5 nL)
Chest x-ray to be reviewed

CONCEPT MAP 3.6 Nursing assessment for Patrice

3.8 PLANNING CARE FOR PNEUMONIA

Planning person-centred care for an individual with pneumonia has the goals of:

- oxygenation
- antibiotics for the lung infection
- patient education.

Patrice is a partner in her care, and in partnership with the nurse participates in formulation and delivery of her care. Part of the care will focus on the discharge planning for Patrice. **Box 3.4** indicates the areas that are targeted in the planning stage of caring for a person with pneumonia.

BOX 3.4   PLANNING CARE FOR PNEUMONIA

- » Self-care
- » Lifestyle modifications
- » Physical activity
- » Medication
- » Respond to severity of symptoms, pain management and airway maintenance
- » Tests – sputum culture and sensitivity, arterial blood gases (ABGs)

Concept map 3.7 outlines a plan for Patrice's care.

3.9 NURSING INTERVENTIONS TO SUPPORT HEALTH CARE FOR PNEUMONIA

Nursing interventions are implemented as part of person-centred care. As pneumonia is a lung infection, the aim of Patrice's care is to reverse the signs and symptoms and the associated pathophysiology of pneumonia. One of the key interventions for a

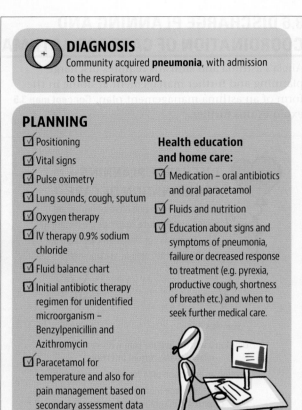

DIAGNOSIS

Community acquired **pneumonia**, with admission to the respiratory ward.

PLANNING

- ☑ Positioning
- ☑ Vital signs
- ☑ Pulse oximetry
- ☑ Lung sounds, cough, sputum
- ☑ Oxygen therapy
- ☑ IV therapy 0.9% sodium chloride
- ☑ Fluid balance chart
- ☑ Initial antibiotic therapy regimen for unidentified microorganism – Benzylpenicillin and Azithromycin
- ☑ Paracetamol for temperature and also for pain management based on secondary assessment data
- ☑ Slow abdominal breathing, deep breathing and coughing
- ☑ Write a Nursing Prioritisation Planner

Health education and home care:

- ☑ Medication – oral antibiotics and oral paracetamol
- ☑ Fluids and nutrition
- ☑ Education about signs and symptoms of pneumonia, failure or decreased response to treatment (e.g. pyrexia, productive cough, shortness of breath etc.) and when to seek further medical care.

CONCEPT MAP 3.7 Diagnosis and planning for Patrice

lung infection is the administration of antibiotics (Broyles et al., 2023).

Concept map 3.8 explores Patrice's journey from the emergency department to the respiratory ward.

INTERVENTIONS

1. Positioning: Fowlers
2. Vital signs 4-hourly
3. Pulse oximetry 4-hourly
4. Lung sounds, cough, sputum 4-hourly assessment
5. Oxygen therapy: nasal prongs 4 L/min
6. IV therapy 0.9% sodium chloride 8/24
7. Benzylpenicillin 1.2 g QID IV
8. Fluid balance chart
9. Azithromycin 500 mg daily IV over 1 hour
10. Paracetamol 1 g QID oral for temperature
11. Slow abdominal breathing, deep breathing and coughing

Health education and home care:

- Medication: oral antibiotics and oral paracetamol
- Fluids and nutrition
- Education about signs and symptoms of pneumonia, including failure or decreased response to treatment and when to seek further medical care.

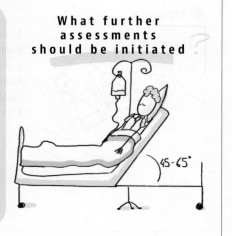

What further assessments should be initiated

45-65°

CONCEPT MAP 3.8 Nursing interventions for Patrice

SAFETY IN NURSING

STANDARD PRECAUTIONS AND DROPLET PRECAUTIONS

Pneumonia that is acquired in the community is considered to be infectious as it is caused by droplet infection. It is therefore essential to follow standard precautions and droplet precautions when managing pneumonia patients so the nurse does not become infected with the respiratory-based pathogen (see Figure 3.1).

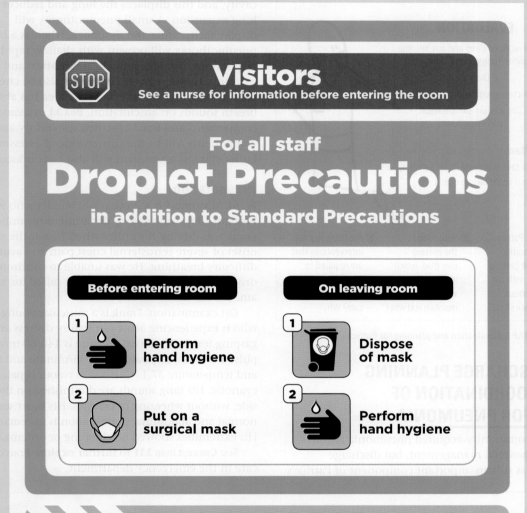

FIGURE 3.1 Standardised infection and control prevention sign: Droplet precautions

SOURCE: REPRODUCED WITH PERMISSION FROM THE APPROACH 1 DROPLET STANDARD PRECAUTIONS PHOTO, DEVELOPED BY THE AUSTRALIAN COMMISSION ON SAFETY AND QUALITY IN HEALTH CARE (ACSQHC). ACSQHC: SYDNEY (2012)

3.10 EVALUATION OF CARE FOR PNEUMONIA

As part of the further assessment of Patrice's presentation, **Concept map 3.9** asks further questions in relation to Patrice's management.

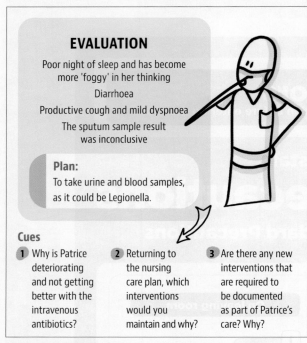

EVALUATION

Poor night of sleep and has become more 'foggy' in her thinking

Diarrhoea

Productive cough and mild dyspnoea

The sputum sample result was inconclusive

Plan:
To take urine and blood samples, as it could be Legionella.

Cues

1. Why is Patrice deteriorating and not getting better with the intravenous antibiotics?

2. Returning to the nursing care plan, which interventions would you maintain and why?

3. Are there any new interventions that are required to be documented as part of Patrice's care? Why?

CONCEPT MAP 3.9 Evaluation and planning for Patrice

3.11 DISCHARGE PLANNING AND COORDINATION OF CARE FOR PNEUMONIA

Patrice's community-acquired pneumonia requires ongoing hospital management, but discharge planning is still an important component of Patrice's care. **Concept map 3.10** explores discharge planning and coordination of care for Patrice.

3.12 ASSESSMENT FOR PNEUMOTHORAX

Pneumothorax involves air entry into the pleural cavity, and this displaces the lung and reduces lung expansion. A small pneumothorax will display tachycardia and dyspnoea, whereas a large pneumothorax will present with shallow rapid respirations, dyspnoea, tracheal deviation and a low oxygen saturation level. There may also be chest pain, cough, and the affected lung area has absent breath sounds on auscultation. **Box 3.1** assessment components and **Box 3.2** focused respiratory assessment components will be the cornerstone of assessment. Other systems assessment will also be conducted.

Presentation

Frank Musumeci is a 26-year-old builder who was brought to the emergency department by ambulance. Frank was driving his utility when he felt the sudden onset of severe retrosternal chest pain and acute difficulty breathing. He was unable to continue driving and pulled off the road. He called for an ambulance on his mobile phone.

On examination, Frank is a muscular young man who is experiencing acute respiratory distress and is gasping for air. His blood pressure is 140/80 mmHg, pulse 100 bpm, respiratory rate 35/minute and shallow and temperature 37.1 °C. His skin colour is pale, but not cyanotic. His lung sounds are diminished on the right side, without wheezing or crackles. His heart sounds are normal and abdominal examination is unremarkable. His extremities showed no clubbing or oedema.

See **Concept map 3.11** to further explore Frank's initial care in the emergency department.

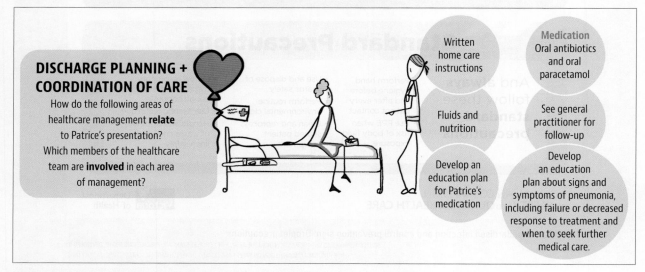

DISCHARGE PLANNING + COORDINATION OF CARE

How do the following areas of healthcare management **relate** to Patrice's presentation? Which members of the healthcare team are **involved** in each area of management?

Written home care instructions

Medication
Oral antibiotics and oral paracetamol

Fluids and nutrition

See general practitioner for follow-up

Develop an education plan for Patrice's medication

Develop an education plan about signs and symptoms of pneumonia, including failure or decreased response to treatment and when to seek further medical care.

CONCEPT MAP 3.10 Discharge planning and coordination of care for Patrice

PHx

Frank has no past medical history of asthma, pneumonia, lung or heart disease, and cannot recall recent trauma. He is not taking medications and has no allergies. He has smoked one packet of cigarettes per day for the last 3 years, and drinks one stubby of beer each night before dinner. His family history does not indicate cardiovascular disease.

 ASSESSMENT

Primary survey

A: Clear
B: RR 35, gasping for air, SpO$_2$ 93% on room air (RA), pleuritic chest pain 6/10 pain scale at rest, pale skin, diminished R side lung sounds
C: HR 100 bpm, BP 140/80 mmHg
D: Alert and orientated
E: 37.1 °C

Cues

1 What is the relationship between the chest pain and respiratory distress?

2 What do the diminished lung sounds indicate?

3 What tests should be obtained to confirm a diagnosis of pneumothorax?

CONCEPT MAP 3.11 Nursing assessment for Frank

3.13 PLANNING CARE FOR A PERSON WITH A PNEUMOTHORAX

The planning of person-centred care for a person with a pneumothorax will have the goals of:

- relieving positive air pressure in the pleural space
- increasing oxygenation
- relieving pain
- providing rest.

Frank is a partner in the planning of his care. **Box 3.5** indicates the areas that are targeted in the planning stage of pneumothorax care.

BOX 3.5 PLANNING FOR CARE OF A PERSON WITH A PNEUMOTHORAX

- Signed informed consent for intercostal catheter insertion
- RN assists with set-up and management of intercostal catheter (ICC)
- Provision of oxygen

> Medication
> Post-insertion ICC chest X-ray
> Self-care

Concept map 3.12 outlines a plan for Frank's care.

 DIAGNOSIS

Right-sided **pneumothorax** with 35% lung bleb that requires transfer to the respiratory ward

PLANNING

☑ Insertion of right intercostal catheter
☑ Chest x-ray
☑ ABGs
☑ Vital signs
☑ Pulse oximetry
☑ Underwater seal drainage system
☑ Positioning
☑ Pain medication – for chest tube insertion, for maintenance of drainage system and chest tube removal
☑ Oxygen therapy
☑ Incentive spirometry
☑ Deep breathing exercises
☑ Write a Nursing Prioritisation Planner

Health education and home care:

☑ Cessation of smoking
☑ Wound care
☑ Signs and symptoms of return of spontaneous pneumothorax and when to return to hospital
☑ Individuals who have had a spontaneous pneumothorax will require a series of follow-up chest X-Rays by their GP in the community.

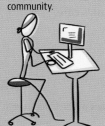

CONCEPT MAP 3.12 Diagnosis and planning for Frank

3.14 NURSING INTERVENTIONS TO SUPPORT HEALTH CARE FOR PNEUMOTHORAX

Nursing interventions are implemented as part of person-centred care, and in the case of a pneumothorax are to reverse signs and symptoms of air collection in the pleural cavity. **Concept map 3.13** explores Frank's admission to the emergency department and the respiratory ward.

REFLECTIVE PRACTICE

In the observation of the underwater seal drainage system, which indicator should be the first to be observed: bubble, swing or drainage?

INTERVENTIONS

1 Insertion of right intercostal catheter and attachment of underwater drainage system

2 Chest x-ray

3 ABGs

4 Vital signs – every 15 minutes first hour, hourly for the next four hours, then 4 hourly

5 Pulse oximetry and lung sounds – as above with vital signs

6 Underwater seal drainage system – checked hourly for bubble, swing, drainage, and gauze and occlusive dressing

7 Positioning – high Fowlers

8 Check chest tube insertion site gauze and occlusive dressing 8 hourly

Pain management:

9 Chest tube insertion – 1% lignocaine + 1:10 000 adrenaline SC

10 Chest tube maintenance – for example, tramadol and diclofenac

11 Chest tube removal – for example, tramadol

Health education and home care:

- Cease smoking to reduce risk of reoccurrence
- Monitor catheter insertion site
- Provide patient education about dressing and need for it to remain intact and dry
- Provide patient education on underwater drainage system and movement of the device.

What further assessments should be initiated

CONCEPT MAP 3.13 Nursing interventions for Frank

3.15 EVALUATION OF CARE FOR PNEUMOTHORAX

As part of the further assessment of Frank's presentation, **Concept map 3.14** asks further questions in relation to the intercostal catheter no longer required in Frank's care.

EVALUATION

Frank will be transferred to the respiratory ward for monitoring while his pneumothorax resolves.

Plan:
Discharge Frank when his intercostal catheter has been removed for more than 24 hours without adverse effect.

Cues

1 What additional information should we obtain to ensure that Frank's right lung is reinflated? Why is this important?

CONCEPT MAP 3.14 Evaluation and planning for Frank

3.16 DISCHARGE PLANNING AND COORDINATION OF CARE FOR PNEUMOTHORAX

What discharge planning is required for Frank's ongoing recovery at home? **Concept map 3.15** explores discharge planning and coordination of care.

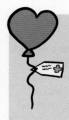

DISCHARGE PLANNING + COORDINATION OF CARE
How do the following areas of healthcare management **relate** to Frank's presentation? Which members of the healthcare team are **involved** in each area of management?

Written home care instructions

Medication
Oral paracetamol

Fluids and nutrition

See general practitioner for follow-up.

Develop an education plan for Frank, including:
- signs and symptoms of return of pneumothorax
- no heavy lifting, running, swimming, exposure to high altitudes for 4-6 weeks after resolution of pneumothorax
- ceasing smoking to reduce risk of recurrence.

CONCEPT MAP 3.15 Discharge planning and coordination of care for Frank

SUMMARY

The lungs are an essential organ to enable individuals to provide self-care in varying environments. When providing care for a person who has decreased respiratory function, the nurse has the additional challenge of providing care to an individual whose activity levels are curtailed and self-care is challenged due to oxygen levels.

CLINICAL SKILLS IN RESPIRATORY HEALTH

The following clinical skills are required when managing a person with respiratory conditions; consult your Clinical Skills resources, such as Tollefson and Hillman (2022), *Clinical Psychomotor Skills* (8th ed.).

- Temperature, pulse and respiration measurement
- Blood pressure measurement
- Monitoring pulse oximetry
- Pain assessment

- Focused respiratory health history and physical assessment
- Inhaled medication
- Oral medication
- Intravenous medication administration
- Oxygen therapy via nasal cannula or various masks
- Oropharyngeal and nasopharyngeal suctioning
- Chest drainage system assessment and management

PROBLEM-SOLVING SCENARIO

Using a concept map approach, how would you care for baby Carlos in the paediatric unit?

Carlos Romero is a 9-month-old boy who has had a history of mild nasal congestion for the last three days. All of the family are currently recovering from head colds. Overnight Carlos has been coughing, and in turn is not feeding well. He is lethargic and has a respiratory rate of 80 breaths per minute with mild intercostal retractions and nasal flaring.

A chest x-ray shows some hyperinflation. The diagnosis of bronchiolitis is made.

1   What are the causes of bronchiolitis?
2   What are the associated signs and symptoms of bronchiolitis?
3   Why are infants admitted to hospital with bronchiolitis?
4   What is the management for bronchiolitis?

PORTFOLIO DEVELOPMENT

As humans we require oxygen to live. This means that our lungs must be functioning to a level that promotes cellular oxygenation. Specific knowledge is required to provide safe nursing care for a person with a respiratory condition.

The websites below will assist in meeting continuing professional development activities to enhance respiratory care and meet the NMBA yearly registration requirements for a Registered Nurse.

USEFUL WEBSITES

Asthma Australia
https://asthma.org.au/about-us

Lung Foundation Australia
https://lungfoundation.com.au/about/who-we-are

The Thoracic Society of Australia and New Zealand
https://www.thoracic.org.au/about-us/about-us

Nursing and Midwifery Board of Australia, Decision-making framework for nursing and midwifery (2020)
https://www.nursingmidwiferyboard.gov.au/codes-guidelines-statements/frameworks.aspx

REFERENCES AND FURTHER READING

Australian Commission on Safety and Quality in Health Care. (2021). *2.1 Chronic obstructive pulmonary disease (COPD)*. https://www.safetyandquality.gov.au/our-work/healthcare-variation/fourth-atlas-2021/chronic-disease-and-infection-potentially-preventable-hospitalisations/21-chronic-obstructive-pulmonary-disease-copd

Australian Institute of Health and Welfare (AIHW). (2023, 30 June). Chronic respiratory conditions: Asthma. https://www.aihw.gov.au/reports/chronic-respiratory-conditions/asthma

Bidder, T. M. (2019). Effective management of adult patients with asthma. *Nursing Standard, 34*(8), 43–49. DOI:10.7748/ns.2019.e11411

Broyles, B., Reiss, B., Evans, M., Pleunik, S., Page, R., & Badoer, E. (2023). *Pharmacology in nursing* (4th ANZ ed.). Cengage Learning Australia.

Calleja, P., Theobald, K., & Harvey, T. (2024). *Estes Health assessment and physical examination* (3rd ed.). Cengage Learning Australia.

DeLaune, S., Ladner, P., McTier, L., Tollefson, J., & Lawrence, J. (2024). *Fundamentals of nursing* (3rd ed.). Cengage Learning Australia.

Holmes, L. J. (2017). Nurses' role in improving outcomes for patients with severe asthma. *Nursing Times, 113*(4), 22–25.

Moreton, T., & Preston, W. (2019). Challenges of diagnosing and managing pneumonia in primary care. *Nursing Times, 115*(9), 36–40.

Neighbors, M., & Tannehill-Jones, R. (2023). *Human diseases* (6th ed.). Cengage.

South Australia Health. (2021). *Community acquired pneumonia (adults) clinical guideline*, https://www.sahealth.sa.gov.au/wps/wcm/connect/9da8d680432af0a6a631f 68cd21c605e/CAP+Clinical+Guideline+%28Adults%29_v2_FINAL_Jan2021+%282%29.pdf

Tarhan, M., Gokduman, S. A., Aryan, A., & Dalar, L. (2016). Nurses' knowledge levels of chest drain management: A descriptive study. *Eurasian Journal of Pulmonology, 18*, 153–159. DOI:10.5152/ejp.2016.97269

Tollefson, J., & Hillman, E. (2022). *Clinical psychomotor skills: Assessment tools for nurses* (8th ed.). Cengage Learning Australia.

CHAPTER 4

CARDIOVASCULAR SYSTEM

The most common types of cardiovascular disease in Australia include coronary heart disease, atrial fibrillation, peripheral arterial disease and cardiac valve disease. Aboriginal and Torres Strait Islander peoples have a higher mortality rate than non-Aboriginal and Torres Strait Islanders from cardiovascular disease. Cardiovascular disease causes more deaths in women than any other disease. Aboriginal and Torres Strait Islander women are twice as likely to die from coronary heart disease as non-Aboriginal and Torres Strait Islander women (Australian Institute of Health and Welfare, 2019).

LEARNING OBJECTIVES

After reading this chapter, you should have an understanding of the:

1 assessment required for a person with a cardiac condition
2 prioritisation of key components in the development of plans of care for a person with the cardiac conditions of:
   – acute myocardial infarction
   – atrial fibrillation and deep vein thrombosis
   – heart valve disease – mitral regurgitation
3 prioritised and targeted nursing interventions required to promote recovery or prevent further deterioration of people presenting with the cardiac conditions of acute myocardial infarction, atrial fibrillation and deep vein thrombosis, and heart valve disease – mitral regurgitation
4 evaluation phase and how the prioritised and targeted nursing interventions inform further assessment of the person, planning of care and collaboration with the healthcare team
5 discharge planning and coordination of care required when preparing the person for discharge and subsequent continuity of care between the person and their healthcare providers.

INTRODUCTION

The cardiovascular system consists of the heart and blood vessels. The heart pumps oxygenated blood within arteries, arterioles and capillaries; deoxygenated blood is removed via the capillaries, venules and veins to be returned to the heart and the arterial system, and in turn oxygenated by the lungs. Health problems of the cardiovascular system invariably disrupt the person's activity levels and decrease their sense of wellbeing, which in turn impacts on their quality of life and lifespan. Whether the condition is newly diagnosed or is long term and considered chronic in presentation, the concepts of person-centred care are the same, with the goal of maintaining cardiovascular function so the individual can maintain a level of activities of daily living and a quality of life that represents their situation.

Common problems of the cardiovascular system can be divided into vascular disorders (hypertension, peripheral vascular disease, aneurysms, thrombus formation and shock), coronary heart disease (atherosclerosis and acute coronary syndrome), heart failure, valvular disease and dysrhythmias.

4.1 ASSESSMENT OF CARDIAC PROBLEMS

In the collection of subjective data, previous and current person-reported information is important in the determination of cardiac symptoms. See **Box 4.1** for the health assessment data collection areas.

BOX 4.1   SUBJECTIVE ASSESSMENT

- ➤ History of illness
- ➤ Past health history
- ➤ Medications
- ➤ Surgery

Functional health patterns:
- – Health perception and management
- – Nutritional and metabolic
- – Elimination
- – Activity and exercise
- – Sleep and rest
- – Cognitive and perceptual
- – Self-perception and concept
- – Role relationship
- – Sexuality and reproductive
- – Coping and stress
- – Values and beliefs
- ➤ Risk calculation

The collection of objective data is informed by the subjective data, and also enables the delineation of both cardiovascular and other organ problems. The respiratory, renal, haematological and neurological systems are often impacted by cardiovascular disease, and in turn manifestations of organ dysfunction within these systems is also observed in the physical assessment and diagnostic studies results (see **Box 4.2**) of the person.

BOX 4.2   OBJECTIVE ASSESSMENT

Peripheral vascular system:
- ➤ Inspect skin, nail beds and large neck veins
- ➤ Palpate upper and lower extremities, pulses in neck and extremities, and capillary refill
- ➤ Auscultate major arteries

Thorax:
- ➤ Inspect and palpate thorax, cardiac valves and auscultatory areas of the aorta, pulmonic, tricuspid, mitral and Erb's point, and PMI
- ➤ Inspect and palpate epigastric area, particularly abdominal aorta (if able)

- ➤ Auscultation of heart sounds
- ➤ Inspection of the thorax
- ➤ Diagnostic test – cardiac biomarkers, electrolytes, renal function, blood glucose, full blood count, serum lipids, homocysteine, chest x-ray, 12-lead ECG, exercise testing, echocardiography, nuclear imaging, magnetic resonance imaging, computed tomography, invasive studies
- ➤ Other body systems as appropriate

4.2 ASSESSMENT FOR ACUTE MYOCARDIAL INFARCTION

During the health assessment for a person presenting with an acute myocardial infarction, the components in **Box 4.1** and **Box 4.2** are applied.

Presentation

Wesley Shapiro is a 58-year-old man who was assisting his friend in the launching of a small boat from a boat trailer when he started to feel sore in the chest. He thought the soreness was due to pulling a muscle, but this pain spread to down his left arm and upper jaw. He mentioned the pain to his friend who then decided to put the boat back on the trailer and drive Wesley to the local hospital.

See **Concept map 4.1** to further explore Wesley's initial care in the emergency department.

4.3 PLANNING CARE FOR ACUTE MYOCARDIAL INFARCTION

The planning for the nursing care of a person with an acute myocardial infarction has the goals of:
- ■ maintaining circulation and oxygenation
- ■ pain relief
- ■ collecting physical assessment data including pathology and radiographic investigations
- ■ reperfusion therapy
- ■ patient education
- ■ cardiac rehabilitation
- ■ adverse effects of therapy.

Wesley is a partner in his care plan and contributes to his health care by following his plan of care and managing his condition in the home environment. **Box 4.3** indicates the areas that are targeted in the planning stage of acute myocardial infarction management.

→

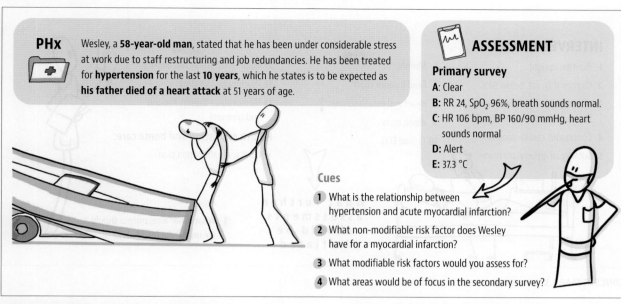

PHx Wesley, a **58-year-old man**, stated that he has been under considerable stress at work due to staff restructuring and job redundancies. He has been treated for **hypertension** for the last **10 years**, which he states is to be expected as **his father died of a heart attack** at 51 years of age.

ASSESSMENT

Primary survey

A: Clear

B: RR 24, SpO$_2$ 96%, breath sounds normal.

C: HR 106 bpm, BP 160/90 mmHg, heart sounds normal

D: Alert

E: 37.3 °C

Cues

1 What is the relationship between hypertension and acute myocardial infarction?

2 What non-modifiable risk factor does Wesley have for a myocardial infarction?

3 What modifiable risk factors would you assess for?

4 What areas would be of focus in the secondary survey?

CONCEPT MAP 4.1 Nursing assessment for Wesley

BOX 4.3   PLANNING CARE FOR ACUTE MYOCARDIAL INFARCTION

➤ Cardiovascular function
➤ Pain relief
➤ Oxygenation
➤ Tests
➤ Reperfusion therapy
➤ Medication
➤ Self-care

Concept map 4.2 outlines a plan for Wesley's care.

4.4 NURSING INTERVENTIONS TO SUPPORT HEALTH CARE FOR ACUTE MYOCARDIAL INFARCTION

Nursing interventions are implemented as part of person-centred care to reduce or reverse signs and symptoms and address the associated pathophysiology of myocardial infarction, which includes reperfusion (Neighbors & Tannehill-Jones, 2023) and pain management (Broyles et al., 2023).

Concept map 4.3 explores Wesley's journey in the emergency department and transfer to the coronary care unit.

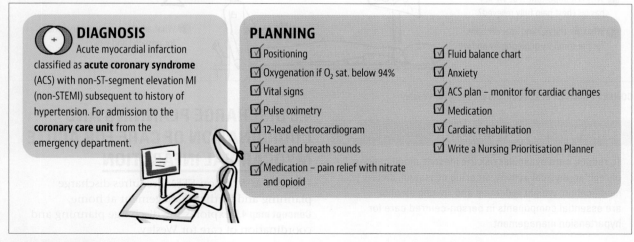

DIAGNOSIS

Acute myocardial infarction classified as **acute coronary syndrome** (ACS) with non-ST-segment elevation MI (non-STEMI) subsequent to history of hypertension. For admission to the **coronary care unit** from the emergency department.

PLANNING

☑ Positioning
☑ Oxygenation if O$_2$ sat. below 94%
☑ Vital signs
☑ Pulse oximetry
☑ 12-lead electrocardiogram
☑ Heart and breath sounds
☑ Medication – pain relief with nitrate and opioid

☑ Fluid balance chart
☑ Anxiety
☑ ACS plan – monitor for cardiac changes
☑ Medication
☑ Cardiac rehabilitation
☑ Write a Nursing Prioritisation Planner

CONCEPT MAP 4.2 Diagnosis and planning for Wesley

INTERVENTIONS

1 Position upright
2 Oxygen if O₂ sat. below 94%
3 Vital signs and pulse oximetry, frequency as determined by ADDS
4 Continuous cardiac monitoring
5 Sublingual glyceryl trinitrate
6 Morphine
7 Fluid balance chart
8 Heart and breath sounds
9 Blood tests
10 12-lead ECG
11 Monitor for stress and anxiety
12 Psychosocial support
13 Medication – aspirin, heparin and captopril

Health education and home care:
• Cardiac rehabilitation plan

What further assessments should be initiated

Cues
1 What other assessments should we undertake for Wesley?

CONCEPT MAP 4.3 Nursing interventions for Wesley

4.5 EVALUATION OF CARE FOR ACUTE MYOCARDIAL INFARCTION

As part of the further assessment of Wesley's presentation, **Concept map 4.4** asks further questions in relation to Wesley's management.

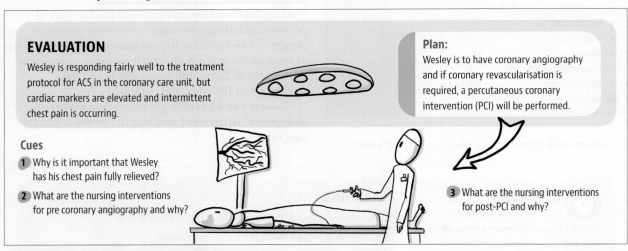

EVALUATION

Wesley is responding fairly well to the treatment protocol for ACS in the coronary care unit, but cardiac markers are elevated and intermittent chest pain is occurring.

Cues
1 Why is it important that Wesley has his chest pain fully relieved?
2 What are the nursing interventions for pre coronary angiography and why?

Plan:
Wesley is to have coronary angiography and if coronary revascularisation is required, a percutaneous coronary intervention (PCI) will be performed.

3 What are the nursing interventions for post-PCI and why?

CONCEPT MAP 4.4 Evaluation and planning for Wesley

EVIDENCE-BASED PRACTICE

To reduce cardiovascular risk the lifestyle modifications of regular physical activity, smoking cessation, dietary modification, weight reduction and limiting alcohol are essential components in person-centred care for hypertension management.

4.6 DISCHARGE PLANNING AND COORDINATION OF CARE FOR ACUTE MYOCARDIAL INFARCTION

Wesley's ACS of non-STEMI requires discharge planning and further management at home. **Concept map 4.5** explores the discharge planning and coordination of care for Wesley.

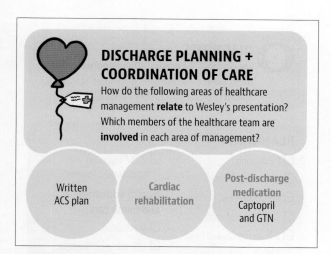

DISCHARGE PLANNING + COORDINATION OF CARE

How do the following areas of healthcare management **relate** to Wesley's presentation? Which members of the healthcare team are **involved** in each area of management?

Written ACS plan

Cardiac rehabilitation

Post-discharge medication Captopril and GTN

CONCEPT MAP 4.5 Discharge planning and coordination of care for Wesley

4.7 ASSESSMENT FOR ATRIAL FIBRILLATION AND DEEP VEIN THROMBOSIS

Please refer to **Box 4.1** and **Box 4.2** regarding a focused health assessment for Margaret Dungala Pierce. Recall also **Boxes 3.1** and **3.2** to guide your respiratory assessment. Margaret is experiencing dyspnoea, hence the respiratory system as well as the cardiovascular system will be prominent in the assessment of the body systems in an objective assessment.

Presentation

Margaret Dungala Pierce is a 65-year-old widow and a proud Yorta Yorta woman and was admitted to the emergency department (ED) with a past history of an anterior acute myocardial infarction (AMI) six years ago and mild heart failure controlled by enalapril with atorvastatin. She has had dyspnoea on exertion for the past two weeks, and her general practitioner (GP) ordered a 12-lead electrocardiogram which displayed atrial fibrillation (AF) with a ventricular rate of 80 beats per minute.

See **Concept map 4.6** to further explore Margaret's initial care in the emergency department, before transfer to the coronary care unit for further care.

4.8 PLANNING CARE FOR ATRIAL FIBRILLATION AND DEEP VEIN THROMBOSIS

Planning person-centred care for an individual with atrial fibrillation and deep vein thrombosis has the goals of:

- maintaining circulation and oxygenation
- pain relief
- collecting physical assessment data including pathology and radiographic investigations
- patient education
- cardiac rehabilitation
- adverse effects of therapy.

PHx

Margaret has a past history of an anterior acute myocardial infarction six years ago and mild heart failure controlled by enalapril and atorvastatin. She has had dyspnoea on exertion for the past two weeks, and a 12-lead electrocardiogram taken at the general practice today revealed atrial fibrillation with a ventricular rate of 80 beats per minute.

Cues

1. What is the relationship between acute myocardial infarction and heart failure?

2. What is the relationship between dyspnoea and heart failure?

3. What is the relationship between dyspnoea and atrial fibrillation?

4. What is the relationship between heart failure and reduced peripheral circulation?

ASSESSMENT

Primary survey

A: Clear

B: RR 24, dyspnoea on exertion, SaO₂ 96% on room air, chest x-ray shows enlarged heart with clear lungs

C: HR 90 bpm, BP 150/95 mmHg, pedal pulses present but weak to palpate. A 12-lead electrocardiogram showed an old anterior AMI, atrial fibrillation and no pulmonary hypertension

D: Alert and orientated. No pain

E: 36.8 °C

Secondary survey

CNS: Alert and orientated

CVS: BP 165/90 mmHg, HR 110 bpm, T 36.8 °C, cap return >2 seconds

Resp: RR 26, SaO₂ 96%.

GIT: Tolerating food and fluids. Bowel sounds present with a non-tender abdomen.

Renal: 50 mL/hr and no abnormalities detected.

Metabolic: BGL 5.7 mmol/L

Integumentary: Cool feet with slight oedema

BMI: 31.1

Musculoskeletal: Equal limb strength

CONCEPT MAP 4.6 Nursing assessment for Margaret

Margaret is a partner in her care plan and can contribute by discussing her plan of care and managing her recovery in the home environment. **Box 4.4** indicates the areas that are targeted in the planning stage for caring for a person with atrial fibrillation and deep vein thrombosis.

BOX 4.4 PLANNING FOR CARE OF A PERSON WITH ATRIAL FIBRILLATION AND DEEP VEIN THROMBOSIS

➤ Cardiac monitoring
➤ Daily weight
➤ Medication
➤ Monitor blood pressure and weight gain
➤ Sodium-restricted diet
➤ Fowler's position
➤ Vital signs
➤ Fluid balance chart
➤ Medication therapy

Health education and home care:

➤ Lifestyle modifications
➤ Self-care
➤ Physical activity
➤ Medication

Concept map 4.7 outlines a plan for Margaret's care.

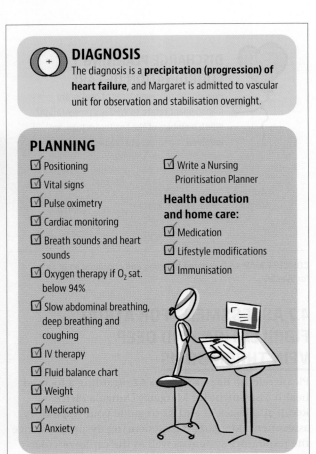

DIAGNOSIS

The diagnosis is a **precipitation (progression) of heart failure**, and Margaret is admitted to vascular unit for observation and stabilisation overnight.

PLANNING

☑ Positioning
☑ Vital signs
☑ Pulse oximetry
☑ Cardiac monitoring
☑ Breath sounds and heart sounds
☑ Oxygen therapy if O₂ sat. below 94%
☑ Slow abdominal breathing, deep breathing and coughing
☑ IV therapy
☑ Fluid balance chart
☑ Weight
☑ Medication
☑ Anxiety

☑ Write a Nursing Prioritisation Planner

Health education and home care:
☑ Medication
☑ Lifestyle modifications
☑ Immunisation

CONCEPT MAP 4.7 Diagnosis and planning for Margaret

4.9 NURSING INTERVENTIONS TO SUPPORT HEALTH CARE FOR ATRIAL FIBRILLATION AND DEEP VEIN THROMBOSIS

Nursing interventions are implemented as part of person-centred care and also to reduce or reverse signs and symptoms of atrial fibrillation and deep vein thrombosis and to address the associated pathophysiology of heart failure. Atrial fibrillation is a risk factor for deep vein thrombosis, and as such, both atrial fibrillation and deep vein thrombosis are treated simultaneously to prevent a recurrence of blood clots and stabilise the cardiac rhythm (Neighbors & Tannehill-Jones, 2023).

Concept map 4.8 explores Margaret's journey from the emergency department to the coronary care unit.

INTERVENTIONS

1 Positioning – Fowlers
2 Vital signs 4 hourly
3 Pulse oximetry 4 hourly
4 Cardiac monitor for arrhythmia detection
5 Breath and lung sounds assessment 4 hourly
6 Oxygen therapy if O₂ sat. below 94%
7 Slow abdominal breathing, deep breathing and coughing
8 IV therapy 0.9% sodium chloride 8/24

9 Fluid balance chart hourly
10 Medication enalapril, atorvastatin, diltiazem and warfarin
11 Low fat and sodium diet
12 Relieve anxiety

Health education and home care:

• Medication – enalapril, atorvastatin, diltiazem and warfarin
• Lifestyle modification

What further assessments should be initiated

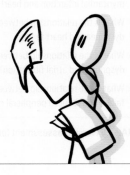

CONCEPT MAP 4.8 Nursing interventions for Margaret

SAFETY IN NURSING

ATRIAL FIBRILLATION AND DEEP VEIN THROMBOSIS

When a patient is taking warfarin to reduce the incidence of blood clots due to atrial fibrillation, regular INR levels are required (Broyles et al., 2023) and to observe the patient for bruising and bleeding.

4.10 EVALUATION OF CARE FOR ATRIAL FIBRILLATION AND DEEP VEIN THROMBOSIS

As part of the further assessment of Margaret's presentation, **Concept map 4.9** asks further questions in relation to Margaret's management.

EVALUATION

The night shift handover stated that Margaret is stable. Just as the handover was completed Margaret rang the call bell for an extra blanket as her left lower leg was painful. The blanket was brought to the bed and it was observed that her left calf had a reddened appearance and was slightly oedematous. Margaret had a pain scale of 4 out of 10.

Plan:

To contact the medical team and facilitate further assessment. Advise Margaret to rest in bed until medical review. Notify RN in-charge of shift of Margaret's deterioration. Document assessment findings and nursing actions taken in Margaret's health record.

Cues

1 Why does Margaret describe her left lower leg as painful?

2 Why does the calf look reddened and slightly oedematous?

3 What has precipitated the presentation in the left calf?

4 What further assessments are required?

The medical team have been notified of Margaret's left calf and other observations remain unchanged.
While Margaret was being prepared to have an ultrasound, she complains of muscle spasms in the left calf.

5 Which blood tests should be ordered for Margaret and why?

6 Does this newly diagnosed condition relate to Margaret's reason for admission?

7 How will this newly diagnosed condition be managed and why? Consider medical and nursing management.

CONCEPT MAP 4.9 Evaluation and planning for Margaret

4.11 DISCHARGE PLANNING AND COORDINATION OF CARE FOR ATRIAL FIBRILLATION AND DEEP VEIN THROMBOSIS

The discharge planning for Margaret's atrial fibrillation and deep vein thrombosis has the foci of further management at home and follow-up appointments with her GP and Practice Nurse. **Concept map 4.10** explores the discharge planning and coordination of care for Margaret.

DISCHARGE PLANNING + COORDINATION OF CARE

How do the following areas of healthcare management **relate** to Margaret's presentation? Which members of the healthcare team are **involved** in each area of management?

Written home care instructions

Medication

INR tests

BP monitoring

Compression stockings

See GP and Practice Nurse for follow-up

Lifestyle modification:

Weight reduction, low fat and sodium diet, exercise

CONCEPT MAP 4.10 Discharge planning and coordination of care for Margaret

4.12 ASSESSMENT FOR HEART VALVE DISEASE – MITRAL REGURGITATION

In the health assessment for a person with heart valve disease, the subjective and objective assessment components in **Box 4.1** and **Box 4.2** are employed.

Presentation

David Lee Chew is a 36-year-old chef who was brought to the emergency department by his wife. David has become fatigued over the last two months, is breathless on occasions and today has developed palpitations.

See **Concept map 4.11** to further explore David's initial care in the emergency department.

PHx

David has no past medical history of heart or lung problems, although he did have rheumatic fever when he was 6 years old. He is not taking medications and has no allergies. He drinks an occasional glass of whisky, as he has been under a lot of stress at work. His family history does not indicate cardiovascular disease.

Cues

1. What is the relationship between David's feelings of fatigue, breathlessness and palpitations?

2. What initial tests should be obtained to confirm a diagnosis of heart valve disease – mitral regurgitation?

3. What areas would be of focus during the secondary survey?

ASSESSMENT

Primary survey

A: Clear

B: RR 30, normal breath sounds, oxygenation saturation 98%

C: HR 120 bpm, BP 145/95 mmHg, peripheral pulses present but not strong, extremities cool but perfused, perfusion time of 3 seconds, pan systolic murmurs

D: Alert and orientated

E: 37.1 °C

CONCEPT MAP 4.11 Nursing assessment for David

4.13 PLANNING CARE FOR A PERSON WITH A HEART VALVE DISEASE – MITRAL REGURGITATION

The planning of person-centred care for an individual with a heart valve disease – mitral regurgitation will have the goals of:

- maintaining circulation and oxygenation
- pain relief
- collecting physical assessment data including pathology and radiographic investigations
- patient education
- surgery
- cardiac rehabilitation
- adverse effects of therapy.

David is a partner in the planning of his care. **Box 4.5** indicates the areas that are targeted in the planning stage of heart valve disease – mitral regurgitation care.

BOX 4.5 PLANNING FOR CARE OF A PERSON WITH HEART VALVE DISEASE – MITRAL REGURGITATION

- » Positioning
- » Medication
- » Further tests
- » Admission to coronary care unit
- » Surgery
- » Health education and home care

Concept map 4.12 outlines a plan for David's care.

DIAGNOSIS
Right sided **heart valve disease – mitral regurgitation**

PLANNING

- ☑ Position-high Fowlers
- ☑ Vital signs
- ☑ Pulse oximetry
- ☑ Cardiac monitoring
- ☑ Medication – ACE inhibitor
- ☑ Fluid balance chart
- ☑ Echocardiogram
- ☑ Further radiology tests
- ☑ Further blood tests
- ☑ Transfer to coronary care unit for further management
- ☑ Surgical referral

- ☑ Write a Nursing Prioritisation Planner
- ☑ Health education and home care

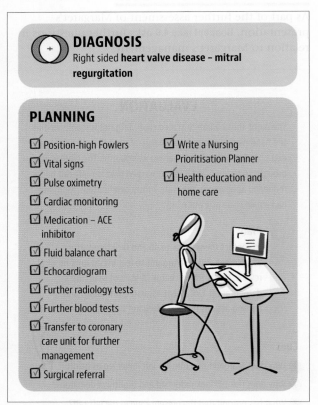

CONCEPT MAP 4.12 Diagnosis and planning for David

4.14 NURSING INTERVENTIONS TO SUPPORT HEALTH CARE FOR HEART VALVE DISEASE – MITRAL REGURGITATION

Nursing interventions are implemented as part of person-centred care to reduce the signs and symptoms of mitral valve regurgitation and address the associated pathophysiology of heart valve disease (Neighbors & Tannehill-Jones, 2023).

Concept map 4.13 explores David's journey in the emergency department before transfer to the coronary care unit.

INTERVENTIONS

1 Positioning – high Fowlers
2 Vital signs, frequency as determined by ADDS
3 Pulse oximetry and heart sounds
4 12-lead ECG
5 Medication – ACE inhibitors
6 Fluid balance chart
7 Blood tests

8 Radiology tests
9 Cardiology consultation
10 Surgical consultation

Health education and home care:

• Medication – ACE inhibitors
• Prophylactic antibiotics for surgical procedures

What further assessments should be initiated

CONCEPT MAP 4.13 Nursing interventions for David

4.15 EVALUATION OF CARE FOR HEART VALVE DISEASE – MITRAL REGURGITATION

As part of the further assessment of David's presentation, **Concept map 4.14** asks further questions in relation to the proposed mitral valve replacement.

EVALUATION

David's stay in the emergency department for monitoring and further care for his heart valve disease – mitral regurgitation.

Plan:
Transfer David to the coronary care unit. Surgical team recommending a mitral valve replacement?

Cues 1 Why would a mitral valve replacement be considered as part of David's care?

CONCEPT MAP 4.14 Evaluation and planning for David

EVIDENCE-BASED PRACTICE

When oxygen levels are less than 94% saturation, supplemental oxygen therapy is required. Increasing oxygen levels means that the heart rate is reduced and the heart as a pump is under less stress to oxygenate the body via the circulation.

4.16 DISCHARGE PLANNING AND COORDINATION OF CARE FOR HEART VALVE DISEASE – MITRAL REGURGITATION

David's condition requires ongoing hospital management, but discharge planning is still an important component of David's care. **Concept map 4.15** explores discharge planning and coordination of care for David.

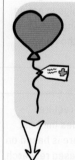

DISCHARGE PLANNING + COORDINATION OF CARE
How do the following areas of healthcare management **relate** to David's presentation? Which members of the healthcare team are **involved** in each area of management?

Written home care instructions

Medication

Cardiac rehabilitation
See GP for follow-up

Discharge planning
Prophylactic ABs may be required for some people with MV replacement who require dental work undertaken

CONCEPT MAP 4.15 Discharge planning and coordination of care for David

REFLECTIVE PRACTICE

Always consider that pharmacological interventions may produce adverse effects. Thrombolytic therapy may produce reperfusion arrhythmias and reduce cardiac output which is the opposite to the intention of the therapy. Bleeding from thrombolytic therapy can impact on cardiac output. Antihypertensive drugs can lower blood pressure too much and unintentionally reduce cardiac output.

SUMMARY

Health problems of the cardiovascular system invariably disrupt the person's activity levels and may decrease their sense of wellbeing, which in turn impacts their quality of life and lifespan. When providing care for a person who has decreased cardiac function, the nurse has the additional challenge of providing care to an individual whose activity levels are curtailed and self-care may be challenged due to blood flow and oxygen levels.

CLINICAL SKILLS IN CARDIAC HEALTH

The following clinical skills are required when managing a person with cardiac conditions; consult your Clinical Skills resources, such as Tollefson and Hillman (2022), *Clinical Psychomotor Skills* (8th ed.).

- Temperature, pulse and respiration measurement
- Blood pressure measurement
- Monitoring pulse oximetry
- Height, weight and waist circumference measurements
- Blood glucose measurement

- Pain assessment
- Focused cardiovascular health history and physical assessment
- 12-lead electrocardiogram
- Oral medication
- Topical medication
- Intravenous medication administration
- Oxygen therapy via nasal cannula or various masks

PROBLEM-SOLVING SCENARIO

Using a concept map approach, how would you assist Alfonso Polimeni?

Alfonso Polimeni's heart failure has become progressively worse to be classified as chronic heart failure. Alfonso is quite often breathless at rest, this is more noticable if 'he forgets to take his tablets'. Alfonso also does like to indulge in eating salami, olives and cheeses at night while watching television. As Alfonso wishes to remain at home, what are the nursing

interventions that you would put in place to maintain Alfonso's care at home? Some areas to consider are:

- lifestyle modifications
- oxygen therapy
- medication therapy
- cardiac rehabilitation
- home health nursing
- palliative and end-of-life care.

PORTFOLIO DEVELOPMENT

Caring for people with cardiovascular disorders requires current evidence-based nursing care that provides the best possible outcomes for the patient. As cardiac care is based on evidence-based practice and ongoing clinical-based research, engaging in continuing professional development activities will enable the nurse to provide contemporary healthcare practice

for patients with cardiac conditions. The Heart Foundation (Australia) is an organisation that provides professional development activities for healthcare professionals to complement the Heart Foundation's best practice guidelines for patient care.

USEFUL WEBSITES

Cardiac Society of Australia and New Zealand https://www.csanz.edu.au/for-professionals/position-statements-and-practice-guidelines
Heart Foundation https://www.heartfoundation.org.au

Nursing and Midwifery Board of Australia, Decision-making framework for nursing and midwifery (2020) https://www.nursingmidwiferyboard.gov.au/codes-guidelines-statements/frameworks.aspx

REFERENCES AND FURTHER READING

Australian Institute of Health and Welfare (AIHW). (2019, 22 July). *Cardiovascular disease in women*. https://www.aihw.gov.au/reports/heart-stroke-vascular-diseases/cardiovascular-disease-in-women-main/summary

Bidder, T. M. (2019). Effective management of adult patients with acute myocardial infarction. *Nursing Standard, 34*(8), 43–49. DOI:10.7748/ns.2019.e11411
Broyles, B., Reiss, B., Evans, M., Pleunik, S., Page, R., & Badoer, E. (2023).

Pharmacology in nursing (4th ANZ ed.). Cengage Learning Australia.
DeLaune, S., Ladner, P., McTier, L., Tollefson, J., & Lawrence, J. (2024). *Fundamentals of nursing* (3rd ed.). Cengage Learning Australia.

El Hussein, M., Blayney, S., & Clark, N. (2020). ABCs of heart failure management: A guide for nurse practitioners. *The Journal for Nurse Practitioners, 16*, 243–248. https://doi.org/10.1016/j.nurpra.2019. 12.021

Holmes, L. J. (2017). Nurses' role in improving outcomes for patients with severe acute myocardial infarction. *Nursing Times, 113*(4), 22–25.

Moreton, T., & Preston, W. (2019). Challenges of diagnosing and managing atrial fibrillation and deep vein thrombosis in primary care. *Nursing Times, 115*(9), 36–40.

National Acute Myocardial Infarction Council of Australia. (2019). *Acute myocardial infarction, version 2.* https://www.acute myocardial infarctionhandbook.org.au/ static/files/Australian-Acute myocardial infarction-Handbook-v2.0-Acute-acute myocardial infarction.pdf

Neighbors, M., & Tannehill-Jones, R. (2023). *Human diseases* (6th ed.). Cengage.

Oliver-McNeil, S. (2019). Management of valvular heart disease in adults: Implications for nurse practitioner practice. *The Journal for Nurse Practitioners, 15*(1), 65–72. https://doi. org/10.1016/j.nurpra.2018.08.029

Pagnesi, M., Adamo, M., Sama, I., Anker, S., Cleland, J., Dickstein, K., Filippatos, G., Lang, C., Ng, L., Ponikowski, P., Ravera, A., Samani, N., Zannad, F., van Veldhuisen, D., Voors, A., & Mtra, M. (2021). Impact of mitral regurgitation in patients with worsening heart failure: insights from BIOSTAT-CHF. *European Journal of Heart Failure, 23*, 1750–1758. https://doi. org/10.1002/ehhf.2276

Tollefson, J., & Hillman, E. (2022). *Clinical psychomotor skills: Assessment tools for nurses* (8th ed.). Cengage Learning Australia.

CHAPTER 5

HAEMATOLOGICAL SYSTEM

Within Australia, around 19000 people are newly diagnosed with blood cancers such as leukaemia, myeloma or lymphoma annually. This means around one person every 27 minutes is diagnosed with blood cancer. The incidence of these types of cancers has increased by 47 per cent in the past ten years (Leukaemia Foundation, 2022).

LEARNING OBJECTIVES

After reading this chapter, you should have an understanding of the:

1 assessment required for a person with a haematological condition
2 prioritisation of key components in the development of a plan of care for a person with:
   – anaemia
   – haematoma (post-surgery)
3 prioritised and targeted nursing interventions required to promote recovery or prevent further deterioration for anaemia and haematoma (post-surgery)
4 evaluation phase and how the prioritised and targeted nursing interventions inform further assessment, planning of care and collaboration with the healthcare team
5 discharge planning and coordination of care required when preparing the person for discharge and subsequent continuity of care between the person and their healthcare providers.

INTRODUCTION

The haematological system is responsible for the delivery of all nutrients and oxygen necessary for survival through blood circulating. Red blood cells provide oxygen and, importantly, remove carbon dioxide, while maintaining acid-base balance. Blood contains a transport system for platelets, white blood cells, hormones, electrolytes and proteins (see **Figure 5.1**) – a significant role considering how innately blood is tied in response to homeostasis. The circulating blood volume is around 4.5–6 litres in adults.

The haematological system is comprised predominantly of blood, and includes bone marrow, the spleen, liver and kidneys. Blood is essential for homeostasis, and without it performing its three main functions – regulation, transportation and protection – this is unable to be maintained. To understand the significance of the haematological system, let's look at the three functions in more detail:

- regulation – maintenance of the fluid and electrolyte balance, body temperature, oncotic pressure and the acid-base balance
- transportation – movement of hormones from endocrine glands to the relevant tissues/cells; waste products (carbon dioxide, ammonia, etc.) from the cells to the lungs for exhalation; nutrients from the gastrointestinal tract to cells where they are needed
- protection – response to invasion or pathogens within the body (sending white blood cells, etc.) and maintenance of homeostasis and coagulation or clotting of blood (Brown et al., 2019; Craft & Gordon, 2019).

Alterations of the haematological system are related to either insufficient or excessive numbers of red blood cells (RBCs) in the circulating volume. This can impact upon haemostasis also, which is when blood clots to prevent bleeding (Brown et al., 2019; Craft & Gordon, 2019). Patients who present with haematological disorders are likely to have vague or diverse symptoms such as:

- fatigue
- frequent infections
- swollen glands
- bleeding tendencies.

This requires the nurse to ensure that a systematic physical examination is undertaken, utilising the subjective data from the patient and any available diagnostic findings. Haematological conditions generally require laboratory/pathology investigations to determine the cause or the impact upon the person (Bryant et al., 2019; Craft & Gordon, 2019; Waugh & Grant, 2023).

There are many common haematological conditions. These include:

- anaemia
- thalassaemia
- haemochromatosis
- thrombocytopaenia
- disseminated intravascular coagulation
- neutropaenia
- leukaemia
- lymphomas.

Each of these conditions will 'look' different on every person. Again, focus on the holistic physical assessment of your patient, coupled with subjective data, and investigative reports, particularly in haematological conditions, to aid your evaluation and planning.

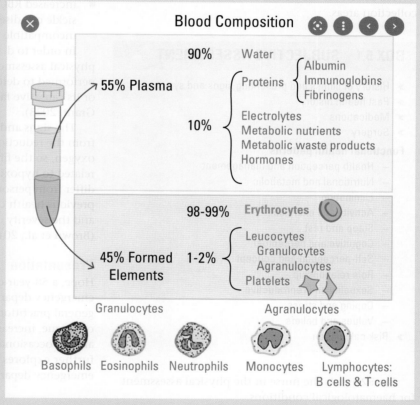

Blood Composition

90% Water

55% Plasma

Proteins { Albumin, Immunoglobins, Fibrinogens }

10% { Electrolytes, Metabolic nutrients, Metabolic waste products, Hormones }

98–99% **Erythrocytes**

45% Formed Elements   1–2% { Leucocytes, Granulocytes, Agranulocytes, Platelets }

Granulocytes   Agranulocytes

Basophils   Eosinophils   Neutrophils   Monocytes   Lymphocytes: B cells & T cells

FIGURE 5.1 Composition of blood

SOURCE: <TBC>

Blood transfusion/blood component therapy

The most common types of blood components for patient administration include:

- fresh components – red cells, platelets
- frozen components – fresh frozen plasma, cryoprecipitate, cryodepleted plasma
- fractionated plasma products – albumin, prothrombinex, immunoglobulins and factor concentrates.

Blood and blood products within Australia are biological products – meaning they come from donors. The risk for reaction to blood does not decrease with each exposure to a blood transfusion, rather it remains the same. Unlike penicillin or any other medication, blood and blood products are not made in a laboratory and therefore the risk of reaction remains unchanged. Fresh blood products are administered to manage symptomatic anaemia or to maintain intravascular volume during critical bleeding. Frozen components are used to manage clotting factors or other immunocompromised conditions. One unit of RBCs costs $430, platelets cost $300 per unit and plasma costs $185–280 per unit (Australian Red Cross, 2022).

It should be noted that the transfusion of any blood component only temporarily supports the patient until the underlying issue is corrected. Pouring blood into someone who is bleeding out is not an effective use of blood as it is not being circulated (Brown et al., 2019).

5.1 ASSESSMENT FOR HAEMATOLOGICAL CONDITIONS

All patients with a haematological dysfunction or condition will present with various symptoms, requiring investigation and assessment to determine the best and safest course of action. The presentation, be it anaemia or a clotting disorder, could also exacerbate other underlying medical conditions.

It is important to note that a haematological condition can be induced by trauma, shock, burns or bleeding, for example, which is not related directly to the haematological system, but rather to the impact upon homeostasis from the loss of the circulating blood volume.

See **Box 5.1** for the health assessment data collection areas.

BOX 5.1   SUBJECTIVE ASSESSMENT

- ➤ History of illness and presenting signs and symptoms
- ➤ Past health history
- ➤ Medications
- ➤ Surgery

Functional health patterns
- – Health perception and management
- – Nutritional and metabolic
- – Elimination
- – Activity and exercise
- – Sleep and rest
- – Cognitive and perceptual
- – Self-perception and concept
- – Role relationship
- – Sexuality and reproductive
- – Coping and stress
- – Values and beliefs
- ➤ Risk calculation

Box 5.2 assists the nurse in the physical assessment for haematological conditions.

BOX 5.2   PHYSICAL ASSESSMENT

- ➤ Glasgow Coma Scale (GCS), including pupillary assessment
- ➤ Vital signs
- ➤ Blood tests such as full blood count
- ➤ Blood glucose level (BGL)
- ➤ Electrocardiogram
- ➤ Pain assessment
- ➤ Capillary refill
- ➤ Neurovascular assessment
- ➤ Abdominal assessment
- ➤ Cardiovascuar assessment
- ➤ Respiratory assessment

5.2 ASSESSMENT FOR ANAEMIA

One of the most common presentations or reasons for hospitalisation is anaemia. Anaemia is the deficiency in the number of RBCs, the quality of haemoglobin (Hb) and the volume of packed RBCs (referred to as haematocrit). It can be caused by many factors, and it should be noted that it is not a disease, but a pathological process due to the loss of RBCs. This means that it is not something the person may experience for the 'rest of their life' (Brown et al., 2019).

Anaemia can be caused by:
- ■ decreased RBC production – which can be a deficiency in nutrients, erythropoietin, or iron availability
- ■ blood loss
- ■ increased RBC destruction – through trauma, sickle cell disease, medication or administration of incompatible blood.

In order to diagnose anaemia, aside from a full physical assessment, a full blood count needs to be performed to determine the specific type of anaemia or its causative factors (Brown et al., 2019; Waugh & Grant, 2023).

The signs and symptoms of anaemia are caused from the reduction in circulating RBCs, which carry oxygen, so the first observable sign/symptom is related to hypoxia. The presenting symptoms will differ from person to person and will be reliant upon previous health conditions, pre-existing conditions and the severity of the anaemia (and the cause) (Brown et al., 2019).

Presentation

Hope, a 58-year-old female, was admitted via the emergency department following referral from her general practitioner (GP). Hope reports a 2/52 history of fatigue, increased shortness of breath, headaches and an occasional 'racing heart'. **Concept map 5.1** further explores Hope's presentation in the emergency department.

5.3 PLANNING CARE FOR ANAEMIA

Planning for management of haematological conditions is broad as the causative factor needs to be identified. In any planning, the person is a partner in their care plan and needs to be able to contribute to their health care in being able to follow their plan of care and manage their condition in the home environment. **Box 5.3** indicates the areas that are targeted in the planning stage for care of haematological conditions.

PHx

Hope, a 58-year-old female presents with 2/52 history of fatigue, increased SOB, headaches and palpitations. Alcohol 2–3 standard drinks/week, never smoked/ vaped, menstrual history – 28–35 day cycle, OTC – Vitamin D, Calcium, denies illicit drug use.
PMHx: NKDA, Hypertension, dysmenorrhoea.
Meds: OCP, Metoprolol 25 mg, Atorvastatin 40 mg, Esomeprazole 20 mg.

ASSESSMENT

Primary survey

A: Patent airway
B: RR 20
C: Centrally warm and peripherally cooler
D: Alert
E: T 36.9°C
F: Nil in, HNPU
G: BGL 7.5 mmol

Secondary survey

CNS: E 4 V 5 M 6 = 15 PEARLLA 3 mm
PAIN: C/o frontal headache, dull, rated as 3/10
CVS: HR 90 bpm, BP 160/90 mmHg, T 36.9°C

RESP: RR 20, patent airway – spontaneous breathing, increasing SOB, SpO$_2$ 94% RA, AE = on auscultation.
GIT (Input): BS present in all four quadrants, NBM currently, IVC to be placed, currently nothing running.
RENAL (Output): HNPU since admission 4 hours ago, Pt does not report any blood in urine.
SKIN/INTEG: Centrally warm and peripherally cooler. Cap refill > 4 secs.
MUSCULOSKELETAL (Mobility): C/o dizziness at times prior to admission – RIB.
BMI: 26.5

Cues

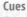

1 What are your priorities with this patient?
2 What other vital signs or bedside investigations would you perform?
3 What is the relationship between anaemia and increased SOB/hypoxia?
4 What is the pathophysiological relationship between hypoxia and homeostasis?
5 What are some concerns in relation to the integumentary assessment for this patient?
6 What physiological impact do low circulating RBCs have on the body?
7 What investigative or diagnostic procedures do you think would be relevant for this patient?

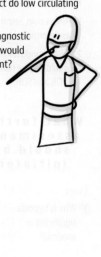

CONCEPT MAP 5.1 Nursing assessment for Hope

BOX 5.3   PLANNING FOR CARE OF HAEMATOLOGICAL CONDITIONS

➤ Lifestyle modifications
➤ Diet
➤ Iron supplementation – including dietary advice
➤ Physical activity
➤ Medication/s interactions, including OTC and prescribed medications
➤ Monitor blood pressure

In any acute care setting your observational skills will be the most important clinical skill you use – patient assessment is paramount – and this includes reassessment, re-evaluation and escalation of care. Remember that all haematological conditions will affect patients differently and their response to treatment will also differ. See **Concept map 5.2** for an outline of Hope's care plan.

DIAGNOSIS

The diagnosis is **anaemia secondary to iron deficiency**.

PLANNING

☑ Vital signs – at least hourly
☑ Monitor oxygen saturation – consider supplemental oxygen if CRT is > 4 secs
☑ Fluid balance chart
☑ Medication therapy
☑ Pathology – FBC, MCV, RBC, Hct, Fe
☑ BGL
☑ 12-lead ECG, pt has reported palpitations
☑ Insertion of a peripheral intravenous cannula (PIVC)
☑ Write a Nursing Prioritisation Planner

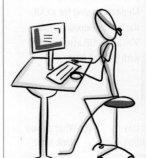

CONCEPT MAP 5.2 Diagnosis and planning for Hope

5.4 NURSING INTERVENTIONS TO SUPPORT HEALTH CARE FOR ANAEMIA

Nursing interventions are implemented as part of person-centered care to reduce or reverse signs and symptoms and the associated condition. Interventions are based upon your assessment findings and collaboration with the treating team – medical officers, nurse practitioners and other healthcare professionals. **Concept map 5.3** explores the nursing interventions and cues for Hope.

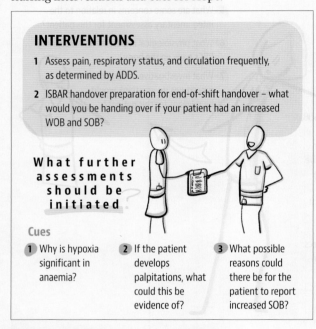

INTERVENTIONS

1 Assess pain, respiratory status, and circulation frequently, as determined by ADDS.

2 ISBAR handover preparation for end-of-shift handover – what would you be handing over if your patient had an increased WOB and SOB?

What further assessments should be initiated?

Cues

1 Why is hypoxia significant in anaemia?

2 If the patient develops palpitations, what could this be evidence of?

3 What possible reasons could there be for the patient to report increased SOB?

CONCEPT MAP 5.3 Nursing interventions for Hope

5.5 EVALUATION OF CARE FOR ANAEMIA

As part of the further assessment of Hope's presentation, **Concept map 5.4** asks further questions in relation to her management.

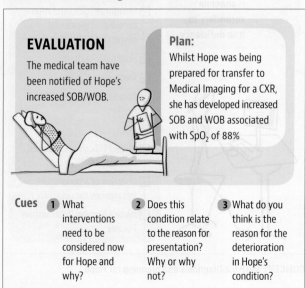

EVALUATION

The medical team have been notified of Hope's increased SOB/WOB.

Plan:
Whilst Hope was being prepared for transfer to Medical Imaging for a CXR, she has developed increased SOB and WOB associated with SpO_2 of 88%

Cues

1 What interventions need to be considered now for Hope and why?

2 Does this condition relate to the reason for presentation? Why or why not?

3 What do you think is the reason for the deterioration in Hope's condition?

CONCEPT MAP 5.4 Evaluate and planning for Hope

Ageing and the haematological system

Ageing does not alter the composition of blood – surprisingly. As we age, however, erythrocytes are replenished more slowly after bleeding – generally due to iron depletion (rather than deficiency). Iron deficiency is often the reason for lower haemoglobin levels noted in older adults. The impact of other chronic conditions, such as renal insufficiency, heart disease and chronic inflammation, also affects the rate of erythropoietin production, which impacts directly on the production of RBCs.

Also associated with ageing is the decrease in lymphocyte function, which means that older people are more susceptible or vulnerable to viruses. It also inhibits uptake of vaccinations, often requiring frequent 'boosters'.

Much of this information will continue to be updated with the impact of the ageing population living longer being observed. It is based on findings such as these that older people are placed in a vulnerable category for exposure to disease/s and when you look at the decline in function you can see why (Craft & Gordon, 2019; Waugh & Grant, 2023).

5.6 DISCHARGE PLANNING AND COORDINATION OF CARE FOR ANAEMIA

For conditions such as anaemia, your patient may have previously experienced it, or it may be the very first presentation. Regardless, your role will include planning care with the patient alongside the medical and allied healthcare team. The patient and their family will likely have many questions, and this is where you will need to consider the impact the condition will have on the patient and plan your care around this, particularly if it is an ongoing haematological condition that requires lifestyle changes or modifications.

Hope is being discharged and has three main areas for planning and nursing care. See **Concept map 5.5**.

5.7 ASSESSMENT FOR HAEMATOMA (POST-SURGERY)

The next patient journey will be a patient who is several hours postoperative and requires transfusion of packed red blood cells (PRBCs).

Presentation

Jason Jenkins is a 52-year-old male who is three hours post-femoral popliteal bypass graft. He has a past medical history of PTSD, type II diabetes mellitus and peripheral vascular disease.

Concept map 5.6 explores Jason's presentation with a haematoma after surgery.

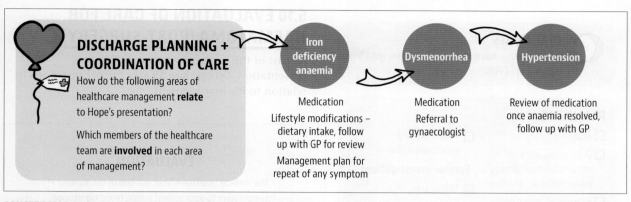

DISCHARGE PLANNING + COORDINATION OF CARE

How do the following areas of healthcare management **relate** to Hope's presentation?

Which members of the healthcare team are **involved** in each area of management?

Iron deficiency anaemia

Medication

Lifestyle modifications – dietary intake, follow up with GP for review

Management plan for repeat of any symptom

Dysmenorrhea

Medication

Referral to gynaecologist

Hypertension

Review of medication once anaemia resolved, follow up with GP

CONCEPT MAP 5.5 Discharge planning and coordination of care for Hope

 PHx

Jason, a 52-year-old male, is 3 hours postoperative, following L Femoral popliteal bypass graft. (L FPBG)
PMHx: PTSD, T2DM, PVD, HTN, GORD, Hyperlipidaemia
NKDA. No alcohol or cigarettes/ illicit drugs
Meds: Escitalopram 20 mg, atorvastatin 40 mg, esomeprazole 20 mg, prazosin 2 mg, metformin 500XR

 ASSESSMENT

CNS: E4 V5 M6 = 15 PEARLA 4 mm
T: 36.4 °C
PAIN: C/o pain behind left knee. Rating as 8/10, burning, sharp, sudden onset
CVS: HR 115 bpm, regular. BP 100/65 mmHg. Centrally warm, peripherally cooler. CAP refill <3 secs, popliteal

pulses DP R present, L only via Doppler, PT R present, L absent
RESP: RR 20, chest on auscultation clear throughout R = L. Nil cough. SpO$_2$ 98% RA
GIT: BS Audible in all quadrants. BGL 6.5 mmol/L
RENAL (Output): HNPU as yet

SKIN/INTEG: Surgical dressing intact with nil strike through ooze visible on the dressing
MUSCULOSKELETAL (Mobility): Strict RIB, with VTE prophylaxis - combination as documented
BMI: 24.0

Cues

1. What are your priorities with this patient?
2. What is the significance of the increase in pain and rigidity behind the knee?
3. What is the significance of VTE prophylaxis?
4. What is the pathophysiological relationship between PVD and the need for this surgery?
5. What are some concerns regarding the patient's observations?
6. What investigative or diagnostic procedures would you think would be relevant for this patient?

CONCEPT MAP 5.6 Nursing assessment for Jason

5.8 PLANNING CARE FOR HAEMATOMA (POST-SURGERY)

Concept map 5.7 explores the planning of Jason's care.

5.9 NURSING INTERVENTIONS TO SUPPORT HEALTH CARE FOR HAEMATOMA (POST-SURGERY)

Nursing interventions for Jason are explored in **Concept map 5.8.**

DIAGNOSIS

The diagnosis is **haematoma** post-surgery, requiring transfusion of PRBC

PLANNING

- ☑ Analgesia
- ☑ Order group and hold/ cross match if not already performed prior to surgery
- ☑ Insertion of second PIVC if not already in situ for blood transfusion
- ☑ Consent form check
- ☑ Blood product – confirm availability
- ☑ IV fluid with monitoring of fluid input and output
- ☑ Documentation – vital signs, fluid balance chart, PIVC
- ☑ VTE Prophylaxis
- ☑ Bloods and pathology
- ☑ Full physical assessment

- ☑ Write a Nursing Prioritisation Planner

Further investigations:

- ☑ 12-lead ECG
- ☑ Baseline observations prior to blood transfusion
- ☑ Surgical evacuation of haematoma?

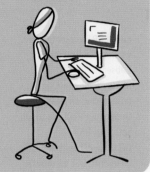

CONCEPT MAP 5.7 Diagnosis and planning for Jason

INTERVENTIONS

1 Assess pain, surgical site, blood transfusion observations, patient observations – including development of urticaria, rash, etc.

2 ISBAR handover preparation for end-of-shift handover – what would you be handing over if Jason had developed a fever during the blood transfusion?

What further assessments should be initiated

Cues

1 What further questions or information would you like to know from Jason?

2 What is the deterioration or change in patient status here?

What is it related to pathophysiologically?

3 What clinical observations would alert you to a reaction to the PRBCs?

CONCEPT MAP 5.8 Nursing interventions for Jason

5.10 EVALUATION OF CARE FOR HAEMATOMA (POST-SURGERY)

As part of the further assessment of Jason's presentation, **Concept map 5.9** asks further questions in relation to his management.

EVALUATION

The medical team have been notified of the increase in temperature to your patient during blood transfusion.

Plan:
Medical officer has requested you to hold the PRBC infusion for 30 minutes.

Cues

1 What interventions need to be considered now for your patient and why? What is your priority here?

2 If the PRBC was prescribed to be administered over four hours, and you are ceasing it for 30 mins does this impact the life of the product? What will you need to do to ensure no loss of blood product?

3 What do you think is the reasoning for increase in temperature? Is this a significant reaction and why?

CONCEPT MAP 5.9 Evaluation and planning for Jason

5.11 DISCHARGE PLANNING AND COORDINATION OF CARE FOR HAEMATOMA (POST-SURGERY)

Further information for Jason's discharge planning can be found in **Concept map 5.10**.

SAFETY IN NURSING

ADVERSE EVENTS IN BLOOD TRANSFUSIONS

Within blood transfusions there are four classifications of adverse reactions:

- immunological acute (occurring within 24 hours)
- non-immunological acute (occurring within 24 hours)
- immunological delayed (>24 hours)
- non-immunological delayed (>24 hours)

Immunological acute adverse events are the most severe, with significant impact upon the patient such as transfusion-related acute lung injury (TRALI) or even anaphylaxis.

Anaphylaxis generally occurs within a few minutes after the start of the transfusion and can be fatal. Patients can present with an incredibly sudden onset of cough, bronchospasm, severe hypotension, angioedema, urticaria and loss of consciousness. Anaphylaxis occurs in 1:20 adverse reactions.

The significance of transfusion reactions is often related to the incorrect product or patient and most facilities will require nursing staff to complete the haemovigilance program for patient safety, as well as adherence to the NSQHS Standard for Blood Management.

More information regarding adverse reactions and the incidence of them can be found here https://www.lifeblood.com.au/health-professionals/clinical-practice/adverse-events/classification-incidence.

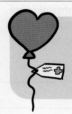

DISCHARGE PLANNING + COORDINATION OF CARE

How do the following areas of healthcare management **relate** to the patient presentation? Which members of the healthcare team are **involved** in each area of management?

Post-op bleed – reaction to PRBC	Mobility postoperatively	Type 2 Diabetes	Wound and vascular follow–up
Management and education to patient on delayed blood transfusion reactions. Follow up with GP in one week	Gait assessment – Physiotherapist Management of wound site and haematoma – assessment of home surroundings for ADLs – may need OT referral also.	Patient education and health promotion regarding type 2 diabetes postoperatively – expectation of BGLs etc. – what to report.	Follow-up by wound care nurse in community. OPD appointment with vascular surgeon Review by GP for removal of staples 14 days post-op.

CONCEPT MAP 5.10 Discharge planning and coordination of care for Jason

SUMMARY

The haematological system is incredibly complex, and nursing patients with disorders of this system is also complex. Haematological nursing is a specialty and focuses on caring for patients with blood disorders such as anaemia or thrombocytopaenia, to more complicated conditions such as leukaemia and lymphoma. The primary goal, as with any body system or condition, is to manage symptoms, support the patient and their family and assess the patient.

CLINICAL SKILLS IN HAEMATOLOGICAL HEALTH

The following clinical skills are required when managing a person with haematological health issues; consult your Clinical Skills resources, such as Tollefson and Hillman (2022), *Clinical Psychomotor Skills* (8th ed.).

- Temperature, pulse and respiration measurement
- Blood pressure measurement
- Monitoring pulse oximetry
- Pain assessment

- Focused cardiovascular health history and physical assessment
- Focused respiratory health history and physical assessment
- Neurovascular assessment
- 12-lead electrocardiogram
- Blood glucose measurement
- Oral medication
- Intravenous medication administration
- Venipuncture

PROBLEM-SOLVING SCENARIO

Jenny Bennett has presented with palpitations, dizziness and a 3/7 history of black stools. She has a previous history of a gastric ulcer and has no known allergies. She has recently lost 5 kg, and has increased her alcohol intake.

1 With this information, what are some pathophysiological processes in place that could be occurring here?
2 What nursing considerations would you have for Jenny?

PORTFOLIO DEVELOPMENT

BloodSafe is an eLearning transfusion practice and patient blood management provider. It is peer reviewed and regularly updated. It can be found here https://bloodsafelearning.org.au.

USEFUL WEBSITES

Registered Nurse Standards for Practice
The Registered Nurse Standards for Practice consist of seven crucial standards that all nurses must follow. Download and review the standards at the following link. https://www.nursingmidwiferyboard.gov.au/Codes-Guidelines-Statements/Professional-standards/registered-nurse-standards-for-practice.aspx

Australian Red Cross – Lifeblood
The Australian Red Cross has a comprehensive guide accessible through the internet and via an app for blood transfusion practice. https://www.lifeblood.com.au

Australian Commission on Safety and Quality in Health Care
The National Safety and Quality Health Service (NSQHS) has a standard dedicated to the safe management of blood and transfusion practices. It is a requirement of all hospitals to abide by this standard. https://www.safetyandquality.gov.au/standards/nsqhs-standards/blood-management-standard

National Blood Authority
This website has best practice principles for treatment and management of haematological disorders, including anaemia. It is peer reviewed and evidence based. https://www.blood.gov.au/best-practice

REFERENCES AND FURTHER READING

Australian Red Cross. (2022). *Health professionals*. https://www.lifeblood.com.au/health-professionals

Brown, D., Edwards, H., Buckley, T., Aitken, R. L., Lewis, S. L., Bucher, L., McLean Heitkemper, M., Harding, M. M., Kwong, J., & Roberts, D. (2019). *Lewis's medical-surgical nursing ANZ* (5th ed.). Elsevier.

Bryant, B. K., Darroch, S., & Rowland, A. (2019). *Pharmacology for health professionals* (5th ed.). Elsevier.

Craft, J., & Gordon, C. (2019). *Understanding pathophysiology* (3rd ed.). Elsevier Australia.

Leukaemia Foundation. (2022). *Blood cancer facts and figures*. https://www.leukaemia.org.au/blood-cancer/understanding-your-blood/blood-cancer-facts-and-figures

Tollefson, J., & Hillman, E. (2022). *Clinical psychomotor skills: Assessment tools for nurses* (8th ed.). Cengage Learning Australia.

Waugh, A., & Grant, A. (2023). *Ross & Wilson anatomy and physiology in health and illness* (14th ed.). Elsevier.

CHAPTER 6

CENTRAL NERVOUS SYSTEM

During 2021–2022 in Australia there were 8.8 million presentations to hospital emergency departments nationally (Australian Institute of Health and Welfare (AIHW), 2023). Over 800 000 of these presentations were triaged as 'non-urgent'. There are many reasons for this number of non-urgent presentations, including after-hours need for medical assistance, free access to medical services (e.g. x-ray, pathology and physiotherapy), though most patients presented to emergency with acute illness or injury. According to the AIHW (2023), the top five presentations to emergency departments for 2021–2022 were:
- symptoms, signs and abnormal clinical and laboratory findings (25%)
- injury, poisoning or other 'consequences' of external causes (22%)
- diseases of the respiratory system (6%)
- diseases of the digestive system (5%)
- certain infectious and parasitic diseases (5%).

LEARNING OBJECTIVES
After reading this chapter, you should have an understanding of the:
1 assessment required for a person with an acute neurological condition
2 prioritisation of key components in the development of a plan of care for a person with a neurological condition
3 prioritised and targeted nursing interventions required to promote recovery or prevent further deterioration
4 evaluation phase and how the prioritised and targeted nursing interventions inform further assessment, planning and collaboration with the healthcare team
5 discharge planning and coordination of care required when preparing the person for discharge and subsequent continuity of care between the person and their healthcare providers.

INTRODUCTION

There are a vast number of acute health conditions that affect every system of our body. Visualising the effects of acute neurological health conditions will greatly assist with your consolidation of learning. Acute neurological conditions are those which are sudden in onset and nature.

There will be many conditions that you will gain exposure to and experience with across not only your clinical placement but also your nursing career. Acute care nursing should assess the client for urgent and emergency conditions, using both physiologically and technologically derived data, to evaluate for physiological instability and potential life-threatening conditions.

The myriad of conditions and injuries that are acutely caused is too exhaustive to list. Common acute neurological conditions are the result of accident or injury, with systematic neurological conditions resulting from autoimmune disorders such as myasthenia gravis or Guillain-Barré syndrome. Systemic acute neurological conditions can be the result of an infective process such as meningitis. There are systemic responses to acute injury, such as hypovolaemic shock, that occur due to volume depletion. Volume depletion can occur for many reasons – bleeding, both internal and external, fluid loss through diarrhoea and vomiting, and multiple injuries.

The nervous system
The nervous system is composed of the central nervous system (CNS) and the peripheral nervous system (PNS). The CNS contains the brain and spinal cord, and the PNS consists of the nerves that relay messages from the

brain and spinal cord. The neurological system is crucial in maintaining voluntary and involuntary body activities. Breathing/respiration and our heart beating are both involuntary activities. When the brain is significantly damaged these functions are not able to be regulated involuntarily – which is related to brain death (Croft et al., 2021; Marieb & Hoehn, 2021; Rizzo, 2015).

The CNS houses the brain and spinal cord, which is one structure continually joined and extends from the skull through to the spine. The cerebrum is the largest part of the brain and has two distinct lobes – the outer is the grey matter and the inner is the white matter. The brain is mirrored, so the left side of the brain controls the function of the right side of the body and vice versa. The other major aspect of the brain is the cerebellum, which coordinates movement/muscle activity and balance. The cerebellum is connected to the brain stem which is the centre for controlling involuntary movements – respirations, pulse and vital organ movement (e.g. peristalsis). If a head injury occurs, initially the meninges will attempt to soften the blow, but if the head injury is traumatic, or blunt force, then the impact cannot be softened. The spinal cord is also responsible for the secretion of cerebrospinal fluid. In a client with a head injury, it is prudent to assess ears and nose for CSF leaking (Croft et al., 2021; Rizzo, 2015).

There are many common neurological conditions, including:

- fractures
- cerebrovascular accident (stroke)
- meningitis
- meningococcal
- lacerations
- Guillain-Barré syndrome
- migraine
- head injury – traumatic – open or closed
- contusion
- subarachnoid haemorrhage
- subdural haematoma
- concussion
- cerebral oedema
- epilepsy
- anoxic injury
- overdose/ingestion of medications/illicit substances

You will need to rely upon your foundation anatomy and physiology and the application of this to your patient's condition. Some conditions will be unusual or 'weird' – you will need to source information regarding treatment methods or the pathophysiological process of the condition. Some overdoses or ingestions of medicines or poisons can occur rarely or infrequently, so staff may not be aware of the impact and need to source information. Within every state and territory in Australia there is a dedicated 24-hour poisons information line. Health professionals have a direct link to a toxicologist who can provide information regarding the toxicology of the ingested medications.

SAFETY IN NURSING ⚠

CLINICAL TOXICOLOGY

Medicines are readily available to many Australians, both legal and illicit. Within nursing, it is crucial to not rely on memory for the treatment of overdose or ingestion of medications. There are dedicated services in each state and territory that provide up-to-date and evidence-based treatment guidelines. Almost all states and territories have dedicated webpages for healthcare professionals to access information. These services are necessary when you consider the vast geographcial locations and make-up of Australia. Not all regional, rural or remote hositals have specialists on hand to answer these intricate questions.

For some examples, please refer to the following websites:
- Austin Health, Melbourne, Clinical Toxicology Guidelines, https://www.austin.org.au/page?ID=1779
- Queensland Poisons Information Centre, https://www.childrens.health.qld.gov.au/chq/our-services/queensland-poisons-information-centre/
- Western Australia, https://ww2.health.wa.gov.au/Articles/N_R/Poisoning-advice-for-health-professionals
- New South Wales, https://www.poisonsinfo.nsw.gov.au/
- Health Direct site has information for all of Australia, https://www.healthdirect.gov.au/poisoning

6.1 ASSESSMENT FOR AN ACUTE NEUROLOGICAL CONDITION

All patients with acute health conditions will commence their hospital journey through the emergency department; some patients may, however, begin treatment in a primary healthcare setting but will still require acute care intervention. Upon admission, you will need to perform and document a complete, system-focused or symptom-specific physical assessment. A patient, for instance, may be presenting for a closed head injury. The nurse needs to assess the health status of the affected region, but also of the whole body. For example, this patient may have an associated respiratory condition that will increase the risk in the operative and postoperative phase.

Although other medical problems are not often the priority of the admission, it is important to understand how they will impact on the present treatments. The current acute episode could also exacerbate other underlying medical conditions.

In the collection of subjective data, previous and current person-reported information is important in the determination of symptoms. See **Box 6.1** for the health assessment data collection areas.

BOX 6.1   SUBJECTIVE ASSESSMENT

- ➤ History of illness
- ➤ Past health history
- ➤ Medications
- ➤ Surgery

Functional health patterns

- – Health perception and management
- – Nutritional and metabolic
- – Elimination
- – Activity and exercise
- – Sleep and rest
- – Cognitive and perceptual
- – Self-perception and concept
- – Role relationship
- – Sexuality and reproductive
- – Coping and stress
- – Values and beliefs
- ➤ Risk calculation

The collection of objective data is informed by the subjective data and enables the delineation of both neurological and any other potential organ problems. The respiratory, renal, haematological and neurological systems are often impacted by neurological or central nervous system injury/illness. In turn, manifestations of organ dysfunction within these systems are also observed in the physical assessment and diagnostic studies results of the person (see Box 6.2).

BOX 6.2   PHYSICAL ASSESSMENT

- ➤ Glasgow Coma Scale (GCS), including pupillary assessment
- ➤ Vital signs
- ➤ Perfusion
- ➤ Response to stimuli (reflexes, and brain-stem testing)
- ➤ Diagnostic investigations, such as MRI or CT
- ➤ Blood tests such as full blood count, liver function tests, urea, etc.
- ➤ Electrolytes such as potassium, calcium, magnesium
- ➤ Blood glucose level (BGL)
- ➤ Renal function
- ➤ Electrocardiogram

Now that we have outlined an assessment, let us move on to the presentation of a patient with neurological dysfunction.

Presentation

Steven, an 18-year-old male, was admitted via emergency department with a base of skull fracture sustained in a high-speed MVA. He was the passenger and was wearing a seat belt. Other injuries include a fractured clavicle and closed head injury.

Concept map 6.1 further explores Steven's presentation in the emergency department.

Other considerations for Steven's head injury would include:

- ■ ensure patent airway
- ■ C-spine precautions/protection
- ■ peripheral IV access
- ■ 'less than 8 intubate' – GCS lower than 8 has potential for significant airway compromise
- ■ assess scalp for lacerations, fractures or skull depression
- ■ assess for battle signs/raccoon eyes
- ■ assess for pupillary response.

6.2 PLANNING CARE FOR AN ACUTE NEUROLOGICAL CONDITION

In planning for neurological injury, key considerations are blood pressure control and temperature control. Box 6.3 indicates the areas that are targeted in the planning stage for neurological injury. Any patient who sustains a head injury has the risk of an increased intracranial pressure (ICP), which can be catastrophic for CNS function. Other conditions, such as cerebrovascular accident, subarachnoid haemorrhage, subdural haemorrhage, mass occupying leasion/s or cranial/cerebral infections also place the patient at a risk of a raised ICP. ICP is not solely related to an acute head injury and needs to be considered for all conditions that affect the neurological system (Brown et al., 2019; Marieb & Hoehn, 2021).

BOX 6.3   PLANNING FOR AN ACUTE NEUROLOGICAL CONDITION

- ➤ Previous medical history
- ➤ Previous surgical history
- ➤ Nature of injury – accelerant, blunt force
- ➤ C-spine precautions
- ➤ Serum sodium levels and electrolytes
- ➤ Alcohol – BAL
- ➤ Substances of abuse screening
- ➤ LOC/GCS/pupillary response
- ➤ Medication
- ➤ Monitor blood pressure
- ➤ Thermoregulation
- ➤ Secondary assessment – other injuries to review

Your observational skills will be the most important clinical skill you will use in patient care – patient assessment is paramount as no two injuries are the same. You could have two patients with exactly the same mechanism of injury who will respond to it completely differently. They will have different levels of pain (as pain is personal, and as such is subjective), different amounts of bleeding and inflammation and different recovery time. Even when comparing an operation; for example, laparoscopic appendicectomy, each patient will have varying levels of postoperative pain, varying

PHx

Steven, an **18-year-old male** was admitted via the emergency department with a **base of skull fracture** sustained in an **MVA** at high speed (>140 km/hr). He was the front seat passenger and was wearing a seat belt. He was not ejected from the vehicle. Extricated by emergency services. Other injuries include a **fractured left clavicle**, and **closed head injury**.

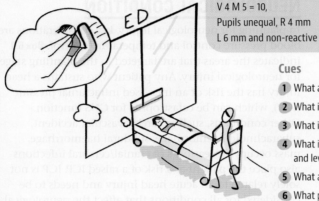

 ASSESSMENT

Primary survey
A: Patent
B: RR 14
C: Warm
D: ALOC
E: T 38.5 °C
F: IVF 166 ml/hr; IDC 50 ml/hr
G: BGL 4.6 mmol/L

Secondary survey
GCS: E 1 (Swollen shut) V 4 M 5 = 10, Pupils unequal, R 4 mm L 6 mm and non-reactive

PAIN: Responding to painful stimuli
CVS: HR 90 bpm, BP 180/95 mmHg, pedal pulses bounding. A 12-lead electrocardiogram showed a sinus rhythm with no abnormalities.
T: 38.5 °C
RESP: RR 14, patent airway – spontaneous breathing, not laborious
GIT (Input): IVF 166 mL/hr, NGT for gut decompression –

bile aspirate, strong ETOH smell, abdo soft, BS in all quadrants
RENAL (Output): IDC in situ 50 mL/hr – no sediment, straw coloured
SKIN/INTEG: Centrally and peripherally warm and well perfused.
MUSCULOSKELETAL (Mobility): Strict RIB, with chemical VTE prophylaxis
BMI: 22.4

Cues

1. What are your priorities with this patient? ABC.
2. What is the significance of the temperature in a closed head injury?
3. What is the relationship between head injury and pupillary response/s?
4. What is the pathophysiological relationship between base of skull fractures and level of consciousness?
5. What are some concerns in relation to the GCS assessment in this patient?
6. What physiological impact does a high-speed impact have on the body?
7. What investigative or diagnostic procedures do you think would be relevant for this patient?

CONCEPT MAP 6.1 Nursing assessment for Steven

levels of nausea and vomiting post-anaesthesia and varying differences in mobility postoperatively. See **Concept map 6.2** for an outline of Steven's care plan.

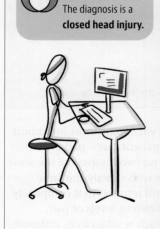 **DIAGNOSIS**
The diagnosis is a **closed head injury**.

PLANNING
☑ Neurological observations – at least hourly
☑ Monitor blood pressure closely
☑ Pupillary response – ensure this is completed hourly with GCS
☑ Monitor neurovascular observations in relation to clavicle
☑ Vital signs
☑ Fluid balance chart
☑ Medication therapy
☑ Write a Nursing Prioritisation Planner

CONCEPT MAP 6.2 Diagnosis and planning for Steven

6.3 NURSING INTERVENTIONS TO SUPPORT HEALTH CARE FOR AN ACUTE NEUROLOGICAL CONDITION

Nursing interventions are implemented as part of person-centred care to reduce or reverse signs and symptoms and the associated acute condition. When planning interventions, not just for neurological injury but for any CNS health condition, it is imperative that you are focused on the patient, and not the tasks. Subjective data can be obtained even if the patient has a varied level of consciousness. Physiological signs of pain can be evident, as can body posturing. Planning your care is always rewarding, especially ticking off the 'done stuff'; but the differentiating factor between nurses and list makers is that nurses must consistently add their assessment and interventions and evaluate the findings, not just tick them off.

In continuing with the closed head injury for Steven, there has been a decrease in his GCS (see **Concept map 6.3**). Your recent observations have given the following:

- GCS – E 1 V 3 M 5 = 9/15. Pupils R 4 mm and reactive, L 6 mm and non-reactive.

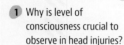

INTERVENTIONS

1   Assess pain, level of consciousness and GCS frequently.

2   ISBAR handover preparation for end-of-shift handover – what would you be handing over if your patient had a GCS: E 1 V 3 M 5 = 9/15. Pupils R 4 mm and reactive, L 6 mm and non-reactive.

3   Prepare patient for urgent imaging/scanning due to decrease in GCS.

4   Elevate head of bed to 30–45 degrees if tolerated and not contraindicated (check with Buddy RN).

What further assessments should be initiated

Cues   **1** Why is level of consciousness crucial to observe in head injuries?   **2** What is the deterioration here? What is the significance of the GCS change?

CONCEPT MAP 6.3 Nursing interventions for Steven

Interventions need to be evaluated. For instance, this GCS is a decline from previous assessments. The decline in GCS is significant in an obvious head injury and can indicate cerebral oedema, raised ICP, and decreased cerebral perfusion. Decreased cerebral perfusion indicates that there is less oxygenated blood available, and without oxygen, function is altered.

Head injuries are intricate and incredibly unique. Sure, there are similarities, but patients who have a traumatic closed head injury do not follow the same recovery pathway.

REFLECTIVE PRACTICE

Coward's punches

Coward's punches are a 'one hit/punch' that causes death. There were 127 deaths because of the coward punch in Australia between 2000–2016. All these deaths were preventable; 94 per cent of victims were males, with an average age of 37 years. In more than 70 per cent of fatalities, alcohol was involved. These deaths commonly occur over the weekend, are associated with binge drinking, and occur between 12 pm and 3 am (Schuman, 2019). The actual numbers would be higher, as some perpetrators have gone on to kick, repeatedly punch or inflict other injuries, meaning it was not recorded as a coward/one punch death.

Sadly, there are many more one-punch victims who do not die but end up permanently impaired physically and mentally. These patients often have had extensive ICU admissions and neurosurgical interventions, coupled with extensive rehabilitation and ongoing care.

One such case, which can be reviewed here https://www.abc.net.au/news/2019-07-09/one-punch-death-brisbane-man-

sentenced/11290704 outlines the catastrophic impact of one punch, with the death of a 40-year-old man.

The confronting aspect of these types of deaths is that they occur in public places, meaning that many people potentially witness the last moments of someone's life.

Questions

1   After reviewing the news article, what would be the causative factor in his death? What do you think was 'happening' in his brain?

2   If you had to explain traumatic brain injury from a coward punch, how would you explain it to a student RN? A family member? What actually causes death?

6.4 EVALUATION OF CARE FOR AN ACUTE NEUROLOGICAL CONDITION

Evaluation is an ongoing process. In any nursing intervention you will be assessing the impact or outcome in the patient. For instance, if you administer analgesia, there is no point in administering it if you do not reassess and evaluate the impact of the analgesia. Did the patient's pain score reduce? What effect did the analgesia have? This is all information that is unique to the patient and your documentation and evaluation of the assessment.

Concept map 6.4 asks further questions in relation to Steven's management.

EVALUATION

The medical team have been notified of Steven's **decreased level of consciousness**, and **alteration in pupillary shape** (now ovoid).

Plan:
Whilst Steven is being prepared to have a repeat CT head for the change in GCS, he becomes drowsy, his speech is very difficult to understand and his GCS drops further – E 2 V 2 M 4 = 8 PEARL 5 mm, non-reactive, ovoid.

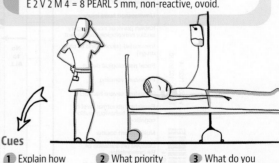

Cues

1 Explain how Steven's clinical deterioration relates to his initial closed head injury diagnosis.

2 What priority interventions need to be considered now for Steven? Justify your priorities of care here.

3 What do you think is the reason for this significant deterioration?

CONCEPT MAP 6.4 Evaluation and planning for Steven

EVIDENCE-BASED PRACTICE

Clinical pathways

Clinical pathways exist not to replace clinical judgement, but to ensure that every person, regardless of what hospital they are at, gets the same treatment/interventions. Clinical pathways are based on evidence and research to ensure the best possible outcome. They are generally only 1–2 pages and facilitate the early intervention, for instance, if the patient has serious risks. Clinical pathways enable accountability for not only nursing staff, but medical and other healthcare professionals.

Another factor to consider when using clinical pathways is that they are a short document to transfer if a patient requires transport to another hospital. This is crucial as often with patient transfers there can be the potential for information to be lost in the process. Clinical pathways ensure that all information and data are available for all healthcare professionals.

Figure 6.1 is an example of a closed head injury pathway from the Clinical Excellence Commission, Queensland Health.

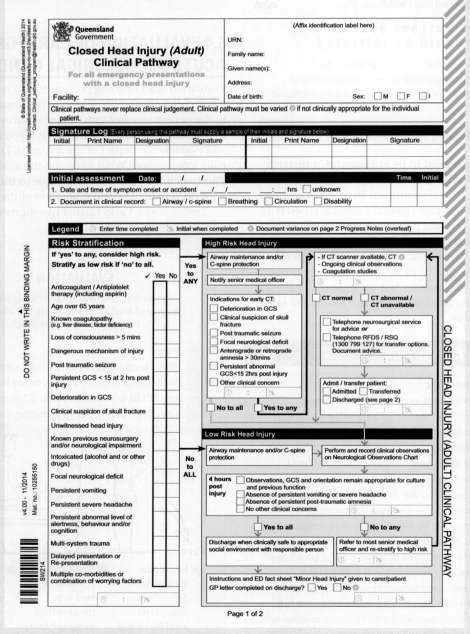

FIGURE 6.1 Closed head injury (adult) clinical pathway

6.5 DISCHARGE PLANNING AND COORDINATION OF CARE FOR AN ACUTE NEUROLOGICAL CONDITION

The nature of any injury and illness is diverse. Almost all illnesses and/or injuries are unexpected. This generally means that the patient and their family will not be prepared for the impact of the health condition – imagine driving home from your day's work and getting a call that a family member has had an accident or needed an operation – that would be frightening.

Your role will include discussing the processes and planned care with the patient alongside the medical and allied healthcare team; and doing so with empathy – it might be an everyday occurrence for us as nurses to see accidents, trauma or surgery, but for most Australians this is not a normal day. Patients and their families will most likely have many questions, and this is where you will need to consider the impact the injury or illness can have on the patient and plan your care around this.

Discharge planning around CNS conditions will vary greatly and be dependent upon the impact of the injury/illness that has occurred. You may be providing care for three patients all of whom have suffered a cerebrovascular accident (CVA), with all three having different outcomes in their prognosis and abilities

post-CVA. Planning discharge and liaising with other healthcare professionals will require a person-centred approach, and also a holistic and inclusive one.

REFLECTIVE PRACTICE

Unexpected injury or illness

'Some of the most challenging shifts in my nursing career have been because of the nature of the injury or illness. Families and the patient do not have time to prepare, everything is all new, all frightening and there are always so many questions. Someone having an accident on the way home from work is potentially devastating to a family. There are many emotions, and it is always not just about the patient. The family will call, they will attend, and they will have so many questions. I always think that if it were me in that situation, I would want someone to answer all of my questions, so I really try to be empathetic and as patient as possible, because every single one of us reacts differently to stress.'

Kerrie, 40, RN.

The final component of Steven's care is in **Concept map 6.5**. Here you can see the appropriate referrals and multidisciplinary approach for his holistic care.

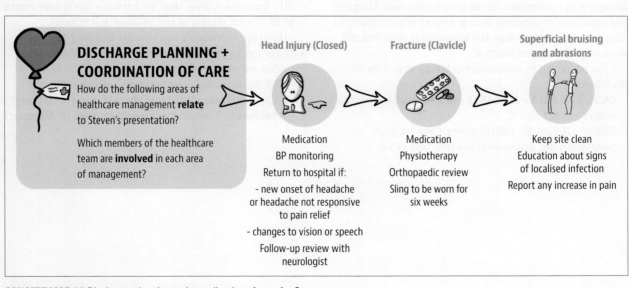

DISCHARGE PLANNING + COORDINATION OF CARE

How do the following areas of healthcare management **relate** to Steven's presentation?

Which members of the healthcare team are **involved** in each area of management?

Head Injury (Closed)

Medication

BP monitoring

Return to hospital if:

- new onset of headache or headache not responsive to pain relief

- changes to vision or speech

Follow-up review with neurologist

Fracture (Clavicle)

Medication

Physiotherapy

Orthopaedic review

Sling to be worn for six weeks

Superficial bruising and abrasions

Keep site clean

Education about signs of localised infection

Report any increase in pain

CONCEPT MAP 6.5 Discharge planning and coordination of care for Steven

SUMMARY

Neurological assessment and nursing care is a specialty, but you will need to possess basic assessment skills as any patient at any time can have a neurological condition. Patients who are postoperative can experience a cerebrovascular accident (CVA) or a subarachnoid haemorrhage (SAH). Hypertension can also cause stroke or an embolism. Primary and secondary surveys will ensure you have a constant checkpoint or algorithm to establish patient safety.

CLINICAL SKILLS IN NEUROLOGICAL NURSING

The following clinical skills are required when managing a person with neurological health issues; consult your Clinical Skills resources, such as Tollefson and Hillman (2022), *Clinical Psychomotor Skills* (8th ed.).

- Temperature, pulse, and respiration measurement
- Blood pressure measurement
- Monitoring pulse oximetry
- Pain assessment
- Focused health history and physical assessment
- 12-lead electrocardiogram
- Neurovascular observations
- Height, weight and waist circumference measurements (weight measurement required for some medications)
- Blood glucose measurement

- Oral medication
- Intravenous medication
- Venipuncture
- C-spine management
- Airway management associated with altered level of consciousness (ALOC)
- Assess level of consciousness (Glasgow Coma Scale)

Your clinical assessment skills will improve with practice and experience. This is true for all nurses. No-one starts knowing exactly how to hear the Korotkoff sounds or how to assess a GCS in full – or more importantly, why. Try not to focus on how long an assessment is taking you – there are no shortcuts in patient assessment that are safe for patients.

PROBLEM-SOLVING SCENARIO

Using the concept map approach, consider the following scenario.

Margaret Jason is a 22-year-old female who as been brought in by housemates for her erratic behaviour. Margaret has consumed an unknown dose or amount of amphetamines (Ice) over the past few days. Her housemates state that she does not 'shoot up, just snorts it'.

You undertake an assessment of Margaret and identify the following:

- CNS – E 4 V 4 M 5 = 13 PEARL 6 mm + agitated, not compliant with requests T 39.0 °C
- CVS HR 138 bpm, BP 180/110 mmHg. Centrally cool, peripherally hot, diaphoretic, cap refill time <4 sec

- RESP – RR 24 bpm SpO$_2$ 92% (RA) (poor trace due to tremors)
- GIT – Hyperactive BS, no guarding
- GU – Incontinent, urine clear, almost water-like in appearance
- SKIN – Intact, picking at arm however. Hot to touch.

Using the toxicology guide from the website https://www.austin.org.au/page?ID=1780, plan your care for Margaret.

1 What are your priorities here?
2 With this ingestion, what are some pathophysiological processes in place that could affect Margaret's recovery?
3 What nursing considerations would you have for Margaret?

Amphetamines and Amphetamine-type substances (includes 'ice', MDMA/ecstasy)   Austin Health

Amphetamines can produce life threatening hyperthermia + neurological, cardiovascular, and metabolic toxicity.

Toxicity / Risk Assessment	Management: Decontamination: There is no role for administration of activated charcoal
Dose-dependent sympathomimetic +/- serotonergic stimulation	**Rapid titration of benzodiazepines (and rapid cooling) is the mainstay of treatment.**
Can be ingested, snorted, injected or smoked	Diazepam 5-10 mg IV every 5-10 mins to achieve sedation; less severe cases: use oral diazepam q30 mins
Clinical features:	**Agitation** - Droperidol 10 mg IM / 5-10 mg IV initially. Continued agitation may require titrated
- Clinical effects of amphetamines occur rapidly	doses of droperidol 5 mg IV increments or diazepam 5 mg IV increments to achieve gentle sedation
- **Hyperthermia and multi-organ failure**	**Excited Delirium** – *MEDICAL EMERGENCY. Treat aggressively as extreme catecholamine excess can lead to*
- **CNS:** Anxiety, agitation, aggression, euphoria, seizures	*death. Consider ketamine sedation or RSI / general anesthetic / intubation*
- **Excited Delirium:** (delirium, psychomotor agitation,	**Hyperthermia** - *treat aggressively as temperatures > 40⁰C can rapidly lead to death*
marked physiological excitation) = **medical emergency**	- If T > 39⁰C rapid cooling measures (fanning, tepid sponging, ice). May require intubation and paralysis.
- **CVS:** ↑HR+BP, arrhythmias, pulmonary oedema,	**Seizures** - Diazepam 5-10 mg IV every 5-10 mins
acute coronary syndrome (ACS) – vasospasm +/-	**Continued seizures or altered mental status**
thrombosis, aortic dissection,	- Check sodium concentration for possible hyponatraemia (treat as below). CT brain to exclude ICH.
- **Metabolic:** lactic acidosis	- General anesthetic sedation with propofol, midazolam or barbiturates
- **SIADH** (Syndrome of Inappropriate Anti-Diuretic	**Hypertension/Tachycardia** – *Beta-blockers are contra-indicated due to unopposed alpha effects*
Hormone): substituted amphetamines including MDMA	- Diazepam: if refractory – IV GTN infusion +/- calcium channel antagonist (seek expert advice)
/Ecstasy can cause SIADH, increasing the likelihood of	**Acute Coronary Syndrome**
hyponatraemia	- Manage along conventional lines, but avoid beta blockers; PCI is preferred over thrombolysis
- **Other:** Diaphoresis, tremor, mesenteric ischaemia,	**Hyponatraemia** - *beware hyponatraemia secondary to SIADH +/- excess H₂O intake*
intracranial haemorrhage, rhabdomyolysis	- Euvolaemic fluid overload: fluid restrict. If Na+ conc. < 120 mmol/L, consider 3% NaCl. (1-2 mL/ kg IV)
	Observe all ingestions for at least 4 hours, and all exposures until toxicity resolves

AUSTIN CLINICAL TOXICOLOGY SERVICE GUIDELINE   POISONS INFORMATION CENTRE: 13 11 26

Version 3: Published 3/2021. Review 3/2024

FIGURE 6.2 Austin Clinical Toxicology Service Guidelines
The recommendations contained in these guidelines do not indicate an exclusive course of action, or serve as a standard of medical care. Variations, taking individual circumstances into account, may be appropriate.
These guidelines are designed for doctors and healthcare professionals. They are not intended for use by patients or the general public. Always seek the advice of a healthcare professional when using these guidelines and before making any medical decisions.

SOURCE: AUSTIN HEALTH, AMPHETAMINE CLINICAL GUIDELINES

PORTFOLIO DEVELOPMENT

Ongoing education and professional development will be necessary in the specialised field of neurological nursing. Even if your interest lies in paediatric nursing, neurological assessment will still be required. Head injury can have an incredible impact upon a person, and age (young or old) can further impact this. Professional development includes workshops, in-services and conferences. This is not always possible in person due to times and distance, but there are many options in the virtual world for ongoing professional development.

There are many guidelines for specialised age groups for head injury. The following is a detailed overview of head injury management in children. https://www.childrens.health.qld.gov. au/guideline-head-injury-emergency-management-in-children

The following website has information relevant to portfolio development which you will require in your nursing career. https://healthtimes.com.au/hub/nurse-education/41/practice/ hw/professional-nursing-portfolios/4538

USEFUL WEBSITES

Registered Nurse Standards for Practice
The Registered Nurse Standards for Practice consist of seven crucial standards that all nurses must follow. Download and review the standards at the following link. https://www. nursingmidwiferyboard.gov.au/Codes-Guidelines-Statements/ Professional-standards/registered-nurse-standards-for-practice.aspx

Clinical resources – SA Health
The clinical resources here are evidence-based guidelines and resources for a multitude of clinical conditions.

https://www.sahealth.sa.gov.au/wps/wcm/connect/ public+content/sa+health+internet/clinical+resources

Austin Health – Clinical toxicology guidelines
There is an A–Z reference for specific and common overdoses and ingestions. All are evidence-based and peer-reviewed. https://www.austin.org.au/clinical-toxicology-guidelines

Brain Trauma Foundation
Specialised clinical resources and an organisation that undertakes research into traumatic brain injuries. Peer-reviewed. https://www.braintrauma.org

REFERENCES AND FURTHER READING

Australian Institute of Health and Welfare (AIHW). (2023). *Emergency department care.* https://www.aihw.gov.au/reports-data/myhospitals/sectors/emergency-department-care

Brown, D., Edwards, H., Buckley, T., Aitken, R. L., Lewis, S. L., Bucher, L., McLean Heitkemper, M., Harding, M. M., Kwong, J., & Roberts, D. (2019). *Lewis's medical-surgical nursing ANZ* (5th ed.). Elsevier.

Crisp, J., & Taylor, C. (2021). *Potter and Perry's fundamentals of nursing* (4th ed.). Elsevier.

Croft, H., Moloney, A., Pitkin, J., & Dee, D. (2021). *The Australian carer* (5th ed.). Cengage Learning Australia.

DeLaune, S., Ladner, P., McTier, L., Tollefson, J., & Lawrence, J. (2024). *Fundamentals of nursing* (3rd ed.). Cengage Learning Australia.

Gray, S., Ferris, L., White, L. E., Duncan, G., & Baumle, W. (2019). *Foundations of nursing: Enrolled nurses* (2nd ANZ ed.). Cengage Learning Australia.

Joustra, C., & Moloney, A. (2019). *Clinical placement manual.* Cengage Learning Australia.

Marieb, E. N., & Hoehn, K. N. (2021). *Human anatomy & physiology* (9th ed.). Pearson.

Rizzo, D. C. (2015). *Fundamentals of anatomy and physiology* (4th ed.). Cengage Learning.

Schuman, J. (2019). *Australian deaths involving coward's punches: Research update.* Victorian Institute of Forensic Medicine. https://www.vifm.org/wp-content/uploads/Cowards-Punch-Research-Update-2019.pdf

Tollefson, J., Watson, G., Jelly, E., & Tambree, K. (2022). *Essential clinical skills: Enrolled nurses* (5th ANZ ed.). Cengage Learning Australia.

CHAPTER **7**

PAIN MANAGEMENT

Pain has a significant impact on Australians' health and wellbeing, with 1 in 5 Australians aged 45 and over experiencing chronic pain. Chronic pain is generally defined as pain that is persistent, ongoing and lasts beyond normal healing times associated with the injury or illness (usually 3–6 months). Chronic pain results from surgery, arthritis, medical conditions (such as cancer) or, sometimes, there is no clear physical cause. Pain impacts the ability of people to continue their normal activities of daily living, including sleep patterns, attending work, exercise or social interactions (Australian Institute of Health and Welfare (AIHW), 2020).

Chronic pain currently affects more than 3.2 million Australians. The cost or financial burden of pain in Australia in 2018 (chronic pain only) was $73.2 billion which included:
- $48.3 billion for productivity costs (impact on the person's ability to work)
- $12.2 billion for direct health system costs.

It is estimated that by 2050, the annual cost of chronic pain will rise to $215.6 billion in part due to an ageing population (AIHW, 2020).

LEARNING OBJECTIVES

After reading this chapter, you should have an understanding of the:
1. assessment required for a person with pain
2. prioritisation of key components in the development of a plan of care
3. prioritised and targeted nursing interventions required to promote recovery or prevent further deterioration
4. evaluation phase and how the prioritised and targeted nursing interventions inform further assessment, planning and collaboration with the healthcare team
5. discharge planning and coordination of care required when preparing the person for discharge and subsequent continuity of care between the person and their healthcare providers.

INTRODUCTION

Pain is a deeply personal experience. Pain can be acute, chronic, situational or a combination of all three. Nursing care is based on subjective and objective assessment, and pain falls into the subjective category (Crisp & Taylor, 2021; DeLaune et al., 2024). In 1968, Margo McCaffery (an RN in pain management) provided a definition regarding pain and patient's reporting of it as 'whatever the person experiencing the pain says it is, existing whenever the person says it does' (Brown et al., 2019).

The National Strategic Action Plan for Pain Management outlines five categories of pain –
1. acute pain
2. subacute pain
3. recurrent pain
4. chronic pain
5. cancer-related pain (Department of Health, 2021).

These five categories are based upon the definition of pain and the following from the International Association for the Study of Pain (IASP, 2020): 'Pain is an unpleasant sensory and emotional experience, associated with, or resembling that associated with, actual or potential tissue damage' (Sonneborn & Williams, 2020).

Nurses are the most consistent factor in any patient journey in hospital, and as such, have the most contact with the patient. This places nurses as being well equipped to assess, manage and record pain holistically.

There are many reasons for pain in patients both in and out of hospitals. These can include:

- fractures
- myocardial infarction
- trauma
- lacerations
- migraines
- falls
- sporting injuries
- accident – land vehicle
- slips/trips
- chronic pain – conditions such as arthritis, cancer (palliative), previous injury to an area (back pain, joint pain, etc.), abdominal pain (cause not always determined) (AIHW, 2020; Department of Health, 2021).

You will need to rely upon your foundation anatomy and physiology and the application of this to your patient's condition. For example, it would be expected that there would be abdominal pain postoperatively if the patient had undergone a laparoscopic cholecystectomy.

Acute and chronic pain can be distinguished in terms of cause, treatment, progression of pain and symptoms. Acute pain is related to, generally, a precipitating event – an injury, surgery or illness. With chronic pain the origin or basis for the pain may not be known.

Acute pain generally decreases over time and will disappear when the person has recovered. Chronic pain does not go away and has periods of worsening pain with a high baseline pain level.

Acute pain directly impacts the central nervous system and homeostatic response – through increasing blood pressure, heart rate and respiratory rate. Patients will often also experience diaphoresis and pallor. Other associated symptoms can be urinary retention, agitation, confusion and anxiety. Acute pain is a 'warning' within our body that something is wrong.

Chronic pain generally causes a flat affect, and ongoing fatigue. There is also a reduction in physical activity, and this can be associated with a withdrawal from social interaction/s. Chronic pain does not generally affect the vital signs/disrupt the homeostatic mechanism as it is ongoing and not relenting. Chronic pain serves no biological purpose – meaning there is no reason for it as with acute pain (Brown et al., 2019; Department of Health, 2021; Crisp & Taylor, 2021; DeLaune et al., 2024).

The impact of chronic pain on acute pain (e.g. a patient who has chronic joint pain is admitted to the hospital for a surgical procedure) is within the length of the hospital stay. Patients who have chronic pain generally spend five days longer admitted in the hospital than people who do not have chronic pain, further increasing patient safety (Australian Institute of Health And Welfare, 2020).

7.1 ASSESSMENT OF ACUTE PAIN

Pain assessment involves not only a subjective assessment from the patient, but clinical judgement based upon these findings, observations and context of the person's pain, and their previous response/s to pain management. An essential component of pain assessment and management is to accept and respect what patients say, intervene to relieve pain, and then reassess to see if the interventions have been effective (Brown et al., 2019).

The most common form of pain assessment is the PQRSTU pain assessment acronym (Brown et al., 2019; Crisp & Taylor, 2021; DeLaune et al., 2024) as defined in **Figure 7.1**.

Other pain assessment scales are used in differing patient populations. For instance, children, neonates, intubated or critically ill patients, elderly, people with cognitive or intellectual disabilities and those who may be non-verbal (Sonneborn & Williams, 2020). Examples of other pain assessment scales include FLACC scale (**Figure 7.2**); Wong-Baker FACES

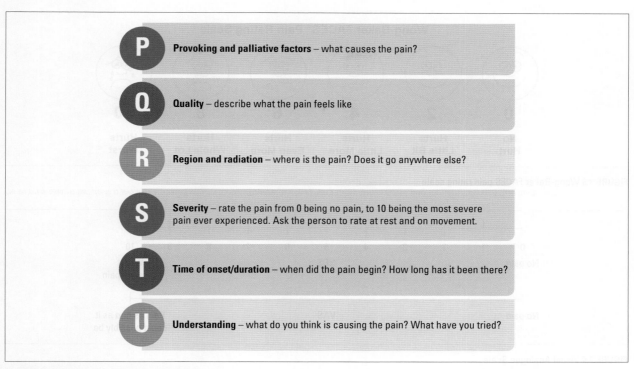

FIGURE 7.1 Pain assessment using PQRSTU

Category	0	1	2
F Face	No Particular expression or smile	Occasional grimace/frown; Withdrawn or disinterested; *appears sad or worried*	Consistent grimace or frown; frequent/constant quivering chin, clenched jaw; *distressed-looking face; expression of fright or panic*
L Legs	Normal position or relaxed; *usual tone and motion to limbs*	Uneasy, restless, tense; *occasional tremors*	Kicking, or legs drawn up; *marked increase in spasticity, constant tremors or jerking*
A Activity	Lying quietly, normal position, moves easily; *regular, rhythmic respirations*	Squirming, shifting back and forth; *tense or guarded movements; mildly agitated (e.g. head back and forth, aggression); shallow, splinting respirations, intermittent sighs*	Arched, rigid or jerking; *severe agitation; head-banging; shivering (not rigors); breath-holding, gasping or sharp intake of breaths, severe splinting*
C Cry	No cry/verbalisation	Moans or whimpers; occasional complaint; *occasional verbal outburst or grunt*	Crying steadily, screams or sobs, frequent complaints; *repeated outbursts, constant grunting*
C Consolability	Context and related	Reassured by occasional touching, hugging, or being talked to, distractable	Difficult to console or comfort; *pushing away caregiver, resisting care or comfort measures*

FIGURE 7.2 FLACC scale

SOURCE: CANADIAN PAEDIATRIC SOCIETY, ADAPTED FROM MALVIYA (2006)

Pain Rating Scale (**Figure 7.3**) and the Visual Analogue Scale (**Figure 7.4**).

Pain is complex – whether it is acute or chronic in nature. It is crucial, in the assessment of chronic pain particularly, that other aspects are considered when assessing the pain. There are bio-psycho-social aspects of pain – where the three determinants here are overlapping, and each has a contributing factor to pain. Physical, psychological and environmental factors are significant in the management and assessment of chronic pain (Department of Health, 2021).

Regardless of the reason for the pain – whether it be acute or chronic, it is the responsibility of all healthcare professionals to assess and effectively manage pain. The ethos of pain management and assessment is that pain is whatever the person says it is.

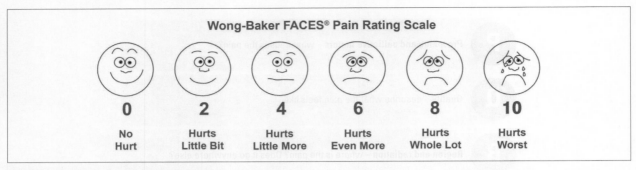

FIGURE 7.3 Wong-Baker FACES pain rating scale

SOURCE: © 1983 WONG-BAKER FACES FOUNDATION. WWW.WONGBAKERFACES.ORG. USED WITH PERMISSION. ORIGINALLY PUBLISHED IN WHALEY & WONG'S NURSING CARE OF INFANTS AND CHILDREN. © ELSEVIER INC.

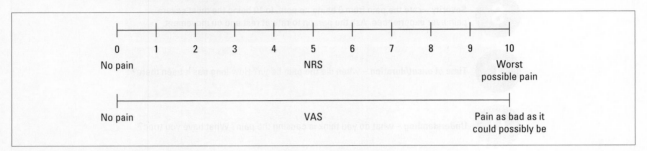

FIGURE 7.4 Visual Analogue Scale

Presentation

Elizabeth, a 39-year-old female, has been hospitalised post an injury sustained to her right shoulder. She presented after three days of trying to manage the pain at home with simple analgesia. She injured her shoulder 'dragging' a heavy bag. **Concept map 7.1** further explores Elizabeth's presentation/admission.

 PHx

Elizabeth, a **39-year-old female** was dragging a suitcase and felt a 'pop' in her right shoulder and immediate pain in the area. She continued to the hotel/destination. Ongoing pain increased over the course of the next 72 hours. Nil previous history of injury to that shoulder/arm. Elizabeth travelled from Fiji to Sydney one day ago.

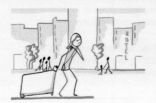

Cues

1. What are your priorities with this patient?
2. What is the significance of hypertension and tachypnoea in a patient with 9/10 pain?
3. What is your immediate course of action in regards to pain assessment? Is there any other information that you would seek?
4. What investigative or diagnostic procedures do you think would be relevant for this patient?

 ASSESSMENT

Primary survey

A: Patent
B: RR 24
C: Warm
D: Alert
E: T 36.9 °C
F: Nil in, HNPU
G: BGL 5.0 mmol/L

Secondary survey

CNS (Cognition): E 4 V 5 M 6 = 15, Pupils equal (PEARLA), 4 mm
PAIN: P – three days ago, pulling a suitcase. Q – stabbing and sharp pain. R – Pain is only in the right shoulder, with no radiation. S – at rest 7/10, movement 9/10. T – pain has been present for 3 days, getting worse. U – paracetamol, RICE, Ibuprofen with little effect.

CVS: HR 90 bpm and reg, BP 160/85 mmHg, pedal pulses bounding.
T: 36.9 °C
RESP: RR 20, patent airway – spontaneous breathing, SpO$_2$ 99% RA
GIT (Input): As tolerated.
RENAL (Output): HNPU over past 6 hours
SKIN/INTEG: Centrally and peripherally well perfused, bruising to right shoulder head, mild localised swelling to right shoulder. Otherwise grossly intact.
MUSCULOSKELETAL (Mobility): Minimal ability to mobilise due to increase in pain. Unable to dress self currently or put bra on.
BMI: 24.2

5. If the patient has already self-administered paracetamol and ibuprofen, could you administer this again? If so, within what time frame?
6. If you note bruising at the right shoulder head, what could this indicate?
7. Is there a risk of DVT in this patient with recent travel?

CONCEPT MAP 7.1 Nursing assessment for Elizabeth

7.2 PLANNING CARE FOR ACUTE PAIN

Planning for a patient's care who has pain requires a person-centred and holistic approach. It is crucial to remember that pain is something that 'looks' different on every single patient. Pain has many associated coping strategies or individual factors such as cultural beliefs, previous experience with pain, and psychological distress that may also worsen the pain. There are different types of pain – nociceptive (damage to the body tissue), neuropathic (occurs following damage to the nervous system) and nociplastic (related to increased nervous system sensitisation rather than clear evidence of tissue damage) (Department of Health, 2021).

In Elizabeth's situation, it would appear that the pain is nociceptive, which is usually responsive to non-opioid and opioid medications (Brown et al., 2019). Nociception is the physiological response by the central nervous system where the tissue damage is communicated from the site/s of injury. There are four processes involved:

1   transduction
2   transmission
3   perception
4   modulation.

Considering this information, we can now plan for Elizabeth's care, with a formal diagnosis and treatment plan for analgesia and ongoing treatment.

See **Concept map 7.2** for an outline of Elizabeth's care plan.

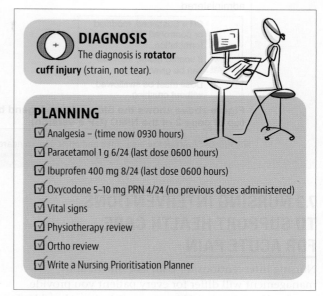

DIAGNOSIS
The diagnosis is **rotator cuff injury** (strain, not tear).

PLANNING
☑ Analgesia – (time now 0930 hours)
☑ Paracetamol 1 g 6/24 (last dose 0600 hours)
☑ Ibuprofen 400 mg 8/24 (last dose 0600 hours)
☑ Oxycodone 5–10 mg PRN 4/24 (no previous doses administered)
☑ Vital signs
☑ Physiotherapy review
☑ Ortho review
☑ Write a Nursing Prioritisation Planner

CONCEPT MAP 7.2 Diagnosis and planning for Elizabeth

SAFETY IN NURSING

OPIOID TOXICITY

Some medications, particularly opioids, are available in multiple forms, including extended or controlled release. This can be referred to as 'sustained release, modified or controlled release formulations'. Such is the risk in administering these medications, that on the National Inpatient Medication Chart (NIMC) there is a standalone box to be checked if the medication is slow release (see **Figure 7.5**) to ensure that this is reviewed prior to administration.

The risk of administering incorrect drugs is one of the safeties aimed to be addressed with the rights of medication administration and the NIMC. In the case of Michael Calder, he was admitted for a headache. Over the course of 53.8 hours, he was administered the equivalent of 535–595 mg of oral morphine due to various medication orders – PRN orders predominantly that differed in the release–slow release and immediate release. From the Coroner's findings:

'He received a complex regime of analgesia including subcutaneous morphine, oxycodone, ordine, MS Contin, Gabapentin, paracetamol, and Ibuprofen. The medication regime adopted large doses of morphine-based medication in both slow release and liquid form … at some point around midnight on 10/11 July, a combination of factors being that of sleep apnoea and with the accumulation of slow-release OxyContin, oral Ordine and gabapentin peaking at around the same time, resulted in an episode of aspiration and respiratory depression to which Michael succumbed'.

The death of this person was avoidable and is a component of safety checks in medication by the prescriber and by the nurse administering the medication.

(The Coronial Investigation can be found here: https://www.courts.qld.gov.au/__data/assets/pdf_file/0008/483497/cif-calder-mj-20160902.pdf)

Slow release medicines and other non-standard formulations
The *Tick if Slow Release* box is included in regular medicine spaces as a prompt to prescribers to consider whether or not the standard release form of the medicine is required. This box must be ticked to indicate a **sustained, modified or controlled** release form of an oral drug (e.g. verapamil SR, Diltiazem CD). If not ticked, then it is understood that the standard release form is to be administered.

Tick if slow release	SR = Sustained, modified or controlled release formulation.
	If scored tablet, then half can be given.
	Dose must be swallowed without crushing.

Figure above shows the Slow release legend box found in the middle of the NIMC and on the top of page 2 of the NIMC (GP e-version).

FIGURE 7.5 Slow release medicines and other non-standard formulations in the NIMC
SOURCE: AUSTRALIAN COMMISSION ON SAFETY AND QUALITY IN HEALTH CARE (2016), NATIONAL INPATIENT MEDICATION CHART USER GUIDE. ACSQHC, SYDNEY.

7.3 NURSING INTERVENTIONS TO SUPPORT HEALTH CARE FOR ACUTE PAIN

Nursing interventions for pain assessment and management will differ for every patient you provide care for. If you were working in a surgical ward and had four postoperative laparoscopic cholecystectomies, each patient would have different perceptions of pain, different experiences of pain, different responses to analgesia, and different recovery times. This is due to the inherent uniqueness of every one of us, but also the physiological processes that drive each one of us. Pain is also influenced by concurrent conditions; for instance, chronic pain, hypertension or diabetes. Pain is not a 'one size fits all' approach and careful assessment and consideration for each patient needs to be undertaken to evaluate, provide interventions and then re-evaluate your patient's pain and progress (AIHW, 2020; Brown

et al., 2019; Crisp & Taylor, 2021; Sonneborn & Williams, 2020).

Concept map 7.3 explores the nursing interventions and cues for Elizabeth.

7.4 EVALUATION OF CARE FOR ACUTE PAIN

As part of the further assessment of Elizabeth's ongoing condition, **Concept map 7.4** asks further questions in relation to her management.

INTERVENTIONS

1 Assess pain, level of consciousness, and observations.

2 ISBAR handover preparation for end-of-shift handover – what would you be handing over if your patient had a pain score of 9/10 post analgesia?

What further assessments should be initiated

Cues

1 What is the physiological link between vital signs and pain?

2 What possible reasons could there be for the patient to report no reduction in their pain?

CONCEPT MAP 7.3 Nursing interventions for Elizabeth

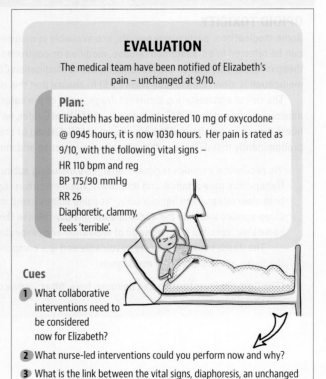

EVALUATION

The medical team have been notified of Elizabeth's pain – unchanged at 9/10.

Plan:

Elizabeth has been administered 10 mg of oxycodone @ 0945 hours, it is now 1030 hours. Her pain is rated as 9/10, with the following vital signs –
HR 110 bpm and reg
BP 175/90 mmHg
RR 26
Diaphoretic, clammy, feels 'terrible'.

Cues

1 What collaborative interventions need to be considered now for Elizabeth?

2 What nurse-led interventions could you perform now and why?

3 What is the link between the vital signs, diaphoresis, an unchanged pain score and her current pain?

CONCEPT MAP 7.4 Evaluate and planning for Elizabeth

7.5 DISCHARGE PLANNING AND COORDINATION OF CARE FOR ACUTE PAIN

The nature of pain and its management is diverse. The nature of recovery and response to pain is also diverse.

In planning for Elizabeth's discharge, **Concept map 7.5** explores the considerations for her care.

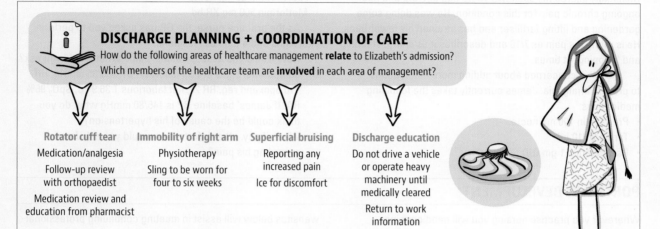

DISCHARGE PLANNING + COORDINATION OF CARE

How do the following areas of healthcare management **relate** to Elizabeth's admission? Which members of the healthcare team are **involved** in each area of management?

Rotator cuff tear	Immobility of right arm	Superficial bruising	Discharge education
Medication/analgesia	Physiotherapy	Reporting any increased pain	Do not drive a vehicle or operate heavy machinery until medically cleared
Follow-up review with orthopaedist	Sling to be worn for four to six weeks	Ice for discomfort	
Medication review and education from pharmacist			Return to work information

CONCEPT MAP 7.5 Discharge planning and coordination of care for Elizabeth

REFLECTIVE PRACTICE

Pain assessment

You are preforming a pain assessment on a new admission to your ward. Michael, a 34-year-old who presented with lower right quadrant pain, rebound tenderness and guarding and is scheduled for a laparoscopic appendicectomy within the next hour. He has not received analgesia for more than two hours. When you walk in, Michael is on his phone and appears calm. When you ask about his pain, he states it is 8/10, and is not getting any better, but feels 'worse'.

Questions

1 If your patient is appearing calm, do you think they have severe pain?
2 What objective data could you collect here to highlight the severe pain?
3 If pain is so deeply personal, how can you as a nurse continue to provide holistic and non-judgemental pain assessment and analgesia?

SUMMARY

Pain is one of the most common causes for presentation to health care – be it primary or acute healthcare settings in Australia. Pain is deeply personal and reliant on many factors – physical, psychological and social.

The impact of pain, be it acute or chronic or a combination, is different for every patient. Ensuring you assess the patient and their subjective data, bearing in mind that pain is whatever the person says it is, will enable holistic person-centred care to be given.

CLINICAL SKILLS IN PAIN MANAGEMENT

Pain management is focused on a clinical assessment to determine as much supporting or objective data as possible. The following clinical skills are required when managing a person with pain; consult your Clinical Skills resources, such as Tollefson and Hillman (2022), *Clinical Psychomotor Skills* (8th ed.).

- Pain assessment
- Physical assessment
- Mental status assessment
- Temperature, pulse and respiration measurement
- Blood pressure measurement

- Monitoring pulse oximetry
- Focused musculoskeletal health history and physical assessment and range of motion exercises (This would

vary between each patient and be dependent upon the mechanism of injury or nature of the person's pain.)

PROBLEM-SOLVING SCENARIO

James Mansfield presents to his GP with increasing back pain. He initially injured his back two years ago at work and has ongoing chronic pain for this condition. He was doing some gardening and lifting fertiliser and has strained his lower back. He is rating his pain as 7/10 and describes it as sharp, stabbing and 'gripping' at times.

His GP is concerned about adding more medications to provide analgesia. James currently takes the following medications:

- Pregabalin 100 mg nocte
- Targin 20/10 bd
- Paracetamol 1 gm QID

- Telmisartan 40 mg mane
- Atorvastatin 20 mg nocte
- Metformin 500 mg XR bd

As the practice nurse, the GP has asked you to perform vital signs and a pain assessment.

1 How would you assess James' pain? What would you ask?
2 James' vital signs are as follows – BP 180/95 mmHg, HR 110 bpm and reg, RR 22, not laborious T 36.9 °C, SpO$_2$ 96% RA. If James' baseline BP is 145/80 mmHg what do you think could be the cause of his hypertension?
3 What, if any, other information would you ask James regarding his pain?

PORTFOLIO DEVELOPMENT

Wherever you practise nursing you will need ongoing continuing professional development to ensure that you are delivering current evidence-based nursing care that provides the best possible outcomes for the patient. The useful

websites below will assist in meeting continuing professional development activities to meet the NMBA yearly registration requirements for a Registered Nurse.

USEFUL WEBSITES

Registered Nurse Standards for Practice
The Registered Nurse Standards for Practice consist of seven crucial standards that all nurses must follow. Download and review the standards at the following link. https://www.nursingmidwiferyboard.gov.au/codes-guidelines-statements/professional-standards/registered-nurse-standards-for-practice.aspx

The Australian Pain Society
https://www.apsoc.org.au

NSW Government – Department of Health
Useful links and materials on chronic pain management. https://www.health.nsw.gov.au/pharmaceutical/doctors/pages/useful-references-medical-practitioners-chronic-pain.aspx

Australian and New Zealand College of Anaesthetists and Faculty of Pain Medicine
Acute pain management: scientific evidence (5th edition, 2020) https://www.anzca.edu.au/getattachment/38ed54b7-fd19-4891-9ece-40d2f03b24f9/acute-pain-management-scientific-evidence-5th-edition#page=

Australian Commission on Safety and Quality in Health Care
The clinical care standards related to acute pain assessment. There is also supporting information for pain assessment and tools to use across various patient populations. https://www.safetyandquality.gov.au/standards/clinical-care-standards/opioid-analgesic-stewardship-acute-pain-clinical-care-standard/quality-statements/quality-statement-2-acute-pain-assessment

Pain assessment and measurement – Clinical Guideline for Nurses
Clinical guidelines for the assessment and measurement of pain in children (acute) with links to tools and further information regarding pain. https://www.rch.org.au/rchcpg/hospital_clinical_guideline_index/Pain_Assessment_and_Measurement/#Pain%20Assessment%20Tool

National Strategic Action Plan for Pain Management
Department of Health in association with Pain Australia's report on the plan for pain management. https://www.health.gov.au/sites/default/files/documents/2021/05/the-national-strategic-action-plan-for-pain-management-the-national-strategic-action-plan-for-pain-management.pdf

REFERENCES AND FURTHER READING

Australian Institute of Health and Welfare (AIHW). (2020). *Chronic pain in Australia.* https://www.aihw.gov.au/reports/chronic-disease/chronic-pain-in-australia/summary

Brown, D., Edwards, H., Buckley, T., Aitken, R. L., Lewis, S. L., Bucher, L., McLean Heitkemper, M., Harding, M. M., Kwong, J., & Roberts, D. (2019). *Lewis's medical-surgical nursing ANZ* (5th ed.). Elsevier.

Crisp, J., & Taylor, C. (2021). *Potter and Perry's fundamentals of nursing* (4th ed.). Elsevier.

DeLaune, S., Ladner, P., McTier, L., Tollefson, J., & Lawrence, J. (2024). *Fundamentals of nursing* (3rd ed.). Cengage Learning Australia.

Department of Health, Australian Government. (2021). *National strategic action plan for pain management.* https://www.health.gov.au/sites/default/files/documents/2021/05/the-national-strategic-action-plan-for-pain-management-the-national-strategic-action-plan-for-pain-management.pdf

International Association for the Study of Pain (IASP). (2020, 16 July). *IASP announces revised definition of pain.* https://www.iasp-pain.org/publications/iasp-news/iasp-announces-revised-definition-of-pain

Malviya, S., Voepel-Lewis, T., Burke, C., Merkel, S., & Tait, A. R. (2006). The revised FLACC observational pain tool: improved reliability and validity for pain assessment in children with cognitive impairment. *Pediatr Anesthesia, 16*(3), 258–65.

Sonneborn, O., & Williams, A. (2020). How does the 2020 revised definition of pain impact nursing practice? *Journal of Perioperative Nursing, 33*(4), 28–28. https://doi.org/https://doi.org/10.26550/2209-1092.1104

INTEGUMENTARY SYSTEMS

Thermal injuries, including burns, occur more frequently in males than females. In 2021–2022, 64 per cent of those admitted to hospital for thermal injuries were male, and of those who died with thermal injuries in 2020–2021, 64 per cent were male. Children under 5 years of age have the highest rate of hospitalisation for thermal injuries, with boys having the highest representation in the age group. Deaths from thermal injuries in 2020–2021 were usually by exposure to fire, smoke and flames and peaked in the winter months (Australian Institute of Health and Welfare [AIHW], 2022).

LEARNING OBJECTIVES

After reading this chapter, you should have an understanding of the:

1 assessment required for a person with a skin condition
2 prioritisation of key components in the development of plans of care for a person with the following skin conditions:
   – erythroderma
   – burn injury
   – wound infection
3 prioritised and targeted nursing interventions required to promote recovery or prevent further deterioration of people presenting with the above skin conditions
4 evaluation phase and how the prioritised and targeted nursing interventions inform further assessment of the person, planning of care and collaboration with the healthcare team
5 discharge planning and coordination of care required in preparing the person for discharge and subsequent continuity of care between the person and their healthcare providers.

INTRODUCTION

The integumentary system includes the skin, hair sensory receptors, nails and oil and sweat glands. The skin is the largest organ of the body (in weight) and accounts for approximately 16 per cent of the total adult weight (McLafferty et al., 2012). The skin differs in thickness depending on the location and function. For example, the skin on the soles of the feet can be up to 4 mm thick, whereas the eyelids may only be 0.5 mm thick (McLafferty et al., 2012). The skin plays a vital functional role in maintaining a person's physical and mental health. Disorders of the skin, such as acute or chronic **erythroderma** or traumatic wounds causing subsequent scarring, can have detrimental effects on physical health (potential for infection) and also alter a person's self-perception.

Nurses need to be knowledgeable about caring for a person with altered skin integrity, and apply a holistic approach to care, with the understanding that the skin is what is seen by others, and therefore plays a role in a person's health perception and subsequently influences post-discharge care.

Skin disorders can include:

- inflammatory skin disorders – erythroderma (dermatitis, psoriasis, acne)
- infectious skin disorders (boils, carbuncles, impetigo, cellulitis, fungal infections, herpes zoster, ectoparasites [scabies, head lice])
- wounds (surgical and non-surgical [trauma, **burns**, **pressure injury**, chronic ulcerations]).

8.1 ASSESSMENT FOR SKIN CONDITIONS

Skin assessment involves all the senses, as by nature skin disorders are visible. As with all nursing assessment, skin assessment involves subjective (patient health history) and objective (physical assessment) data. The nursing assessment should also include information obtained by medical staff, allied health staff and any other health services involved in the care of the person.

Health history (subjective data)

The health history should be given by the person wherever possible; however, it may require the involvement of a family member or carer. Box 8.1 assists the nurse to undertake a focused skin-related health history.

BOX 8.1   SUBJECTIVE ASSESSMENT

- ➤ **Current presentation** – ask the patient 'what made you seek health care today?' This is necessary to determine the priority of care; for example, are there signs of anaphylaxis? Is there a rash which could indicate a highly transmissible infection (meningococcal or measles)?
- ➤ **History of skin disorder** – onset, location, duration, characteristics, associated symptoms, relieving factors (including pharmaceutical or non-pharmaceutical methods), timing and severity of condition (OLD CARTS)
- ➤ **Past health history** – allergies, autoimmune disorders, current medications, previous surgery, previous or current medical conditions
- ➤ **Family history** – skin cancer, autoimmune disorders, other skin-related disorders
- ➤ **Cultural background** – ethnicity, lifestyle and predisposition to skin disorders
- ➤ **Social and lifestyle factors** – alcohol, tobacco, recreational drugs, diet, exercise, sun exposure habits, exposure to toxins and sexual habits
- ➤ **Skin, nail and hair care habits**
- ➤ **Occupational history** – exposure to toxins or sun
- ➤ **Travel history** – history of domestic or international travel in the previous 12 months

---

Physical assessment (objective data)

While a full skin assessment is required to gain an overall picture of the person's presenting problem, the physical assessment is somewhat guided by the person's health history. The physical assessment will most likely require the person to remove their clothes either partly or in full; therefore privacy is required. A gown can be provided should the person be required to remove all their clothes and provide a drape or sheet to cover the person when required (Cole & Gray-Miceli, 2002). The person may be required to be in a sitting, standing or supine position for a complete head-to-toe examination. A room or cubicle with good lighting is necessary (unless other symptoms such as a headache are overriding), and a pen light, ruler and magnifying glass are also required (Moore & O'Brien, 2014).

SAFETY IN NURSING

Appropriate infection prevention and control precautions such as Standard Precautions should be applied, including hand hygiene at the appropriate moments, and the application of gloves and protective eyewear when touching body fluids (Australian Commission on Safety and Quality in Health Care [ACSQHC], 2019). Transmission-based precautions should be applied for suspected or known communicable diseases (National Health and Medical Research Council [NHMRC], 2019).

An initial overall scan of the person's skin should be undertaken to assess changes in colour (erythema, jaundice, cyanosis or pallor) and to assess for localised swelling or oedema. This is followed by a systematic head-to-toe assessment using the techniques of inspection and palpation. Fungal skin infections, necrotic tissue and infected wounds can also emit odours (Manning, 1998), so using the olfactory sense is important.

When inspecting the skin, look for areas of discolouration including bruising, skin moisture (dry/oily), cracks or openings, skin thickness, excoriations, blisters, rashes, scarring, changes in consistency compared to the surrounding skin, and ask the patient about associated symptoms (pain, itchiness, tingling or numbness).

When palpating the skin note the skin turgor and moisture level, check for localised swelling or oedema, compare the skin temperature of the affected areas with non-affected areas, and note any pain on palpation. Remember to assess areas of the body bilaterally, comparing left with right.

Box 8.2 assists the nurse to undertake a focused physical assessment of the skin.

BOX 8.2   OBJECTIVE ASSESSMENT

› **Head, face and neck** – Inspect the hair and scalp (hair loss or excessive hair, texture of hair, presence of ectoparasites (nits), lesions, scales or crusts on the scalp). Inspect the face and neck for sun damage or lesions, and gently palpate lumps. Inspect the mucosal membranes for dryness or lesions.

› **Arms and hands** – Inspect all skin surfaces, paying particular attention to colour, warmth and sensation. Check skin turgor, and inspect web spaces and wrists (scabies). Palpate any localised swelling and oedema, noting the grade of pitting oedema. Assess the nail beds for colour, inspect nails for brittleness, splitting, deformities and splinter haemorrhages.

› **Chest, abdomen, back and buttocks** – Inspect all skin surfaces for colour, warmth and sensation, including under breasts and skin folds (common areas for fungal infections), and pressure points on buttocks and sacrum. Gently palpate localised swelling.

› **Inguinal area** – With permission, inspect the inguinal area for signs of fungal infections, and other rashes or blisters.

› **Legs and feet** – Inspect all skin surfaces, paying particular attention to pressure points such as toes, ankles, heels and lateral aspects of knees. Inspect in between the toes and the soles of the feet. Palpate any localised swelling or oedema and grade any pitting. Note any yellowish diffuse keratoderma on the soles of the feet.

8.2 ASSESSMENT FOR ERYTHRODERMA

Presentation

Mr James Harrison is a 35-year-old male who presented to the emergency department with generalised erythema, itchy warm skin, mildly swollen eyelids and some skin scaling. Mr Harrison also states that he feels 'shivery' at times and tired. He has not experienced generalised erythema before, and Mr Harrison thinks he may have something 'infectious'. **Concept map 8.1** further explores James' presentation/admission.

 PHx

Mr Harrison was diagnosed with **atopic dermatitis** as a child, which has been treated and controlled with topical corticosteroids. He is otherwise fit and well with no other medical or surgical history. Apart from his topical creams, Mr Harrison takes no other medications.

 ASSESSMENT

Primary survey
A: Clear
B: RR 20, SaO₂ 97%, nil wheeze or stridor present
C: HR 90 bpm, BP 130/80 mmHg
D: Alert and orientated complaining of severe generalised itch
E: 37.8 °C

Secondary survey
Head, face and neck: Slight eyelid swelling with mild lymphadenopathy of the neck.

Arms and hands: Generalised erythema with dry flaky skin across all surfaces and pustule-looking lesions on the elbows. Broken skin lesions on elbows and backs of hands where itch is more intense. Some oozing of lesions.
Chest, abdomen, back and buttocks: Generalised erythema across all surfaces, with lesions developing between the buttocks.
Inguinal area: Some pustules developing in

skin folds including under the scrotum, with slight pungent smell noted from these lesions. No lymphadenopathy noted in the inguinal area.
Legs and feet: Generalised erythema with fine scaling present. Lesions noted across thighs, shins and in between the toes where scratching has occurred. Some discharge noted from these lesions.

(Mistry, Gupta, Alavi & Sibbald, 2015)

Cues

1. What are the general signs and symptoms at the skin level for erythroderma?
2. What are the systemic symptoms due to erthryoderma or its underlying cause?
3. What would be two important tests to assist in the diagnosis of erythroderma?
4. What other areas of the secondary survey would be documented, and are there any particular assessments that should be focused on apart from the integumentary system?

CONCEPT MAP 8.1 Nursing assessment for James

8.3 PLANNING CARE FOR ERYTHRODERMA

Planning for the nursing care for acute erythroderma has the goals of:

- normal fluid and electrolyte balance
- normal circulatory status
- afebrile body temperature
- wound repair.

James is a partner in contributing to his care plan, which includes the in-hospital phase and managing his condition in the home environment. **Box 8.3** indicates the areas that are targeted in the planning stage of acute erythroderma management.

BOX 8.3   PLANNING CARE FOR ERYTHRODERMA

➤ Fluid and electrolyte balance
➤ Vital signs
➤ Wound management
➤ Nutrition
➤ Tests
➤ Medication
➤ Self-care

Concept map 8.2 outlines a plan for James' care.

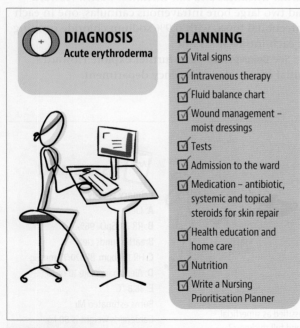

DIAGNOSIS
Acute erythroderma

PLANNING
☑ Vital signs
☑ Intravenous therapy
☑ Fluid balance chart
☑ Wound management – moist dressings
☑ Tests
☑ Admission to the ward
☑ Medication – antibiotic, systemic and topical steroids for skin repair
☑ Health education and home care
☑ Nutrition
☑ Write a Nursing Prioritisation Planner

CONCEPT MAP 8.2 Diagnosis and planning for James

8.4 NURSING INTERVENTIONS TO SUPPORT HEALTH CARE FOR ERYTHRODERMA

Nursing interventions are implemented as part of person-centred care and reverse the signs and symptoms of erythroderma.

Concept map 8.3 explores James' journey in the emergency department and the medical ward.

INTERVENTIONS

1 Vital signs, frequency as determined by ADDS
2 Intravenous therapy
3 Fluid balance chart
4 Wound management – moist dressings
5 Tests
6 Medication – antibiotic, systemic and topical steroids for skin repair

Health education and home care:

- Wound management
- Nutrition

What further assessments should be initiated

Cues

① What other assessments should we undertake for James'?

CONCEPT MAP 8.3 Nursing interventions for James

8.5 EVALUATION OF CARE FOR ERYTHRODERMA

As part of the further assessment of James' presentation, **Concept map 8.4** asks further questions in relation to James' management.

8.6 DISCHARGE PLANNING AND COORDINATION OF CARE FOR ERYTHRODERMA

James' erythroderma requires discharge planning and further management at home. In planning for James' discharge, **Concept map 8.5** explores the considerations for his care.

EVALUATION

James states he feels better as the steroids and wet dressings have made his skin feel less irritated. He also noted that since taking an antibiotic his skin does not smell as much.

Plan:
James will be discharged home, with medication to assist in the repair of his skin.

Cues

1 Why is it important that James practises good wound management?

2 Which medication would James be discharged with and what are the specific roles of the medication?

CONCEPT MAP 8.4 Evaluation and planning for James

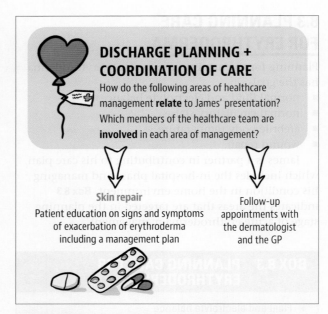

DISCHARGE PLANNING + COORDINATION OF CARE

How do the following areas of healthcare management **relate** to James' presentation? Which members of the healthcare team are **involved** in each area of management?

Skin repair
Patient education on signs and symptoms of exacerbation of erythroderma including a management plan

Follow-up appointments with the dermatologist and the GP

CONCEPT MAP 8.5 Discharge planning and coordination of care for James

8.7 ASSESSMENT FOR BURN INJURY

When undertaking a health assessment for a burn injury, refer to **Box 8.1** and **Box 8.2** for subjective and objective data collection. Further assessment is also required to determine the burn agent (this could be thermal, radiation, chemical, electrical or blast injury), the initial burn treatment (e.g. how was the burn agent removed? first aid?), and the severity of the burn (e.g. depth, skin surface area).

Presentation

Mr Howard Gardener's lawn mower exploded at around 8 a.m. and his wife found him with his clothing on fire and he was rolling on the ground to stop his clothes burning. Mrs Gardener sprayed him with the hose to cool the burns and also called the ambulance service. The paramedic assessment of the burnt skin surface area was approximately 45 per cent burns to his face, arms, front and back of trunk and legs. The burns were a mixture of superficial, partial-thickness and full-thickness burns. Howard had two large bore intravenous cannulas, one in each antecubital fossa, with 0.9% sodium chloride running in each intravenous line.

See **Concept map 8.6** to further explore Howard's initial care in the emergency department.

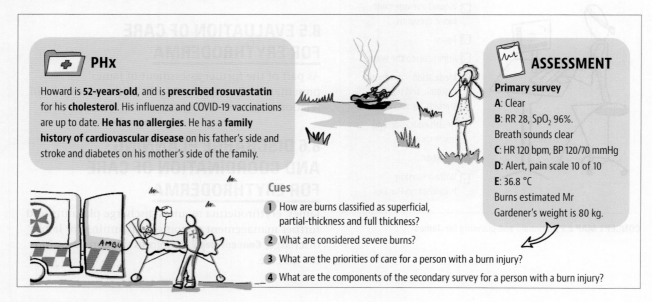

PHx

Howard is **52-years-old**, and is **prescribed rosuvastatin** for his **cholesterol**. His influenza and COVID-19 vaccinations are up to date. **He has no allergies**. He has a **family history of cardiovascular disease** on his father's side and stroke and diabetes on his mother's side of the family.

ASSESSMENT

Primary survey
A: Clear
B: RR 28, SpO$_2$ 96%. Breath sounds clear
C: HR 120 bpm, BP 120/70 mmHg
D: Alert, pain scale 10 of 10
E: 36.8 °C
Burns estimated Mr Gardener's weight is 80 kg.

Cues

1 How are burns classified as superficial, partial-thickness and full thickness?

2 What are considered severe burns?

3 What are the priorities of care for a person with a burn injury?

4 What are the components of the secondary survey for a person with a burn injury?

CONCEPT MAP 8.6 Nursing assessment for Howard

8.8 PLANNING CARE FOR A BURN INJURY

Planning for the nursing care for burn injuries have the goals of:

- continuing regular ongoing primary assessments
- re-establishing and maintaining haemodynamic parameters
- maintaining normothermia
- initiating wound management to reduce fluid volume and heat loss and to reduce to risk of infection
- responding to secondary survey findings.

Box 8.4 indicates the areas that are targeted in the planning stage of severe burns management in the emergency department.

Concept map 8.7 outlines a plan for Howard's care.

8.9 NURSING INTERVENTIONS TO SUPPORT HEALTH CARE FOR A BURN INJURY

Nursing interventions are implemented as part of person-centred care, to promote healing of burn injury. Intravenous fluid resuscitation and maintenance to respond to fluid homeostasis and antibiotic and tetanus prophylaxis (Broyles et al., 2023) are an essential part of the management for burns care.

Concept map 8.8 explores Howard's journey in the emergency department, before admission to the burns unit.

BOX 8.4   PLANNING CARE FOR A BURN INJURY

- Airway maintenance
- High flow oxygen and breathing assessment
- Vital signs
- Assess unburnt skin
- Cardiac monitoring
- Conscious level
- Blood glucose level
- Remove clothing and jewellery, keep warm
- Assess burn extent
- Assess for circumferential burns
- Weight
- Fluid resuscitation
- Fluid maintenance
- Blood tests
- ECG

- Chest x-ray
- Medication, including analgesia
- Fowler's position
- Fluid balance chart
- Urinary catheter
- Urine output 0.5–1 mL/kg/hr
- Wound care
- Elevate burnt area where appropriate
- Prevent heat loss
- Nasogastric tube
- Transfer to burns unit
- Surgery
- Nutrition

Cues:

1   How much health education should be introduced at this time?

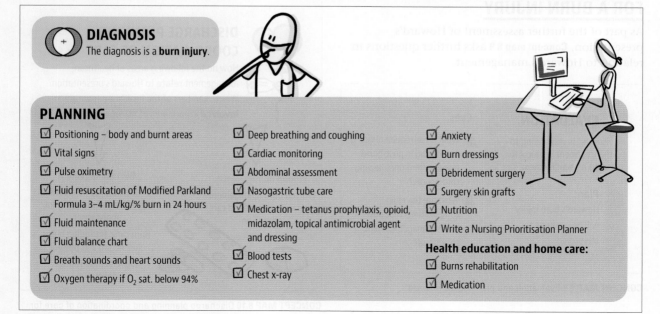

DIAGNOSIS
The diagnosis is a **burn injury**.

PLANNING

- ☑ Positioning – body and burnt areas
- ☑ Vital signs
- ☑ Pulse oximetry
- ☑ Fluid resuscitation of Modified Parkland Formula 3–4 mL/kg/% burn in 24 hours
- ☑ Fluid maintenance
- ☑ Fluid balance chart
- ☑ Breath sounds and heart sounds
- ☑ Oxygen therapy if O_2 sat. below 94%

- ☑ Deep breathing and coughing
- ☑ Cardiac monitoring
- ☑ Abdominal assessment
- ☑ Nasogastric tube care
- ☑ Medication – tetanus prophylaxis, opioid, midazolam, topical antimicrobial agent and dressing
- ☑ Blood tests
- ☑ Chest x-ray

- ☑ Anxiety
- ☑ Burn dressings
- ☑ Debridement surgery
- ☑ Surgery skin grafts
- ☑ Nutrition
- ☑ Write a Nursing Prioritisation Planner

Health education and home care:
- ☑ Burns rehabilitation
- ☑ Medication

CONCEPT MAP 8.7 Diagnosis and planning for Howard

INTERVENTIONS

In the burns unit:

1 Positioning – Fowlers and burns areas

2 Vital signs – hourly

3 Pulse oximetry – hourly

4 Fluid resuscitation of Modified Parkland Formula 3–4 mL/kg/% burn in 24 hours

5 Fluid maintenance – IV fluids

6 Fluid balance chart

7 Oxygen therapy if O_2 sat. below 94%

8 Breath sounds and heart sounds – hourly

9 Deep breathing and coughing – hourly

10 Cardiac monitoring

11 Abdominal assessment – 8 hourly

12 Nasogastric tube care

13 Medication – opioid infusion, midazolam infusion, topical antimicrobial agent and dressing

14 Monitor for anxiety and depression

15 Pain assessment

16 Burns dressings

17 Nutrition

18 Assessment for surgery

19 Scar management

20 Physiotherapy

Health education and home care:

• Burns rehabilitation

• Medication

What further assessments should be initiated?

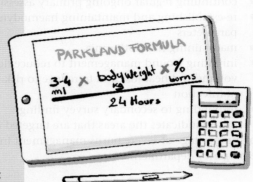

Cues

1 What further tests are required?

2 What are the indications for debridement and skin grafts?

3 By 1600 hours, how much fluid replacement should Howard have received if the Modified Parkland Formula is calculated at 4 mL/kg?

CONCEPT MAP 8.8 Nursing interventions for Howard

EVIDENCE-BASED PRACTICE

Fluid resuscitation is an important component of the management of major burns to prevent hypovolaemia due to fluid shift and loss from injured tissue.

8.10 EVALUATION OF CARE FOR A BURN INJURY

As part of the further assessment of Howard's presentation, **Concept map 8.9** asks further questions in relation to Howard's management.

EVALUATION

Howard is responding to the treatment protocol for burns management.

Plan:
Howard's burn injury will be continue to monitored.

Cues

1 What areas require ongoing monitoring in post-burns management once healing commences?

2 What are the main complications that post-burns management aim to address?

CONCEPT MAP 8.9 Evaluation and planning for Howard

8.11 DISCHARGE PLANNING AND COORDINATION OF CARE FOR A BURN INJURY

Howard's burns management requires discharge planning and further management at home, as shown in **Concept map 8.10**.

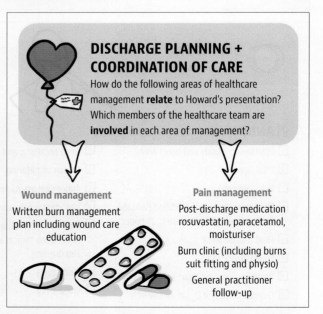

DISCHARGE PLANNING + COORDINATION OF CARE

How do the following areas of healthcare management **relate** to Howard's presentation? Which members of the healthcare team are **involved** in each area of management?

Wound management

Written burn management plan including wound care education

Pain management

Post-discharge medication rosuvastatin, paracetamol, moisturiser

Burn clinic (including burns suit fitting and physio)

General practitioner follow-up

CONCEPT MAP 8.10 Discharge planning and coordination of care for Howard

8.12 ASSESSMENT FOR WOUND INFECTION

As part of Roger's health assessment, refer to **Box 8.1** and **Box 8.2** assessment areas, with a specific focus on dermatological assessment areas. In the assessment of a wound, record tissue colour and appearance, infection/inflammation, odour, exudate, edges, depth, length and width of wound, as well as pain level.

Presentation

Roger Kruger is a 68-year-old man who has been admitted to the intensive care unit post-cardiac surgery. His sternal surgical wound appears to be clean and dry for the first 24 hours. On the third day,

the pm shift assessment of Roger's wound noted the proximal end of his sternal wound is starting to appear to be red, with increased warmth at that site. Roger's temperature is 37.3 °C and his blood glucose reading 11.9 mmol/L. Roger has a history of type 2 diabetes. It was planned to move Roger to the cardiac ward in the next 24 hours, but the infection has occurred and his blood glucose levels have been unstable postoperatively with persistent hyperglycaemia despite a short-acting insulin infusion. Because of this, the decision was made to keep Roger in the intensive care unit to stabilise his blood glucose levels and monitor the sternal wound infection.

See **Concept map 8.11** to further explore Roger's care in the intensive care unit.

 PHx

Roger has had type 2 diabetes for the last 24 years, and the diabetes has been controlled with oral hypoglycaemics.

Cues

1 What other assessments should be made?

 ASSESSMENT

CNS: Alert and orientated
CVS: BP 135/75 mmHg, HR 80 bpm, T: 37.3 °C, peripherally perfused
Resp: Scattered fine crackles at the base of the lungs. RR 24, SaO$_2$ 96%
GIT: Bowel sounds present with a non-tender abdomen
Renal: Urine output approximate 1 mL/kg/hr

Metabolic: BGL 11.9 mmol/L
Integumentary: Warm dry skin
Wound: Length 12 cm, width 0.3 mm, depth 0.5 mm. Currently no exudate, redness to proximal end of wound, with increased warmth at that site
Musculoskeletal: Equal limb strength

CONCEPT MAP 8.11 Nursing assessment for Roger

8.13 PLANNING CARE FOR A WOUND INFECTION

Person-centred goals of care for the individual with a sternal wound infection include blood glucose stabilisation and wound repair. Roger contributes to the plan of care in the intensive care unit, cardiac ward and at home. **Box 8.5** indicates the areas that are targeted in the planning stage for caring for the person with a wound infection. Please refer to

Chapter 21 for coronary artery graft surgery planning, implementation and evaluation of care phases.

Concept map 8.12 outlines a plan for Roger's care.

BOX 8.5	PLANNING CARE FOR A WOUND INFECTION

» Blood glucose measurement
» Wound dressing
» Antibiotic
» Wound culture

 DIAGNOSIS
Sternal wound infection post-coronary artery graft surgery

PLANNING

☑ Wound dressing
☑ Blood glucose measurement
☑ Sliding scale insulin
☑ Flucloxacillin 2 g QID IV wound infection
☑ Write a Nursing Prioritisation Planner

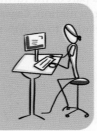

CONCEPT MAP 8.12 Diagnosis and planning for Roger

Wound healing requires good nutrition. Vitamins A, C and E, and minerals zinc and iron play major roles in wound healing. Protein is also an important component in wound healing, and hydration and blood glucose levels require monitoring.

8.14 NURSING INTERVENTIONS TO SUPPORT HEALTH CARE FOR A WOUND INFECTION

Nursing interventions are implemented as part of person-centred care, and prevent the progression of a wound infection, including the stabilisation of blood glucose levels.

Concept map 8.13 explores Roger's journey in the intensive care unit for postoperative care.

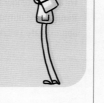

INTERVENTIONS

Postoperative care including for coronary artery graft surgery:

1 Sternal dressing daily

2 Blood glucose measurement 2 hourly

3 Sliding scale insulin

4 Flucloxacillin 2 g QID IV

Health education:

- Medication

- Cardiac rehabilitation

What further assessments should be initiated

CONCEPT MAP 8.13 Nursing interventions for Roger

8.15 EVALUATION OF CARE FOR A WOUND INFECTION

As part of the further assessment of Roger's presentation, **Concept map 8.14** asks further questions in relation to Roger's management.

8.16 DISCHARGE PLANNING AND COORDINATION OF CARE FOR A WOUND INFECTION

The discharge planning for Roger's cardiac surgery, sternal wound and type 2 diabetes includes transfer to the cardiac ward, cardiac rehabilitation, further management at home and a follow-up appointment with his cardiac surgeon and general practitioner (see **Concept map 8.15**).

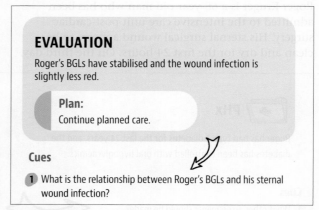

EVALUATION

Roger's BGLs have stabilised and the wound infection is slightly less red.

Plan:
Continue planned care.

Cues

1 What is the relationship between Roger's BGLs and his sternal wound infection?

CONCEPT MAP 8.14 Evaluation and planning for Roger

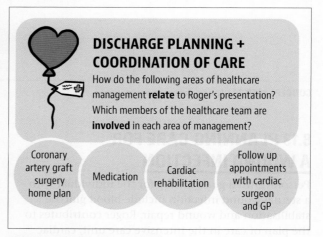

DISCHARGE PLANNING + COORDINATION OF CARE

How do the following areas of healthcare management **relate** to Roger's presentation? Which members of the healthcare team are **involved** in each area of management?

Coronary artery graft surgery home plan

Medication

Cardiac rehabilitation

Follow up appointments with cardiac surgeon and GP

CONCEPT MAP 8.15 Discharge planning and coordination of care for Roger

SUMMARY

The skin, as part of the integumentary system, is the largest organ in the human body and provides the first defence against the environment and assists in the maintenance of body homeostasis. The disruption of the skin barrier can lead to severe and life-threatening illness, and hence the nursing care of the integumentary system is crucial in providing safe person-centred care.

CLINICAL SKILLS FOR INTEGUMENTARY HEALTH

The following clinical skills are required when managing a person with pain; consult your Clinical Skills resources, such as Tollefson and Hillman (2022), *Clinical Psychomotor Skills* (8th ed.).

- Aseptic non-touch technique
- Temperature, pulse and respiration measurement
- Blood pressure measurement
- Monitoring pulse oximetry
- Pain assessment
- Blood glucose measurement
- Oral medication
- Topical medication
- Intravenous medication administration
- Dry dressing technique
- Complex wounds – wound irrigation
- Complex wounds – packing a wound

PROBLEM-SOLVING SCENARIO

Using a concept map approach, how would you assist Mario Focu?

Mario Focu is 85 years old and has had rheumatoid arthritis for the last 35 years. Mario's mobility has decreased considerably in the last two years due to an exacerbation of rheumatoid arthtritis, and he has mainly stayed in bed at his home. Mario's pain from rheumatoid arthritis has increased in the last week, and his wife has noted that the red area on his sacrum has become 'a big sore'. Mario has been admitted to the medical ward for pain and pressure injury management.

1. What are the risk factors for a pressure injury?
2. How do you assess a pressure injury?
3. What is the management for a pressure injury?
4. What role does wound healing and nutrition play in the healing of a pressure injury?

PORTFOLIO DEVELOPMENT

Wherever you practise nursing you will need ongoing continuing professional development to ensure that you are delivering current evidence-based nursing care that provides the best possible outcomes for the patient. As problems of the integumentary system require a specific knowledge base, the useful websites below will assist in meeting continuing professional development activities to meet the NMBA yearly registration requirements for a Registered Nurse.

USEFUL WEBSITES

Nursing and Midwifery Board of Australia, Decision-making framework for nursing and midwifery (2020), https://www.nursingmidwiferyboard.gov.au/codes-guidelines-statements/frameworks.aspx

Alfred Health Burns Service, https://www.alfredhealth.org.au/services/hp/burns

REFERENCES AND FURTHER READING

Australian Commission on Safety and Quality in Health Care (ACSQHC). (2019). *National hand hygiene initiative.* https://www.safetyandquality.gov.au/our-work/infection-prevention-and-control/national-hand-hygiene-initiative

Australian Institute of Health and Welfare (AIHW). (2022). *Injury in Australia: Thermal causes.* https://www.aihw.gov.au/reports/injury/burns-and-other-thermal-causes

Broyles, B., Reiss, B., Evans, M., Pleunik, S., Page, R., & Badoer, E. (2023). *Pharmacology in nursing* (4th ANZ ed.). Cengage Learning Australia.

Cole, J. M., & Gray-Miceli, D. (2002). The necessary elements of a dermatologic history and physical evaluation. *Dermatology Nursing, 14*(6), 377–384.

DeLaune, S., Ladner, P., McTier, L., Tollefson, J., & Lawrence, J. (2024). *Fundamentals of nursing* (3rd ed.). Cengage Learning Australia.

Lender, O., Gobolos, L., Bajwa, G., & Bhatnagar, G. (2022). Sternal wound infections after sternotomy: Risk factors, prevention and management. *Journal of Wound Care, 31*(6).

Manning, M. P. (1998). Metastasis to skin. *Seminars in Oncology Nursing, 14*(3), 240–243.

McLafferty E., Hendry, C., & Farley, A. (2012). The integumentary system: anatomy, physiology and function of skin. *Nursing Standard, 27*(3), 35–42.

Mistry, N., Gupta, A., Alavi, A., & Sibbald, R. G. (2015). A review of the diagnosis and management of erythroderma (generalized red skin). *Advances in Skin and Wound Care, 28*(5), 228–236.

Moore, Z., & O'Brien, J. J. (2014). Nursing care of conditions related to the skin. In

A-M. Brady, C. McCabe, & M. McCann (Eds.), *Fundamentals of medical surgical nursing: A systems approach* (1st ed., pp. 157–173). Wiley Blackwell.

National Health and Medical Research Council (NHMRC). (2019). *Australian guidelines for the prevention and control of infection in healthcare.* https://www.nhmrc.gov.au/sites/default/files/documents/infection-control-guidelines-feb2020.pdf

Neighbors, M., & Tannehill-Jones, R. (2023). *Human diseases* (6th ed.). Cengage.

Tetteh, L., Aziato, L., Mensah, G., Vehvilainen-Julkunen, K., & Kwegyir-Afful, E. (2021). Burns pain management: The role of nurse-patient communication. *Burns, 47*(6), 1416–1423.

Tollefson, J., & Hillman, E. (2022). *Clinical psychomotor skills: Assessment tools for nurses* (8th ed.). Cengage Learning Australia.

CHAPTER 9

URINARY SYSTEM

Kidney infections and urinary tract infections (UTIs) are a common cause of hospitalisation in Australia. In many cases these conditions are preventable. Queensland Health data has identified that UTIs are one of the top ten reasons why people visit emergency departments (Miles, 2021); with over 20 540 people attending emergency departments in 2021 for this very reason.

The Australian Commission on Safety and Quality in Health Care (ACSQHC) identifies that people who attend emergency departments are more likely to be given broad-spectrum antibiotics, which can increase antimicrobial resistance (ACSQHC, 2022). The ACSQHS further asserts that UTIs are a common cause of hospitalisations that are *preventable*.

LEARNING OBJECTIVES
After reading this chapter, you should have an understanding of the:
1 assessment required for a person with urinary conditions or disorders
2 prioritisation of key components in the development of a plan of care for patients with:
   – chronic kidney disease (CKD)
   – hypervolaemia
3 prioritised and targeted nursing interventions required to promote recovery or prevent further deterioration
4 evaluation phase and how the prioritised and targeted nursing interventions inform further assessment, planning and collaboration with the healthcare team
5 discharge planning and coordination of care required in preparing the person for discharge and subsequent continuity of care between the person and their healthcare providers.

INTRODUCTION

The organs of the urinary system include the kidneys, ureters, urinary bladder and the urethra. The kidneys are bean-shaped organs that are located in the back, above the waist and below the ribs in the right lower quadrant (RLQ) and left lower quadrant (LLQ). Kidneys are surprisingly small for the essential daily 'work' they need to undertake to maintain fluid and electrolyte balance. They are around 11 cm long and weigh around 150 g. The nephrons are the filtering units of the kidneys where waste products from the blood and urine are formed. There are over one million of these functional units in each kidney that pass the urine into the collecting ducts to be eventually excreted as urine. The ureters 'attach' the kidney to the urinary bladder and are 25–30 cm in length. Urine is transported down the ureters to the bladder via peristalsis and gravity. The urinary bladder is the collection point for all urine, and as a rule, can hold 350–600 mL of urine. The bladder is smooth muscle, and the bladder walls are thick to enable expansion. The urethra is the thin-walled tube that carries urine from the bladder to the outside of the body via peristalsis. This seemingly 'simple' process of movement of waste and distribution of fluid and electrolytes is something that can be altered from any number of direct or indirect impacts on the person from shock, infection, sepsis to injury, or adverse effect of medication/s (DeLaune et al., 2024).

The primary functions of the kidneys are:
- maintenance of osmolarity – by regulating loss of water and solutes in the urine
- regulation of blood volume – through conserving or eliminating water, the kidneys adjust blood volume and therefore regulate levels of interstitial fluid, blood pressure (increased blood volume – increased blood pressure, decreased blood volume – decreased blood pressure)

- regulation of blood pressure – apart from adjusting the blood volume, the kidneys assist with blood pressure regulation in two ways – by secreting the enzyme renin (which activates the renin-angiotensin pathway) and by adjusting renal resistance (which is the resistance encountered by blood flowing through the kidneys). Blood pressure is increased by either an increase in renin secretion or an increase in renal resistance
- regulation of blood ionic composition – the kidneys assist with the regulation of several ions within the blood – sodium, potassium, calcium, chloride and phosphate
- release of hormones – the kidneys release two hormones – calcitriol (the active form of vitamin D) and erythropoietin (which stimulates red blood cell production)
- excretion of wastes and foreign substances – the formation of urine enables the body to excrete waste – substances that have no useful function in the body
- regulation of blood glucose level – the kidneys deaminate glutamine, which is then used for gluconeogenesis and releases glucose into the blood (Derrickson et al., 2021).

Renal complications or conditions affect each person differently, as so much is reliant upon the fluid and electrolyte balance and management of this. For example, the patient with a UTI would likely be febrile, whereas a person with **chronic kidney disease (CKD)** would likely be hypothermic due to the alteration in homeostasis (Brown et al., 2019; DeLaune et al., 2024). First we'll look at the assessment of the person with CKD. Sections 9.6–9.10 consider a scenario where a person has fluid overload (hypervolaemia).

There are many common urinary conditions/disorders, including:

- urinary tract infection (UTI)
- cystitis
- pyelonephritis
- urethritis
- bladder control problems

- benign prostatic hyperplasia
- renal calculi
- renal failure (acute or chronic)
- chronic kidney disease (CKD)
- glomerulo-nephritis.

You will need to rely upon your foundation anatomy and physiology and the application of this to your patient's condition. Some overdoses or ingestions of medicines or poisons can occur rarely or infrequently, so staff may not be aware of the impact, and you will need to source information. This is particularly relevant to the adverse effects from some medications that impact directly upon the urinary system.

SAFETY IN NURSING

POTENTIALLY NEPHROTOXIC DRUGS

There are many commonly used medications that can and do affect renal function, and the level to which they can affect the kidney depends on age, gender, health status and underlying disease/s. These include:

- diuretics
- beta blockers
- vasodilators
- ACE inhibitors
- NSAIDs
- radio contrast media (contrast dye)
- compound analgesics
- antiviral agents
- lithium
- aminoglycosides.

Within Australia, the Therapeutic Goods Administration (TGA) holds medication safety updates, and recent updates surrounding acute kindey inhjury are in place for clindamycin: https://www.tga.gov.au/publication-issue/clindamycin-capsules-and-injections-acute-kidney-injury.

Medication prescription and administration for a patient needs to take into account any underlying disease/s and acute conditions. There are several medications, such as gentamycin, that have age-related dosage gudielines due to the increased risk of nephrotoxicity.

Your role clinically will be to ensure that you are reviewing medication information relevant for your patient, not just for the medication.

9.1 ASSESSMENT OF A PERSON WITH CHRONIC KIDNEY DISEASE (CKD)

Figure 9.1 shows the progression and loss of kidney function as chronic kidney disease progresses. It also illustrates the impact of this on albumin in the body.

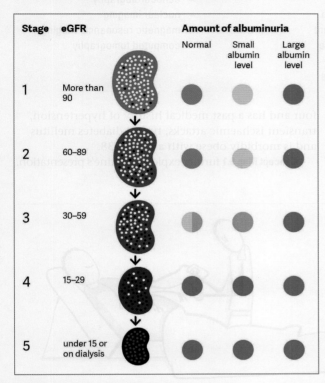

FIGURE 9.1 Five stages of kidney disease

SOURCE: STAGES OF KIDNEY DISEASE. KIDNEY HEALTH AUSTRALIA WEBSITE HTTPS://KIDNEY.ORG.AU/YOUR-KIDNEYS/WHAT-IS-KIDNEY-DISEASE/STAGES-OF-KIDNEY-DISEASE. ACCESSED 29/01/2024.

The assessment of the person with CKD will require the use of both subjective and objective data and will vary for each person. See **Box 9.1** for the health assessment data collection areas.

A focused assessment on the patient with CKD would include the following listed in **Box 9.2**. Throughout this assessment you would identify the stage of CKD your patient is currently 'at' to enable person-centred education and health promotion. Common findings would also include:

- psychosocial issues
- complications or side effects of disease progression
- medications
- self-care issues
- any educational deficits.

Armed with this information you will be able to establish a nursing care plan tailored to your patient. As no two patients are alike – neither are CKD patients, and it's important to remember this in providing care for a chronic disease patient. Some medications or interventions work for some patients, and not for others.

The benefit of this is that person-focused care plans and assessment tools are based on needs analysis and holistic health assessment. These care plans should be developed in conjunction with family members, allied health professionals and, most importantly, the patient. Nursing assessment is the foundation for all of our care provision, so it must be effective.

A final point on holistic nursing assessment – it is what drives our interventions, so if we do not ask relevant and open-ended questions we are not going to have much to work with. With CKD in mind, speaking with not only the patient but their caregivers and significant others will further enhance your holistic care and enable effective care for your patient.

BOX 9.1 SUBJECTIVE ASSESSMENT

- History of illness
- Past health history
- Medications
- Surgery

Functional health patterns
- Health perception and management
- Nutritional and metabolic alterations or interventions
- Elimination
- Activity and exercise
- Sleep and rest
- Cognitive and perceptual insight into management of chronic disease
- Self-perception and concept of death and dying
- Role relationship
- Sexuality and reproductive
- Coping and stress
- Values and beliefs
- Risk calculation

BOX 9.2   OBJECTIVE ASSESSMENT

- ➤ Airway
- ➤ Breathing
- ➤ Circulation
- ➤ Disability
- ➤ Exposure
- ➤ Fluids
- ➤ Glucose (A–G assessment)
- ➤ Vital signs
- ➤ Diagnostic

- ➤ Blood tests such as:
  - – cardiac markers
  - – electrolytes
  - – glucose
  - – renal function
  - – full blood count
  - – clotting profile
  - – cholesterol
  - – homocysteine

- ➤ Electrocardiogram (ECG)
- ➤ Diagnostic imaging such as:
  - – chest x-ray
  - – echocardiography
  - – nuclear imaging
  - – magnetic resonance imaging
  - – computed tomography

Presentation

Maxine Broche is a 48-year-old female who was referred to the local emergency department by her general practitioner as her recent blood tests indicated abnormal renal function. Her GFR is <19. Maxine has CKD, stage four and has a past medical history of hypertension, transient ischaemic attacks, type II diabetes mellitus and is morbidly obese with a BMI of 38.

Concept Map 9.1 further explores Maxine's presentation.

PHx

Maxine is a **48-year-old female**, who has a GFR of <19. She has **CKD, stage four**, and a PMHx of HTN, TIA's, T2DM, and is **morbidly obese** with a BMI of 38.

ASSESSMENT

Primary survey

A: Patent
B: RR 16 bpm
C: Centrally warm
D: Alert
E: Skin coated – white crystals
F: Nil in, HNPU
G: BGL 16.2 mmol/L

Secondary survey

CNS (Cognition): E 4 V 5 M 6 = 15, Pupils equal PEARLA 4 mm
PAIN: currently denies
CVS: HR 60 bpm, BP 195/105 mmHg, pedal pulses bounding. A 12 lead electrocardiogram showed a sinus rhythm with peaked T waves.
T: 35.9 °C
RESP: RR 16, patent airway – spontaneous breathing, not laborious, metallic breath
GIT: Abdo SNT. BGL 16.2 mmol/L (2 hours post prandial)
RENAL: HNPU in >24 hours.
SKIN/INTEG: Centrally warm, peripherally cooler, 'coating' on skin.
MUSCULOSKELETAL (Mobility): Mobile.
BMI: 38

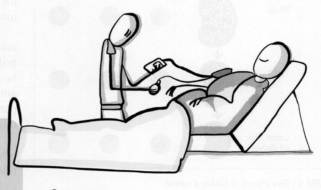

Cues

1. What are your priorities with this patient?
2. What is the significance of peaked T waves?
3. What is the relationship between renal failure and temperature regulation?
4. What is the pathophysiological relationship between blood pressure and CKD?
5. What are some concerns in relation to the skin assessment of this patient?
6. What other assessments would you consider for this patient?
7. What investigative or diagnostic procedures do you think would be relevant for this patient?

CONCEPT MAP 9.1 Nursing assessment for Maxine

9.2 PLANNING CARE FOR A PERSON WITH CKD

Planning for CKD will have the goals of:
- maintenance of blood pressure in normal parameters
- minimal adverse effects of therapy.

The person is a partner in their care plan and is able to contribute to their health care in being able to follow their plan of care and manage their condition in the home environment. **Box 9.3** indicates the areas that are targeted in the planning stage for CKD.

BOX 9.3　PLANNING CARE FOR A PERSON WITH CKD
➤ Lifestyle modifications
➤ Weight reduction
➤ Diet
➤ Sodium reduction
➤ Alcohol
➤ Physical activity
➤ Tobacco
➤ Medication
➤ Monitor blood pressure and weight gain
➤ Vaccinations

See **Concept map 9.2** for an outline of Maxine's care plan.

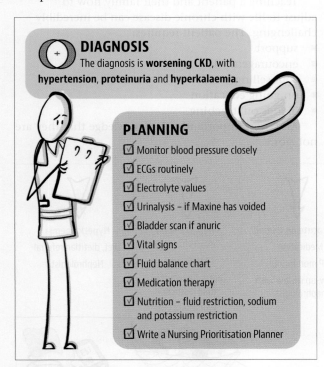

DIAGNOSIS

The diagnosis is **worsening CKD**, with **hypertension**, **proteinuria** and **hyperkalaemia**.

PLANNING

☑ Monitor blood pressure closely
☑ ECGs routinely
☑ Electrolyte values
☑ Urinalysis – if Maxine has voided
☑ Bladder scan if anuric
☑ Vital signs
☑ Fluid balance chart
☑ Medication therapy
☑ Nutrition – fluid restriction, sodium and potassium restriction
☑ Write a Nursing Prioritisation Planner

CONCEPT MAP 9.2 Diagnosis and planning for Maxine

9.3 NURSING INTERVENTIONS TO SUPPORT HEALTH CARE FOR A PERSON WITH CKD

Nursing interventions are implemented as part of person-centred care, and also to reduce or reverse signs and symptoms and the associated acute condition. This can be an acute exacerbation of a chronic condition, just like Maxine's current presentation. The fluid balance or acid base balance of any patient is significant, and urine output needs to be monitored with an aim in functioning kidneys for 0./5–1 mL/kg/hour of urine. This, as well as any other fluid intake or output is measured using a 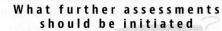 fluid balance chart (FBC).

Concept Map 9.3 further explores Maxine's journey throughout her treatment.

INTERVENTIONS

1 Assess blood pressure, urine, skin and laboratory values regularly.

2 ISBAR handover preparation for end-of-shift handover – what would you be handing over if your patient had peaked T waves, arrythmias intermittently, and anuria?

What further assessments should be initiated

Cues
1 Why is blood pressure important in CKD?
2 What is the deterioration here? What is the significance of the T wave changes?
3 What possible reasons could there be for the uraemic frost on the patient's skin?
4 Does this patient need IV fluids?

CONCEPT MAP 9.3 Nursing interventions for Maxine

9.4 EVALUATION OF CARE FOR A PERSON WITH CKD

As part of the further assessment of Maxine's presentation, **Concept map 9.4** asks further questions in relation to her management.

EVALUATION

The medical team have been notified of Maxine's increasing blood pressure to > 200 systolic, peaked T waves and irregular heart rhythm.

Plan:
Maxine's blood pressure continues to rise, and her HR is irregular, with arrythmia noted on her ECG. She is anuric, and has scaly, dry and crusted skin.

Cues

1. Undertake an A–G assessment of Maxine. What is your priority here?
2. Does this clinical deterioration relate to Maxine's CKD?
3. What do you think is the reason for this significant deterioration?

CONCEPT MAP 9.4 Evaluation and planning for Maxine

9.5 DISCHARGE PLANNING AND COORDINATION OF CARE FOR A PERSON WITH CKD

Maxine has presented with three (3) specific conditions that require discharge planning and further management at home and with assistance from the general practice. How does the management of the three conditions intersect? **Concept Map 9.5** explores the considerations for her care.

If your aim is for self-management, which in CKD it should be, your patient will need to practise with your supervision to receive feedback. Feedback is an essential component of education and teaching – it lets us know 'where we stand' and what we can improve upon. Feedback should be provided in a constructive and educational manner – how can we expect our patients to become self-managing if we are not providing them with assistance and feedback? It's like giving the keys to your car to your child and expecting them to know how to drive. Just because they have seen you drive, does not mean that they are able to.

In the real world, it will not just be one nurse providing the ongoing education and teaching to the patient. This is why it is incredibly important to document your teaching and the patient's response.

To keep track of your patient's education, with not just nursing staff, but allied health staff, or members of the multidisciplinary healthcare team, documentation is essential. Documenting the education, information and teaching you have provided will allow multidisciplinary healthcare team members to ascertain 'where' you are up to with regards to your patient's education.

Your patient, armed with this information, will be able to make informed health decisions and direct their own health care. It is important to remember that the multidisciplinary healthcare team approach is not severed upon discharge. As we have previously mentioned, renal nursing or CKD management is both acute and chronic, and your hospital's management of CKD/renal therapy will affect how the patient is treated from discharge onwards. It's a good idea to find out what the process is at your place of employment.

Teaching a patient and their family how to adjust to life with chronic disease can be incredibly challenging. The patient requires:

- support
- encouragement
- counselling
- on-going education
- 'hands on' teaching.

And most importantly, the knowledge that they are not alone.

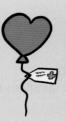

DISCHARGE PLANNING + COORDINATION OF CARE

How do the following areas of healthcare management **relate** to Maxine's presentation?

Which members of the healthcare team are **involved** in each area of management?

CKD – acute on chronic

Medication

BP monitoring

Follow-up review with nephrologist

Hypertension – exacerbation of

Medication

Diet – Na reduction, fluid restriction

Worsening CKD

Hyperkalaemia

Diet, dietitian referral

Nephrologist

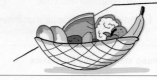

CONCEPT MAP 9.5 Discharge planning and coordination of care for Maxine

9.6 ASSESSMENT OF A PERSON WITH FLUID OVERLOAD – HYPERVOLAEMIA

Fluid overload, hypervolaemia, or fluid retention, refers to excess fluid in the circulatory system. Fluid overload occurs because the kidneys fail to regulate sodium and water balance. Fluid overload can lead to hypertension, pulmonary oedema and peripheral oedema.

Fluid overload may result from excess intake or administration of fluids or an interstitial-to-plasma fluid shift. The goal of treatment is removal of the excess fluid without disrupting the electrolyte balance.

Assessment of the patient who is clinically overloaded will show some, if not all, the following in conjunction with **Box 9.2** objective assessment cues:

- pedal or generalised pitting oedema
- increased central venous pressure (CVP) reading
- hypertension
- decreased urine output
- electrolyte imbalances – hyperkalaemia, hypernatraemia
- low albumin on full blood count
- crackles/creps on chest auscultation
- positive fluid balance – that is, more in than out, usually trending over previous few days
- decreased peripheral perfusion – cool clammy peripheries
- increased jugular venous pressure (JVP)
- full and bounding pulse (Brown et al., 2019; DeLaune et al., 2024; Derrickson et al., 2021).

Hypervolaemia can occur to any patient; it is not specific to those with urinary or kidney conditions. It highlights the importance of completing fluid balance charts and for holistic patient assessment. Changes in blood pressure, oedema, heart rate and respiratory rate are also related to changes in circulating fluid volume (Marieb & Hoehn, 2021; Rizzo, 2015).

Presentation

Jessica is a 24-year-old female who is 2/7 post-laparotomy for a gangrenous appendix. She has developed hypervolaemia. She has no previous medical or surgical history.

Concept map 9.6 explores the assessment of Jessica, and please refer to **Box 9.1** and **Box 9.2** for the key assessment points.

 PHx

Jessica is a 24-year-old female who is 2/7 post-laparotomy for a gangrenous appendix. She has no previous medical or surgical history. In the past 24 hours her fluid balance is +2785 mL, she has IVF @ 125 mL/hr and is NBM.

 ASSESSMENT

Primary survey
A: Patent
B: RR 16 bpm
C: Centrally warm
D: Alert
E: Pitting oedema
F: Nil in, IDC
G: BGL 10.2 mmol/L

Secondary survey
CNS (Cognition): E 4 V 5 M 6 = 15, Pupils equal PEARLA 4 mm
PAIN: 2/10 on movement. PCA running.
CVS: HR 120 bpm, BP 165/85 mmHg. A 12-lead electrocardiogram showed sinus arrhythmia with peaked T waves. T 37.9 °C. Bilateral pitting oedema 3+
RESP: RR 16, patent airway – spontaneous breathing, not laborious bilateral crepitus to mid/lower zones R=L
GIT: Abdo soft, tender on palpation. BS absent
RENAL: IDC in situ urine output for last four hours 42 mL. Sedimented, amber in colour
SKIN/INTEG: Centrally warm, peripherally cooler, oedema to bilateral lower limbs. Has removed ring to right index finger as it was 'tight'. TEDS in situ
MUSCULOSKELETAL (Mobility): Mobile with assistance
BMI: 24

Cues

1 What are the nurse-led priorities for this patient?

2 What are the collaborative priorities of care for Jessica?

CONCEPT MAP 9.6 Nursing assessment for Jessica

9.7 PLANNING CARE FOR HYPERVOLAEMIA

Concept map 9.7 further explores Jessica's presenting condition and diagnosis with clinical cues for planning her care. Refer also to **Box 9.3**.

DIAGNOSIS

The diagnosis is **hypervolaemia**, **hypertension**, **hyperkalaemia** and **hypernatraemia**

PLANNING

- ☑ Monitor blood pressure closely (consider invasive monitoring)
- ☑ ECGs routinely to monitor for T waves
- ☑ Electrolyte values
- ☑ Urinalysis
- ☑ Vital signs
- ☑ Fluid balance chart
- ☑ Medication therapy
- ☑ Remove TEDs due to oedema
- ☑ Neurovascular observations
- ☑ Write a Nursing Prioritisation Planner

CONCEPT MAP 9.7 Diagnosis and planning for Jessica

9.8 NURSING INTERVENTIONS TO SUPPORT HEALTH CARE FOR HYPERVOLAEMIA

Concept map 9.8 explores the nursing interventions for Jessica.

INTERVENTIONS

1 Regular ECGs due to peaked T waves.

2 Strict fluid balance chart monitoring.

3 Assess blood pressure, urine, skin and laboratory values regularly.

4 ISBAR handover preparation for end-of-shift handover – what would your clinical handover include if your patient had pitting oedema, hypertension and creps on auscultation?

What further assessments should be initiated

Cues

1 Why is blood pressure important in hypervolaemia?

2 What is the deterioration here? What is the significance of the urine output?

3 What possible reasons would there be for the creps on auscultation?

4 Does this patient need IV fluids?

5 What would peaked T waves indicate? What are the priorities of care in response to peaked T waves?

CONCEPT MAP 9.8 Nursing interventions for Jessica

9.9 EVALUATION OF CARE FOR HYPERVOLAEMIA

Concept map 9.9 explores the evaluation and further planning for Jessica's care.

EVALUATION

The medical team have been notified of Jessica's developing hypertension and decrease in urine output. Noted also is her increased work of breathing (with associated creps) and arrythmias on 12-lead ECG.

Plan:

Jessica's blood pressure continues to rise, and her HR is irregular, she has worsening shortness of breath and increased work of breathing. Her urine output is 0 mL for the past hour; with 125 mL 'in'. Her fluid balance over the past 24 hours is a positive balance of 2875 mL.

Cues

1 What interventions need to be considered now for Jessica? What is your priority here?

2 Does this clinical deterioration relate to Jessica's surgery?

3 What do you think is the reason for this significant deterioration?

CONCEPT MAP 9.9 Evaluation and planning for Jessica

9.10 DISCHARGE PLANNING AND COORDINATION OF CARE FOR HYPERVOLAEMIA

Concept map 9.10 explores discharge planning and coordination of care for Jessica.

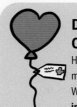

DISCHARGE PLANNING + COORDINATION OF CARE

How do the following areas of healthcare management **relate** to Jessica's presentation? Which members of the healthcare team are **involved** in each area of management?

Hypervolaemia

Medication

BP monitoring

Daily weight, same scales, same time daily

Fluid restriction management

Creps on auscultation

Medication

Hypervolaemia – correction of electrolytes, control of BP

Peripheral oedema

Physiotherapist review – oedema and mobilisation

Occupational therapist review – if ongoing oedema

CONCEPT MAP 9.10 Discharge planning and coordination of care for Jessica

SUMMARY

Assessment of the urinary system is so much more than reviewing a fluid balance chart. The urinary system is responsible for the metabolising of many medications, as well as the electrolyte balance and blood pressure regulation.

Each patient will present with various conditions, but at all times, these can be heavily impacted by blood pressure and fluid volume status. Your physical assessment requires a holistic review of the patient's skin (e.g. to check for oedema) as well as other subjective and objective data.

CLINICAL SKILLS FOR URINARY HEALTH

When assessing the urinary system of the person, there are many factors to consider, as the urinary system is responsible for many aspects of homeostasis and for general health and wellbeing. Assessments are generalised in that skin, blood pressure, urine output and taste can be affected by the dysfunction of the kidneys. The following clinical skills are required when managing a person with a urinary condition or disorder; consult your Clinical Skills resources, such as Tollefson and Hillman (2022), *Clinical Psychomotor Skills* (8th ed.).

- Focused cardiovascular health history and physical assessment
- Focused gastrointestinal health history and abdominal physical assessment
- Continuous bladder irrigation
- Continuous abdominal peritoneal dialysis
- Urinary catheterisation

PROBLEM-SOLVING SCENARIO

Logan Toms is a 63-year-old male who has had recurrent UTIs. He is currently febrile @ 38.9 °C, tachycardiac @ 110 bpm and hypotensive @ 90/62 mmHg. His relevant history is:
- HTN (controlled with medication)
- previously informed he was a 'diet controlled' diabetic; no medications or checking of BGLs
- no STIs

- UTIs × 3 in past four months – treated with PO ABs
- nocturia (× 4–5 times per night).
1   With this medical history, what potentially could impact upon Logan's recovery?
2   What nursing considerations would you have for Logan?
3   What are some patient education points you would need to dicuss with Logan due to the UTIs being recurrent?

PORTFOLIO DEVELOPMENT

You will soon see how much patient assessment is reliant upon the urinary system – the regulation of not only blood pressure, but the impact of fluid and electrolyte balance and the acid base balances within our body. You will need to continue to further your education and clinical currency around

medication regimens for CKD, for example, or treatment for UTIs. The urinary system is significant in the ongoing care of all patients – fluid balance is vital, so ensuring you are up to date and accessing continuing professional development will keep you working with best practice principles.

USEFUL WEBSITES

Registered Nurse Standards for Practice
The Registered Nurse Standards for Practice consist of seven crucial standards that all nurses must follow. Download and review the standards at the following link. https://www.nursingmidwiferyboard.gov.au/Codes-Guidelines-Statements/Professional-standards/registered-nurse-standards-for-practice.aspx

Kidney Health Australia
Kidney Health Australia has resources for both patient and professional alike. There are up-to-date medication and treatment plans for all stages of CKD. https://kidney.org.au

CKD Management in Primary Care Handbook (4th edition)
This is the current version of the primary care handbook for CKD patients. It is used Australia-wide in both primary and secondary health care. https://kidney.org.au/health-professionals/health-professional-resources

REFERENCES AND FURTHER READING

Australian Commission on Safety and Quality in Health Care (ACSQHC). (2022). *Kidney infections and urinary tract infections.* https://www.safetyandquality.gov.au/our-work/healthcare-variation/fourth-atlas-2021/chronic-disease-and-infection-potentially-preventable-hospitalisations/24-kidney-infections-and-urinary-tract-infections

Brown, D., Edwards, H., Buckley, T., Aitken, R. L., Lewis, S. L., Bucher, L., McLean Heitkemper, M., Harding, M. M., Kwong, J., & Roberts, D. (2019). *Lewis's medical-surgical nursing ANZ* (5th ed.). Elsevier.

DeLaune, S., Ladner, P., McTier, L., Tollefson, J., & Lawrence, J. (2024). *Fundamentals of nursing* (3rd ed.). Cengage Learning Australia.

Derrickson, B. H., Burkett, B., Tortora, G. J., Peoples, G., Dye, D., Cooke, J., Diversi, T., McKean, M., Summers, S., Di Pietro, F., Engel, A., Macartney M., & Green, H. (2021). *Principles of anatomy and physiology* (3rd ed.). Wiley and Son.

Marieb, E. N., & Hoehn, K. N. (2021). *Human anatomy & physiology* (9th ed.). Pearson.

Miles, J. (2021, 17 Nov). UTIs are one of the most common reasons people visit emergency departments, but it's easier to consult a GP or pharmacist. *ABC News.* https://www.abc.net.au/news/2021-11-17/utis-gp-pharmacist-emergency-departments-treatment/100624682

Rizzo, D. C. (2015). *Fundamentals of anatomy and physiology* (4th ed.). Cengage Learning.

Tollefson, J., & Hillman, E. (2022). *Clinical psychomotor skills: Assessment tools for nurses* (8th ed.). Cengage Learning Australia.

10

ENDOCRINE SYSTEM

The Australian Institute of Health and Welfare (AIHW) has developed monitoring information regarding diabetes (including type 1, type 2 and gestational diabetes) as the impact is significant upon the healthcare system, and, more importantly, upon the person with diabetes. Diabetes is the most well-known endocrinological disorder, and diabetes affected 1.3 million Australians (4.9% of the population) in 2020. Of note, type 2 diabetes was the 12th largest contributor to Australia's disease burden, with an estimated 3-billion-dollar expenditure in 2018–2019 (2.3% of the health budget).

Diabetes has significant impacts upon other body systems, and management is key. Aboriginal and Torres Strait Islander peoples are almost three times more likely to have diabetes as compared to non-Aboriginal and Torres Strait Islander peoples. This risk is an ongoing component of 'Closing the Gap', with socioeconomic and geographical barriers contributing to some outcomes.

Type 2 diabetes is the most prevalent form of diabetes in Australia, which aligns with international trends of increasing rates of this disease. Fifty-six per cent of deaths from diabetes were related to type 2 diabetes, indicating the impact on other body systems such as cardiovascular and renal being the causative factor in the death. (AIHW, 2022).

> **LEARNING OBJECTIVES**
> After reading this chapter, you should have an understanding of the:
> 1 assessment required for a person with endocrinological conditions
> 2 prioritisation of key components in the development of a plan of care for a person with:
> – hyperglycaemia
> – syndrome of inappropriate antidiuretic hormone (SIADH)
> 3 prioritised and targeted nursing interventions required to promote recovery or prevent further deterioration
> 4 evaluation phase and how the prioritised and targeted nursing interventions inform further assessment, planning and collaboration with the healthcare team
> 5 discharge planning and coordination of care required in preparing the person for discharge and subsequent continuity of care between the person and their healthcare providers.

INTRODUCTION

The endocrine system is made up of many organs and glands that are directly responsible for the secretion and management of hormones. Hormones have a significantly wide role of functioning and are often released at specific times – making the endocrine system heavily reliant upon homeostasis (Brown et al., 2019). Homeostasis is maintained by two main systems – the endocrine system and the autonomic nervous system. The endocrine system is the 'slow' responder, generally providing responses that are much more precise, while the autonomic nervous system produces a rapid or almost immediate change (think 'fight or flight') (Waugh & Grant, 2023).

There are many common endocrine conditions, including:

- acromegaly
- hypopituitarism
- syndrome of inappropriate antidiuretic hormone (SIADH)
- diabetes insipidus
- goitre
- thyroiditis
- Grave's disease
- hyperthyroidism
- cancers.

You will need to rely upon your foundation anatomy and physiology and the application of this to your patient's condition.

10.1 ASSESSMENT FOR ENDOCRINOLOGICAL CONDITIONS

Endocrine dysfunction or alterations are generally the result of hyper or hypo secretion of hormones. Symptoms for various disorders will be specific to the person and may have been present for some time prior to the patient presenting/complaining of these symptoms. Some symptoms with endocrine disorders can seem vague; for example, fatigue, headaches, or sleeplessness, and can be difficult to pinpoint to one condition. A nursing assessment, looking at all aspects of the patient's condition, with subjective and objective data is crucial.

Endocrinological disorders are often difficult to diagnose on physical assessment alone, and require interventional testing (such as blood tests to measure hormone levels in some instances) and as such, many patients are overlooked, or have their symptoms attributed to mood disorders, or other physiological issues such as stress (Brown et al., 2019).

Diabetes

Diabetes is a chronic condition – meaning that it lasts longer than six months and does not 'go away'. Diabetes is a condition that affects many systems in the body, and is related to abnormal insulin production and impaired or altered insulin utilisation, or a combination of both. Diabetes, and particularly type 2 diabetes, is a significant health concern globally, with its prevalence increasing by almost 50 per cent in the past 30 years. There are three types of diabetes:
1 type 1 diabetes
2 type 2 diabetes
3 gestational diabetes.

Diabetes is not just a condition that affects insulin production or utilisation, it has significant impacts and long-term complications on other body systems and is the leading cause of adult blindness (diabetic retinopathy), end stage kidney disease and is a major contributing factor to cerebrovascular accidents (strokes) and heart disease (Brown et al., 2019; Craft & Gordon, 2019).

Type 2 diabetes is the most common form of diabetes within Australia (accounting for upwards of 90% of all cases), and the causative factors are still arguable (AIHW, 2022). Many theories link diabetes to environmental factors which include obesity and see this as one of the largest causes of diabetes and pre-diabetes within Australia (Brown et al., 2019; Craft & Gordon, 2019; Waugh & Grant, 2023).

Type 1 diabetes is an autoimmune condition where there is no production of insulin. It requires the patient to administer insulin frequently to ensure stable glucose levels within the blood/plasma.

Type 1 diabetes also has significant health concerns, particularly around the impact upon blood glucose levels (BGLs) when unwell or injured (Craft & Gordon, 2019).

Box 10.1 and Box 10.2 guide the assessment for a patient with an endocrinological condition such as diabetes.

BOX 10.1   SUBJECTIVE ASSESSMENT

➤ History of illness and presenting signs or symptoms
➤ Past health history
➤ Medications
➤ Surgery
➤ Family history

Functional health patterns:
– Health perception and management
– Nutritional and metabolic
– Elimination
– Activity and exercise
– Sleep and rest
– Cognitive and perceptual
– Self-perception and concept
– Role relationship
– Sexuality and reproductive
– Coping and stress
– Values and beliefs
➤ Risk calculation

BOX 10.2   PHYSICAL ASSESSMENT

➤ Glasgow Coma Scale (GCS), including pupillary assessment
➤ Vital signs
➤ Blood tests such as full blood count, electrolytes
➤ Blood glucose level (BGL)
➤ Electrocardiogram
➤ Abdominal assessment
➤ Renal assessment
➤ Mental health assessment
➤ Neurovascular assessment

Presentation

Wendy Mullins is a 42-year-old woman who has been hospitalised for cellulitis following an insect bite on her right forearm. Wendy initially presented to her general practitioner (GP) for review and was prescribed oral antibiotics. Since commencing these antibiotics, Wendy has developed vaginal thrush, a UTI and her cellulitis has worsened. Her BGL on her home glucometer was 22.4 mmol/L, and Wendy reports feeling 'tired, hot and sweaty, and thirsty'. Concept map 10.1 further explores Wendy's hospitalisation.

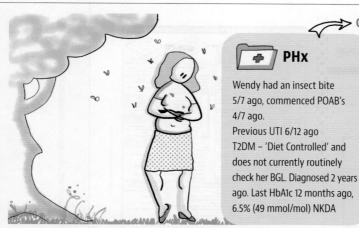

 Cues

PHx

Wendy had an insect bite 5/7 ago, commenced POAB's 4/7 ago.
Previous UTI 6/12 ago
T2DM – 'Diet Controlled' and does not currently routinely check her BGL. Diagnosed 2 years ago. Last HbA1c 12 months ago, 6.5% (49 mmol/mol) NKDA

1 What are your priorities with this patient? ABC

2 What is the significance of the temperature in Wendy's current status?

3 What is the relationship between hyperglycaemia and infection?

4 What is the pathophysiological relationship between inflammation, infection and diabetes (type 2)?

5 What are some concerns in relation to CVS assessment with this patient?

6 What physiological impact does hyperglycaemia have on the patient?

7 What investigative or diagnostic procedures do you think would be relevant for this patient?

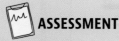 **ASSESSMENT**

Primary survey
A: Patent
B: RR 20
C: Warm
D: Alert
E: T 39.1 °C
F: IVF 166 mL/hr, HNPU
G: BGL 24.8 mmoL

Secondary survey
CNS (Cognition): E 4 V 5 M 6 = 15, Pupils equal, 4 mm, reactive to light (PEARLA)

PAIN: C/o pain on urination, lower abdominal pain to both R and L quadrant.
CVS: HR 105 bpm, BP 140/80 mmHg, pedal pulses bounding. A 12 lead electrocardiograph showed a sinus rhythm with no abnormalities.
T: 39.1 C
RESP: RR 20, patent airway – spontaneous breathing
GIT (Input): IVF 166 mLs/hr, BS present in all quadrants. BGL 24.8 mmol/L via glucometer.

RENAL (Output): Keytones negative. Awaiting urine sample/ward u/a. Patient denies haematuria.
SKIN/INTEG: Centrally and peripherally warm and well perfused – hot to touch.
MUSCULOSKELETAL (Mobility): Strict RIB, with VTE prophylaxis
BMI: 32.4
Wendy is in the general medical ward. She has received one dose of IV ABs; paracetamol is charted but has not yet been administered.

CONCEPT MAP 10.1 Nursing assessment for Wendy

EVIDENCE-BASED PRACTICE

National Subcutaneous Insulin Project
The Australian Commission on Safety and Quality in Health Care have established a guideline/form for the management of subcutaneous insulin adminstration, as well as the consistent documentation of BGLs, using the coloured warning signs seen in other early warning tools to highlight danger areas. This form also has the treatment steps for both hypo- and hyperglycaemia and is used in hospitals Australia wide. **Figure 10.1** is from Queensland Health and is their adaptation of this national form.

10.2 PLANNING CARE FOR A PERSON WITH AN ENDOCRINOLOGICAL CONDITION

Planning for care in any patient with an endocrinological condition/process requires review and understanding of the impact upon homeostasis and functioning (see **Box 10.3**). The body's main fuel storage source is insulin, which is a hormone that removes/facilitates glucose from the blood into the muscle and fat cells through biochemical reactions. It directly impacts storage and useage of carbohydrates, amino acids and fats in the liver, muscle cells and adipose tissue (Bryant et al., 2019). The significant differences between type 1 and type 2 diabetes is in the management of hyperglycaemia and the other involved processes. For example, it is rare for a type 2 diabetic to develop ketoacidosis, whereas for a type 1 diabetic they are prone to this condition. Type 1 diabetics have no insulin resistance, while type 2 diabetics do. It is crucial to undertand the differences between the types of diabetes to ensure safe and effecive patient care is delivered (Brown et al., 2019; Bryant et al., 2019).

Diabetes generally presents with the following pathology:
- hyperglycaemia
- polyphagia
- polydipsia
- polyuria
- ketosis
- fatigue
- abdominal pain.

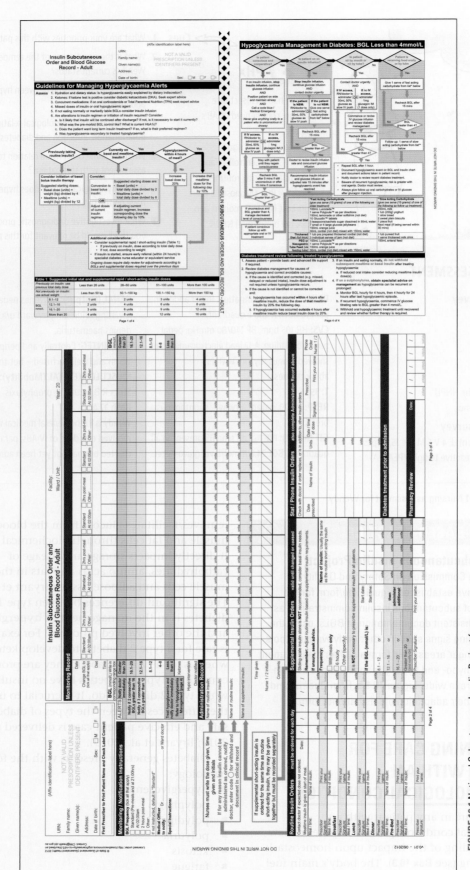

FIGURE 10.1 National Subcutaneous Insulin Project form

PLANNING CARE FOR A PERSON WITH AN ENDOCRINOLOGICAL CONDITION

➤ Physical activity- reduced due to fluctuating BGLs
➤ Medication
➤ Level of consciousness
➤ Monitor vital signs
➤ BGLs – regularly as per orders
➤ Nutrition and hydration status

The general aims of treatment in any endocrinological condition will be to restore homeostasis through either replacing, counteracting or correcting the imbalance. In the situation of diabetes, quite often treatment is focused on administration of insulin, coupled with fluids and other interventions to ensure safe return to normal physiological functioning (Brown et al., 2019; Craft & Gordon, 2019).

See **Concept map 10.2** for an outline of Wendy's care plan.

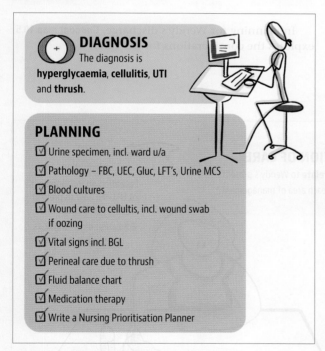

DIAGNOSIS
The diagnosis is **hyperglycaemia**, **cellulitis**, **UTI** and **thrush**.

PLANNING
☑ Urine specimen, incl. ward u/a
☑ Pathology – FBC, UEC, Gluc, LFT's, Urine MCS
☑ Blood cultures
☑ Wound care to cellulitis, incl. wound swab if oozing
☑ Vital signs incl. BGL
☑ Perineal care due to thrush
☑ Fluid balance chart
☑ Medication therapy
☑ Write a Nursing Prioritisation Planner

CONCEPT MAP 10.2 Diagnosis and planning for Wendy

10.3 NURSING INTERVENTIONS TO SUPPORT HEALTH CARE FOR AN ENDOCRINOLOGICAL CONDITION

Nursing interventions in the patient with an endocrinological dysfunction are going to be specific to that person. For example, not every person with type 2 diabetes will respond in the same manner (hyperglycaemia) with a UTI or dental abscess. It is very much reliant upon underlying pathophysiology and the inherent functioning and homeostasis of that person.

Concept map 10.3 outlines a plan for Wendy's care.

INTERVENTIONS

1 Assess BGL and vitals.
2 IV therapy management
3 Insulin administration
4 Fluid balance chart
5 Pain management and assessment

What further assessments should be initiated?

Cues

1 Why is level of consciousness (LOC) crucial to observe in hyperglycaemia?
2 What possible reasons could there be for the patient to report pain?
3 What concerns would you have for the cellulitis and healing factors?
4 What would you hand over clinically if Wendy was still febrile @ 39.1°C with a BGL of 28.6 mmol/L?

CONCEPT MAP 10.3 Nursing interventions for Wendy

10.4 EVALUATION OF CARE FOR AN ENDOCRINOLOGICAL CONDITION

As part of the further assessment of Wendy's presentation, **Concept map 10.4** asks further questions in relation to her management.

10.5 DISCHARGE PLANNING AND COORDINATION OF CARE FOR AN ENDOCRINOLOGICAL CONDITION

The nature of endocrine conditions means that the outcomes and effects that each patient experiences are different. This requires discharge planning and health promotion and education to be a significant focus to ensure safe discharge. But what is more important, however, is patient self-determination and empowerment.

EVALUATION

The medical team have been notified of Wendy's unchanged temperature and worsening hyperglycaemia (increasing BGL).

Plan:

Wendy has been prescribed an insulin infusion. Having not previously been on insulin, and weighing 94 kg, she has been prescribed insulin related to her weight. Her BGL is 28.6 mmol/L which is > 20, meaning she requires (as per the protocol outlined in the Evidence Based Practice box and Figure 10.1) 12 units of a short-acting insulin.

Cues

1 What interventions need to be considered now for Wendy?

2 What is the likely cause for the increasing BGLs?

3 What are some other considerations for Wendy here? How frequently will you need to perform BGLs?

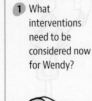

CONCEPT MAP 10.4 Evaluation and planning for Wendy

REFLECTIVE PRACTICE

Ketoacidosis

You are working in a community clinic and Carlie and her mother present for a three-monthly check-up appointment with you. Carlie has had several admissions to hospital with ketoacidosis in the past two years but has been relatively stable in the recent months. You refer to her initial assessment and notice that since that time her entries in her diabetes record book have become very spasmodic and her BGLs are fluctuating with increasing regularity. You ask Carlie about the documentation and she is despondent. She angrily states 'I always stick to my diet and it still makes no difference. My blood glucose levels are always high and I just can't do this anymore'.

You now need to focus your assessment of Carlie in order to collect data that will help you identify what issues may be arising for her.

Questions

1 What questions would you ask Carlie and her mother?
2 What issues might you consider?

In planning for Wendy's discharge, **Concept map 10.5** explores the considerations for her care.

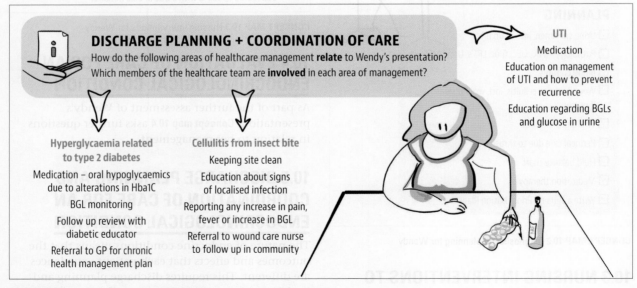

DISCHARGE PLANNING + COORDINATION OF CARE

How do the following areas of healthcare management **relate** to Wendy's presentation? Which members of the healthcare team are **involved** in each area of management?

Hyperglycaemia related to type 2 diabetes

Medication – oral hypoglycaemics due to alterations in Hba1C

BGL monitoring

Follow up review with diabetic educator

Referral to GP for chronic health management plan

Cellulitis from insect bite

Keeping site clean

Education about signs of localised infection

Reporting any increase in pain, fever or increase in BGL

Referral to wound care nurse to follow up in community

UTI

Medication

Education on management of UTI and how to prevent recurrence

Education regarding BGLs and glucose in urine

CONCEPT MAP 10.5 Discharge planning and coordination of care for Wendy

10.6 ASSESSMENT FOR SYNDROME OF INAPPROPRIATE ANTIDIURETIC HORMONE (SIADH)

The second patient condition to be discussed in this chapter will be syndrome of inappropriate antidiuretic hormone (SIADH). This condition is a result of overproduction of antidiuretic hormone (ADH) – which is from either sustained secretion or an abnormally high production of ADH. SIADH involves symptoms such as:

- fluid retention
- dilutional hyponatraemia
- concentrated urine
- hypochloraemia
- normal renal function
- serum hypo-osmolality (Brown et al., 2019).

SIADH is predominantly caused by malignancy, particularly small cell lung cancer. It can also be caused by head trauma or medications, and can also be associated with some metabolic diseases, such as hypothyroidism (Brown et al., 2019; Craft & Gordon, 2019).

The patient with SIADH will experience low urine output and associated weight gain or fluid retention. Serum sodium will fall (often to below 120 mmol/L) and symptoms then become more severe, with associated altered level of consciousness (ALOC), vomiting, nausea, muscle twitching and seizures. Once SIADH is diagnosed, treatment is directed at the underlying cause – so reversing it (Brown et al., 2019; Craft & Gordon, 2019; Waugh & Grant, 2023).

Refer to **Box 10.1** and **Box 10.2** for guidance on the assessment for a patient with an endocrinological condition.

Presentation

Kerry Brouff is a 28-year-old female who has presented with increasing thirst, fatigue and shortness of breath on exertion. She has a history of anxiety and depression and smokes 20–30 cigarettes daily. Kerry has no known allergies.

Concept map 10.6 explores Kerry's condition further.

10.7 PLANNING CARE FOR A PERSON WITH SIADH

For the key areas to be targeted when planning for care, please refer to **Box 10.3**.

Concept map 10.7 explores planning for Kerry's care.

PHx

Kerry, a 28-year-old female has presented with feeling fatigued, SOBOE and thirst.

PMHx: Anxiety, depression. NKDA.

Smokes 20 cigs/day (tobacco)

Meds: Citalopram 20 mg daily, OCP.

ASSESSMENT

CNS: E4 V5 M6 = 15 PEARLA 4 mm.

T: 37.4 °C

PAIN: C/o feeling exhausted. Some muscle twitching/pain but intermittent

CVS: HR 115 bpm, regular. BP 160/70 mmHg. Centrally warm, peripherally cooler. Capillary refill time < 3secs

RESP: RR 22, Increased WOB on exertion, Chest on auscultation clear throughout R=L with crepitus to lower zones bibasally. Nil cough. SpO$_2$ 98% RA.

GIT: BS audible in all quadrants. BGL 6.5 mmol/L. Nausea, reports vomiting prior to presentation

RENAL (Output): HNPU for past 4 hours

SKIN/INTEG: Poor integrity, dry skin, grossly intact. Nil skin tears. Oedema to lower limbs

MUSCULOSKELETAL (Mobility): Strict RIB, with VTE prophylaxis

BMI: 28.0

Cues

1. What are your priorities with this patient?
2. What is the significance of the increased work of breathing?
3. What is the significance of VTE prophylaxis?
4. What is the pathophysiological relationship between SIADH and presenting complaints?
5. What are some concerns in relationship to the patient's presentation?

CONCEPT MAP 10.6 Nursing assessment for Kerry

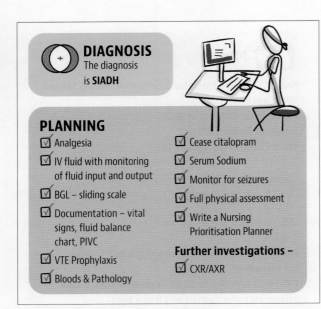

DIAGNOSIS
The diagnosis is **SIADH**

PLANNING

- ☑ Analgesia
- ☑ IV fluid with monitoring of fluid input and output
- ☑ BGL – sliding scale
- ☑ Documentation – vital signs, fluid balance chart, PIVC
- ☑ VTE Prophylaxis
- ☑ Bloods & Pathology
- ☑ Cease citalopram
- ☑ Serum Sodium
- ☑ Monitor for seizures
- ☑ Full physical assessment
- ☑ Write a Nursing Prioritisation Planner

Further investigations –
- ☑ CXR/AXR

CONCEPT MAP 10.7 Diagnosis and planning for Kerry

10.8 NURSING INTERVENTIONS TO SUPPORT HEALTH CARE FOR A PERSON WITH SIADH

Concept Map 10.8 further explores Kerry's journey throughout her treatment.

INTERVENTIONS

1 Assess pain, urine output, peripheral perfusion and vital signs.

2 ISBAR handover preparation for end of shift handover – what would you be handing over if your patient had a decreasing LOC?

What further assessments should be initiated

Cues

1 What further questions or information would you like to know from the patient?

2 What is the deterioration or change in patient status here? What is it related to pathophysiologically?

3 What could be the reason for SIADH occurring?

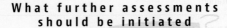

CONCEPT MAP 10.8 Nursing interventions for Kerry

10.9 EVALUATION OF CARE FOR A PERSON WITH SIADH

As part of the further assessment of Kerry's presentation, **Concept map 10.9** asks further questions in relation to her management.

EVALUATION

The medical team have been notified of the decrease in LOC in your patient.

Plan:
Medical officer has requested further pathology (serum Na) and a repeat in vital signs, and changing IV fluids to 3% hypertonic saline.

Cues

1 What interventions need to be considered now for your patient? What is your priority here?

2 The patient has been prescribed 100 mLs of 3% NaCl. What are you nursing considerations here?

3 What do you think is the reasoning for alteration to LOC?

CONCEPT MAP 10.9 Evaluation and planning for Kerry

10.10 DISCHARGE PLANNING AND COORDINATION OF CARE FOR A PERSON WITH SIADH

In planning for Kerry's discharge, **Concept map 10.10** explores the considerations for her care.

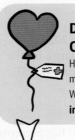

DISCHARGE PLANNING + COORDINATION OF CARE

How do the following areas of healthcare management **relate** to the patient presentation? Which members of the healthcare team are **involved** in each area of management?

SIADH

Medication review – cessation of citalopram

Follow up with GP for repeat bloods (sodium, ADH)

Education on symptoms for SIADH for patient and their family

Development of action plan for management of SIADH

Smoking and alcohol use – so cessation or minimisation of nicotine and alcohol

Medication

Referral (with consent) to AOD team.

QUIT

Anxiety/Depression

Patient education and health promotion regarding reasoning for cessation of citalopram

Review by psychiatrist regarding prescribing medication suitable for patient's anxiety and depression.

CONCEPT MAP 10.10 Discharge planning and coordination of care for Kerry

SUMMARY

Endocrine disorders have varied impacts and effects on people and have a great deal to do with underlying physiology. The impact of diabetes, for example, will affect each person differently when they are faced with infection, surgery or even an injury. Nursing care will need to be person-centred and focused as there will be no 'one size fits all' approach to endocrine disorders. Hormone regulation and management is again specific to each person. We cannot measure how 'stressed' someone is, as it is an internal response with associated hormones and chemicals created in response. Following the assessment, diagnosis, planning and evaluation framework will ensure that patient care is not compromised.

CLINICAL SKILLS FOR ENDOCRINE HEALTH

The following clinical skills are required when managing a person with endocrine health problems; consult your Clinical Skills resources, such as Tollefson and Hillman (2022), *Clinical Psychomotor Skills* (8th ed.).

- Physical assessment
- Mental status assessment
- Blood glucose measurement.

PROBLEM-SOLVING SCENARIO

Using a concept map approach, how would you care for Peter?

Peter Sims is a 21-year-old male who has type 1 diabetes. He has been hospitalised one day prior to an elective inguinal hernia repair. Peter currently takes:

- Novorapid 12u mane
- Novorapid 16u middi
- Novorapid 14u nocte
- Lantus 32u nocte

He has no known allergies, smokes 6–10 cigarettes per day (tobacco) and drinks 4–8 beers per week (tallies). He has a right inguinal hernia for repair.

1 What are some pathophysiological processes in place that could affect Peter's recovery?
2 What nursing considerations would you have for Peter?

PORTFOLIO DEVELOPMENT

To gain continual professional development or ongoing learning regarding diabetes, Diabetes Australia has several resources available to health professionals that are relevant.

They can be accessed here: https://www.diabetesaustralia.com.au/for-health-professionals/tools-elearning.

USEFUL WEBSITES

Registered Nurse Standards for Practice
The Registered Nurse Standards for Practice consist of seven crucial standards that all nurses must follow. Download and review the standards at the following link. https://www.nursingmidwiferyboard.gov.au/Codes-Guidelines-Statements/Professional-standards/registered-nurse-standards-for-practice.aspx

Management of Diabetic Ketoacidosis in Adults
Guidelines for management of DKA from Queensland Health (based on ASCQHC) https://www.health.qld.gov.au/__data/assets/pdf_file/0028/438391/diabetic-ketoacidosis.pdf

Diabetes: Australian facts
Statistics and impact from AIHW regarding diabetes.
https://www.aihw.gov.au/reports/diabetes/diabetes/contents/summary

National Diabetes Nursing Education Framework
Framework for nursing education and patient education within Australia. https://www.ndss.com.au/wp-content/uploads/national-diabetes-nursing-education-framework.pdf

REFERENCES AND FURTHER READING

Australian Institute of Health and Welfare (AIHW). (2022). *Diabetes: Australian facts.* https://www.aihw.gov.au/reports/diabetes/diabetes/contents/about

Brown, D., Edwards, H., Buckley, T., Aitken, R. L., Lewis, S. L., Bucher, L., McLean Heitkemper, M., Harding, M. M., Kwong, J., & Roberts, D. (2019). *Lewis's medical-surgical nursing ANZ* (5th ed.). Elsevier.

Bryant, B. K., Darroch, S., & Rowland, A. (2019). *Pharmacology for health professionals* (5th ed.). Elsevier.

Craft, J., & Gordon, C. (2019). *Understanding pathophysiology* (3rd ed.). Elsevier Australia.

Waugh, A., & Grant, A. (2023). *Ross & Wilson anatomy and physiology in health and illness* (14th ed.). Elsevier.

Tollefson, J., & Hillman, E. (2022). *Clinical psychomotor skills: Assessment tools for nurses* (8th ed.). Cengage Learning Australia.

MENTAL HEALTH AND SUBSTANCE USE

Mental health is a key part of health. Whether the focus is on the presenting problem that may require medical intervention, or a person's recovery and/or progression through their hospital or clinical care, the outcome is going to be more positive when we acknowledge the distress of others. Care planning and intervention considerations need to factor in holistic concepts and acknowledgement that altered mental health impacts upon physical and mental health and the assessment process.

A mental illness can be defined as 'a clinically diagnosable disorder that significantly interferes with a person's cognitive, emotional or social abilities' (COAG Health Council, 2017).

Poor mental health – whether related to disease or disorder, substance use or trauma – has a high impact on the overall health of Australian society. The Australian Institute of Health and Welfare gathers data on burden of disease and estimates 1 in 5 people aged 16–85 experienced a mental disorder in the previous 12 months.

The National Health Survey 2017–2018 estimated that:

- 1 in 5 (20%, or 4.8 million) Australians reported that they had a mental or behavioural condition during the collection period (July 2017 to June 2018)
- females reported a higher proportion of mental or behavioural conditions (22%) than males (18%)
- overall, 15–24 year olds had the highest proportion of mental or behavioural conditions (26%) and 0–14 year olds had the lowest (11%)
- of those participants who had a severe disability, 58 per cent had a mental or behavioural condition compared with 14 per cent of people with no disability or long-term restrictive health condition (Australian Bureau of Statistics (ABS) 2018).

In terms of burden of disease, mental and substance use disorders were the second highest group contributing to non-fatal burden (23%) after musculoskeletal conditions. (25%).

For Aboriginal and Torres Strait Islander peoples, mental and substance use disorders was 2.4 times the rate of non-Aboriginal and Torres Strait Islander people – 57.8 compared with 23.6 (Australian Institute of Health and Welfare [AIHW], 2020).

LEARNING OBJECTIVES

After reading this chapter, you should have an understanding of the:

1 distinction between mental health and mental illness
2 social and cultural determinants of health that contribute to poor physical and mental health
3 assessment required for a person experiencing altered mental health or substance use disorder
4 prioritisation of key components in the development of plans of care for a person with:
   – generalised anxiety disorder
   – depression
   – alcohol-induced sleep disturbance
5 prioritised and targeted nursing interventions required to promote recovery or prevent further deterioration of people presenting with altered mental health or substance use disorder
6 evaluation phase and how the prioritised and targeted nursing interventions inform further assessment of the person, planning of care and collaboration with the healthcare team
7 discharge planning and coordination of care required in preparing the person for discharge and subsequent continuity of care between the person and their healthcare providers.

INTRODUCTION

People with disruptions to their mental health, specifically in relation to mood and substance use, can experience disruption in stress levels, cognition and stigma and discrimination. Whether the condition is newly diagnosed or is long term and considered chronic in presentation, the concepts of person-centred care are the same – with the goal of maintaining a positive experience so the individual can interact at the best level possible with their environment and others. It is important to understand that many people experiencing altered mental health may fear stigma and discrimination (perceived or otherwise) with time constraints, emotional distress, diagnostic overshadowing and labelling being common findings from research (Tyerman et al., 2021).

11.1 MENTAL HEALTH AND MENTAL ILLNESS

Before we begin understanding the concept mapping process of nursing assessment and intervention for mental health and substance use, it is important to understand the distinction between mental health and mental illness. Not everyone we see with altered mental health will have a mental illness or psychiatric disorder as defined by the biomedical model criteria outlined in the diagnostic manuals, *Diagnostic and Statistical Manual of Mental Disorders 5* (DSM-5) (American Psychiatric Association, 2013) and *International Classification of Diseases 11* (ICD-11) (World Health Organization [WHO], 2022a). Also, a person with a mental illness can have good mental health and manage this like any other disease or illness.

The World Health Organization (WHO) constitution states: 'Health is a state of complete physical, mental and social well-being and not merely the absence of disease or infirmity' (WHO, 2023). An important implication of this definition is that mental health is more than just the absence of mental disorders or disabilities.

The WHO also affirm that: 'Mental health is a state of mental well-being that enables people to cope with the stresses of life, realize their abilities, learn well and work well, and contribute to their community' (WHO, 2022b).

So, it's important to remember that although poor physical health, accidents, disease or just the need for medical intervention can temporarily disrupt someone's mental health, this does not mean they have a mental illness. Equally, as we have already identified, people with mental illness experience poor physical health and we must factor the concept of 'diagnostic overshadowing' into our assessment and plan of care. It is helpful to identify the factors required to support good mental health. A great resource is Martin Seligman and the 'pillars of happiness'; these have been identified as core factors to achieving good mental health (in the presence or absence of mental illness) (Seligman, 2011, pp. 16–20). Commonly referred to as PERMA, these factors are listed in **Figure 11.1**.

One of the most important and influential interventions used to support positive mental health, and indeed reduce the severity of distress caused by symptoms, is the recovery model. The recovery model (identified here as the CHIME model, Leamy et al., 2011 – see **Figure 11.2**) complements both the WHO definition of mental health and the pillars of happiness as identified by Seligman. What we can now do as health professionals is adapt this as an approach that is person-centred, offers meaning and begins the process of the therapeutic relationship. Using recovery-based models assists in minimising stigma and the impact stigma and discrimination can have on people accessing care. Recovery uses strength – mental illness

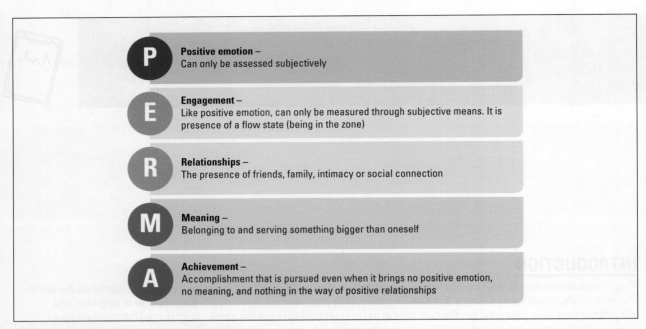

FIGURE 11.1 Seligman's Pillars of Happiness (PERMA)

SOURCE: SELIGMAN (2011), PP. 16–20.

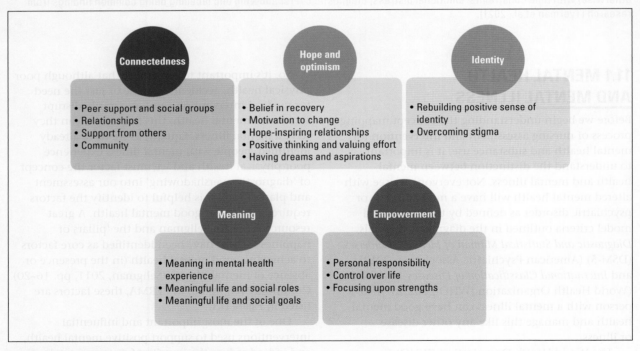

FIGURE 11.2 The CHIME framework for personal recovery

SOURCE: LEAMY ET AL (2011)

is often associated with weakness and despair, and people can end up either avoiding going for treatment as a result of fear and shame or be impacted by self-stigma whereby you believe yourself to be worthless and useless (Jones et al., 2018). An explanation of the CHIME model is illustrated in **Figure 11.2**.

A recovery-orientated model of mental health and mental illness is broader than cure or symptom management as in the biomedical model, though it does complement a clinical approach, as it has more of a focus upon resilience, hope and strength. Many mental disorders can rob people of the ability to think rationally; they can begin to lose their positive sense of self and identity which can impact on their purpose in life. So a key aspect of regaining meaning in life is to keep connection, hope and identity.

A simple definition of recovery is: 'the ability to live well in the presence or absence of one's mental illness' (O'Hagan, 2001, p. 1). So recovery is not about 'curing' or 'fixing', it is about working alongside someone to rebuild meaning.

Cultural safety

The concept of recovery aligns closely with the principles of cultural safety. The principles of cultural safety include reflection, minimising power differentials, communication, understanding and not disempowering or demeaning people (see **Figure 11.3**). This is integral to successful relationships and positive outcomes for people seeking or needing support. Cultural safety is especially important when assessing and caring for Aboriginal and Torres Strait Islander peoples, as their concept of health may differ from yours and/or the service you are representing. Culturally safe care is explored further in Chapter 18, but

it is wise to reflect on the strength and wisdom culture brings to relationships. **Figure 11.3** offers you a depiction of cultural safety principles that were first identified by Dr Irihapeti Ramsden (2002) in response to poor care being received by Indigenous New Zealanders. Cultural safety is determined by the receiver of care and the health practitioner works towards developing cultural competence. The key principles here assist you with assessment, planning, implementation and evaluation through understanding and recognising:

- your own values and perspectives
- the impact history and past policy has on people presenting for care (the process of decolonisation)
- how communication is important to develop relationships and trust
- the power imbalances that may be present.

With mental health this is particularly important as people may be vulnerable to suggestion and open to misinterpretation.

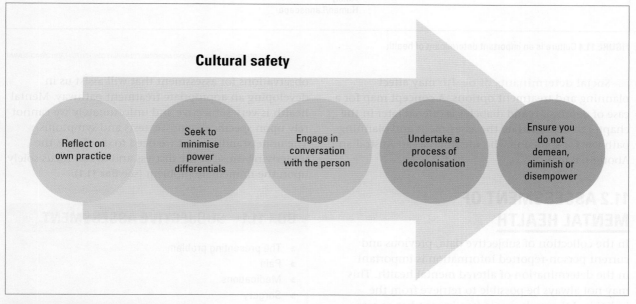

Cultural safety

Reflect on own practice

Seek to minimise power differentials

Engage in conversation with the person

Undertake a process of decolonisation

Ensure you do not demean, diminish or disempower

FIGURE 11.3 Principles of cultural safety

SOURCE: ADAPTED FROM BEST, O. (2018)

Figure 11.4 really demonstrates the close alignment with recovery principles and links cultural determinants such as land, family, country and lore together to create connection, self-determination, identity and meaning.

In many Aboriginal and Torres Strait Islander peoples' cultures, mental health, physical health, spiritual health and social and emotional wellbeing are all interconnected and one cannot be healthy without the others. So when we are considering culture, and the cultural determinants of health, consider the following factors:

- the concept of disease and mental illness may not align with the Western approach to diagnosis and treatment
- the person seeking help may be off Country and in unfamiliar territory and access may be difficult
- the impact of past history and policy may influence trust and engagement with you and the service
- trauma is a very serious consideration (Stolen Generations, stigma and discrimination all contribute to inter-generational trauma)
- other people's health may take priority over their own.

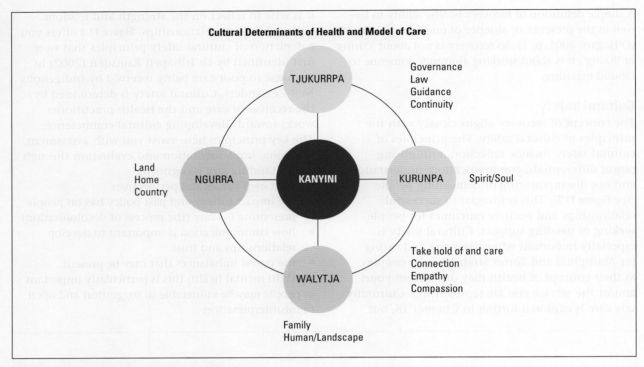

Cultural Determinants of Health and Model of Care

TJUKURRPA

Governance
Law
Guidance
Continuity

NGURRA

Land
Home
Country

KANYINI

KURUNPA

Spirit/Soul

Take hold of and care
Connection
Empathy
Compassion

WALYTJA

Family
Human/Landscape

FIGURE 11.4 Culture is an important determinant of health

SOURCE: BROWN, N. (2013), NACCHO ABORIGINAL COMMUNITY CONTROLLED HEALTH SERVICE SUMMIT.

Social determinants of health may affect planning and treatment options. A concept map for a case of depression and diabetes is offered later in the chapter to demonstrate the assessment and planning pathway for someone who identifies as an Australian Aboriginal male.

11.2 ASSESSMENT OF MENTAL HEALTH

In the collection of subjective data, previous and current person-reported information is important in the determination of altered mental health. This may not always be possible to retrieve from the individual themselves so a family member or care giver can also become part of the assessment process. The holistic assessment in mental health is the same as in other areas of health, and many people who experience altered mental health have higher rates of physical health concerns and hospital admissions than those who don't (Reeves et al., 2018). When considering someone's mental health, nurses and midwives use the Mental Status Examination (MSE) as well as presenting history. It is also important to consider contributing factors such as some of the ones identified with CHIME and PERMA along with physical considerations such as pain, disturbed sleep and fatigue. We can compact these into a series of

observations for assessment that will assist us in developing an appropriate treatment pathway. Mental health is very subjective and unfortunately we cannot rely upon specific diagnostic tests and symptoms. The understanding that we need to develop is the underlying cause of the distress and to not focus solely upon the immediate problem (see **Box 11.1**).

BOX 11.1 SUBJECTIVE ASSESSMENT

➤ The presenting problem
➤ Pain
➤ Medications
➤ Surgery
➤ Nutritional and metabolic
➤ Elimination
➤ Activity and exercise
➤ Sleep and rest
➤ Relationships
➤ Sexuality and reproductive
➤ Coping and stress
➤ Values and beliefs
➤ History of illness/past health history
➤ Family history
➤ Cigarette/nicotine smoking
➤ Substance abuse

The collection of further data with reference to the MSE (see **Box 11.2**) is informed by the subjective data and objective data gathered by you. The MSE is a 'snapshot' in time and is characterised by a series of specific observations relating to appearance, attitude and behaviour. The MSE can be used as a baseline and an ongoing assessment for progression and regression and it generally forms the basis of a clinical formulation that informs care planning. BATOMI is a traditional mnemonic used to remember the MSE; its components may differ from area to area but essentially the main ones are listed in **Box 11.2**. Much of the MSE is objective; for example, you are assessing appearance and congruity – does what they are saying match their facial or bodily expression? The MSE is not used in isolation; as part of the holistic approach we also assess functional inquiry (as per **Box 11.1**) and drug and alcohol use (**Box 11.6**).

BOX 11.2   OBJECTIVE ASSESSMENT

➤ First impressions

Mental Status Examination (MSE)
  – Behaviour and appearance
  – Affect and mood
  – Thought form and thought content
  – Orientation
  – Memory and concentration
  – Insight and judgement

It is good to have an awareness of the common signs and symptoms of mental illness that may present but equally it is important to assess this accurately. Many disorders require the symptoms to be present for at least two weeks or more. If someone is anxious about a procedure and has lost sleep or feeling a bit panicky that is considered to be normal. You need to be able to distinguish between what is a low mood and depression, what is normal anxiety vs an anxiety disorder and the difference between euphoria and mania. **Figure 11.5A-D** advise you on what mental illness looks like, but remember, these symptoms must be present for at least two weeks for a medical diagnosis to be considered. You will find the American Psychiatric Association (APA; 2013) criteria for the major mental disorders you will see in **Figure 11.5A**, **Figure 11.5B** and **Figure 11.5C**. In addition, **Figure 11.5D** gives you an oversight of psychosis which is a symptom, not a diagnosis, and can be caused by many things, so good to keep in mind when you are assessing a patient.

Some of you may confuse psychosis with schizophrenia, but a variety of mental and medical conditions can manifest with psychotic symptoms,

---

Major depressive disorder

Major depressive disorder is classified as a condition in which one or two and at least four of the other symptoms below are present:

1. Depressed mood most of the day, nearly every day
2. Marked diminished interest or pleasure in all, or almost all, activities most of the day, nearly every day (anhedonia)
3. Significant weight loss when not dieting, or weight gain
4. Insomnia or hypersomnia nearly every day
5. Psychomotor agitation or retardation nearly every day
6. Fatigue or loss of energy every day
7. Feelings of worthlessness or excessive or inappropriate guilt nearly every day
8. Diminished ability to think or concentrate, or indecisiveness, nearly every day
9. Recurrent thoughts of death or suicidal ideation

B. The symptoms cause clinically significant distress or impairment in social, occupational, or other important areas of functioning.

C. The episode is not attributable to the physiological effects of a substance or another medical condition.

https://doi.org/10.1176/appi.books.9780890425596.dsm04

FIGURE 11.5A Depression

SOURCE: AMERICAN PSYCHIATRIC ASSOCIATION, DIAGNOSTIC AND STATISTICAL MANUAL OF MENTAL DISORDERS, FIFTH EDITION ONLINE 8 FEBRUARY 2022.

Manic Episode

A distinct period of abnormally and persistently elevated, expansive, or irritable mood and abnormally and persistently increased activity or energy, lasting at least 1 week and present most of the day, nearly every day (or any duration if hospitalization is necessary).

B. During the period of mood disturbance and increased energy or activity, three (or more) of the following symptoms (four if the mood is only irritable) are present to a significant degree and represent a noticeable change from usual behavior:

1. Inflated self-esteem or grandiosity.
2. Decreased need for sleep (e.g., feels rested after only 3 hours of sleep).
3. More talkative than usual or pressure to keep talking.
4. Flight of ideas or subjective experience that thoughts are racing.
5. Distractibility (i.e., attention too easily drawn to unimportant or irrelevant external stimuli), as reported or observed.
6. Increase in goal-directed activity (either socially, at work or school, or sexually) or psychomotor agitation (i.e., purposeless non-goal-directed activity).
7. Excessive involvement in activities that have a high potential for painful consequences (e.g., engaging in unrestrained buying sprees, sexual indiscretions, or foolish business investments).

C. The mood disturbance is sufficiently severe to cause marked impairment in social or occupational functioning or to necessitate hospitalization to prevent harm to self or others, or there are psychotic features.

D. The episode is not attributable to the physiological effects of a substance (e.g., a drug of abuse, a medication, other treatment) or another medical condition.

(Hypomania has the same symptoms but they are only present for up to 4 days)

Mood in a manic episode is often described as euphoric, excessively cheerful, high, or "feeling on top of the world." In some cases, the mood is of such a highly infectious quality that it is easily recognized as excessive and may be characterized by unlimited and haphazard enthusiasm for interpersonal, sexual, or occupational interactions. For example, the individual may spontaneously start extensive conversations with strangers in public. Often the predominant mood is irritable rather than elevated, particularly when the individual's wishes are denied or if the individual has been using substances.

FIGURE 11.5B Mania

SOURCE: AMERICAN PSYCHIATRIC ASSOCIATION, DIAGNOSTIC AND STATISTICAL MANUAL OF MENTAL DISORDERS, FIFTH EDITION ONLINE 8 FEBRUARY 2022.

Generalised anxiety disorder

Definition: 'Excessive anxiety and worry occurring more days than not for a period of at least 6 months, about a number of events or activities. The individual finds it difficult to control the worry.' (APA, 2013, p 472.)

- Also known as free-flowing anxiety.
- Can leave people feeling helpless and depressed
- Typically worry about everyday things
- Heightened startle response
- High co-existence rate with other disorders

The essential feature of generalized anxiety disorder is excessive anxiety and worry (apprehensive expectation) about a number of events or activities. The intensity, duration, or frequency of the anxiety and worry is out of proportion to the actual likelihood or impact of the anticipated event. The individual finds it difficult to control the worry and to keep worrisome thoughts from interfering with attention to tasks at hand. Adults with generalized anxiety disorder often worry about everyday, routine life circumstances, such as possible job responsibilities, health and finances, the health of family members, misfortune to their children, or minor matters (e.g., doing household chores or being late for appointments). Children with generalized anxiety disorder tend to worry excessively about their competence or the quality of their performance. During the course of the disorder, the focus of worry may shift from one concern to another.

FIGURE 11.5C Generalised anxiety disorder

SOURCE: AMERICAN PSYCHIATRIC ASSOCIATION, DIAGNOSTIC AND STATISTICAL MANUAL OF MENTAL DISORDERS, FIFTH EDITION ONLINE 8 FEBRUARY 2022.

Psychosis

According to the DSM-5 (2013; Diagnostic and Statistical Manual of Mental Disorders, fifth edition) Brief Psychotic Disorder is a thought disorder in which a person will experience short term, gross deficits in reality testing, manifested with at least one of the following symptoms:

A. Presence of one (or more) of the following symptoms. At least one of these must be (1), (2), or (3):
   1. Delusions.
   2. Hallucinations.
   3. Disorganized speech (e.g., frequent derailment or incoherence).
   4. Grossly disorganized or catatonic behavior.

Note: Do not include a symptom if it is a culturally sanctioned response.

B. Duration of an episode of the disturbance is at least 1 day but less than 1 month, with eventual full return to premorbid level of functioning.

C. The disturbance is not better explained by major depressive or bipolar disorder with psychotic features or another psychotic disorder such as schizophrenia or catatonia, and is not attributable to the physiological effects of a substance (e.g., a drug of abuse, a medication) or another medical condition.

FIGURE 11.5D Psychosis

SOURCE: AMERICAN PSYCHIATRIC ASSOCIATION, DIAGNOSTIC AND STATISTICAL MANUAL OF MENTAL DISORDERS, FIFTH EDITION ONLINE 8 FEBRUARY 2022.

---

hence the reference to part C in **Figure 11.5D** when diagnosing a brief psychotic disorder. Schizophrenia has all the features of a brief psychotic disorder except the symptoms must be present for a significant portion of time during a one-month period AND for a significant portion of time level of functioning is impaired in areas such as interpersonal relations or self-care AND there have been continuous signs of disturbance for at least six months. The criteria for a diagnosis of schizophrenia are the same as for brief psychotic episode (**Figure 11.5D**, except part B).

You can now begin to see why assessment is important. While nurses, midwives and allied health professionals do not make formal diagnoses, understanding what to look for and what may be going on for an individual is essential for planning and implementing care. As you can see from the APA diagnostic criteria that have been introduced to you here, physical health needs to be assessed too. Physical health and mental health do not function independently of each other – we have to assess them all.

11.3 PHYSICAL ASSESSMENT

Many people presenting to clinical services complaining of physical symptoms may also be experiencing altered mental health. It is important to assess the person from a holistic perspective and consider: Are the physical symptoms causing the distress or is the distress of altered mental health or mental illness causing the physical symptoms? Do not assume; diagnostic overshadowing is a serious clinical error. Physical assessment is important to ascertain the nature of the presenting condition and to also gain an overall picture of health. Many people are unaware that they are experiencing altered mental health but feel uncomfortable and may attribute changes to a physiological process. So, regardless of the presenting problem, conduct a physical assessment as normal. Research has consistently demonstrated that people with serious mental illness have higher rates of poor physical health.

There are many common physical health problems that complicate mental health or may be because of altered mental health; either way they need to be addressed. **Figure 11.6** illustrates some of these common problems.

There are many reasons why a person with a serious mental illness is more likely than other people in the population to develop physical health problems. These include the following:

- **Social factors** People with a serious mental illness experience higher levels of poverty, unemployment, social isolation and exclusion, poor access to, and low uptake of, mainstream health services such as primary care, dental services, ophthalmology, personal health and lifestyle facilities (e.g. gyms and leisure centres).
- **Psychological factors** People with a serious mental illness experience low self-esteem, self-stigma, lack of personal assertiveness.
- **Mental illness-related factors** People with a serious mental illness experience unwanted side effects or complications of the medication used to treat serious mental illness. There also seems to be a decreased awareness in consumers that their physical health and wellbeing is important, perhaps due to the focus that is placed upon their mental state by health professionals. Another factor arises from the negative symptoms of schizophrenia, including a lack of motivation and self-neglect.

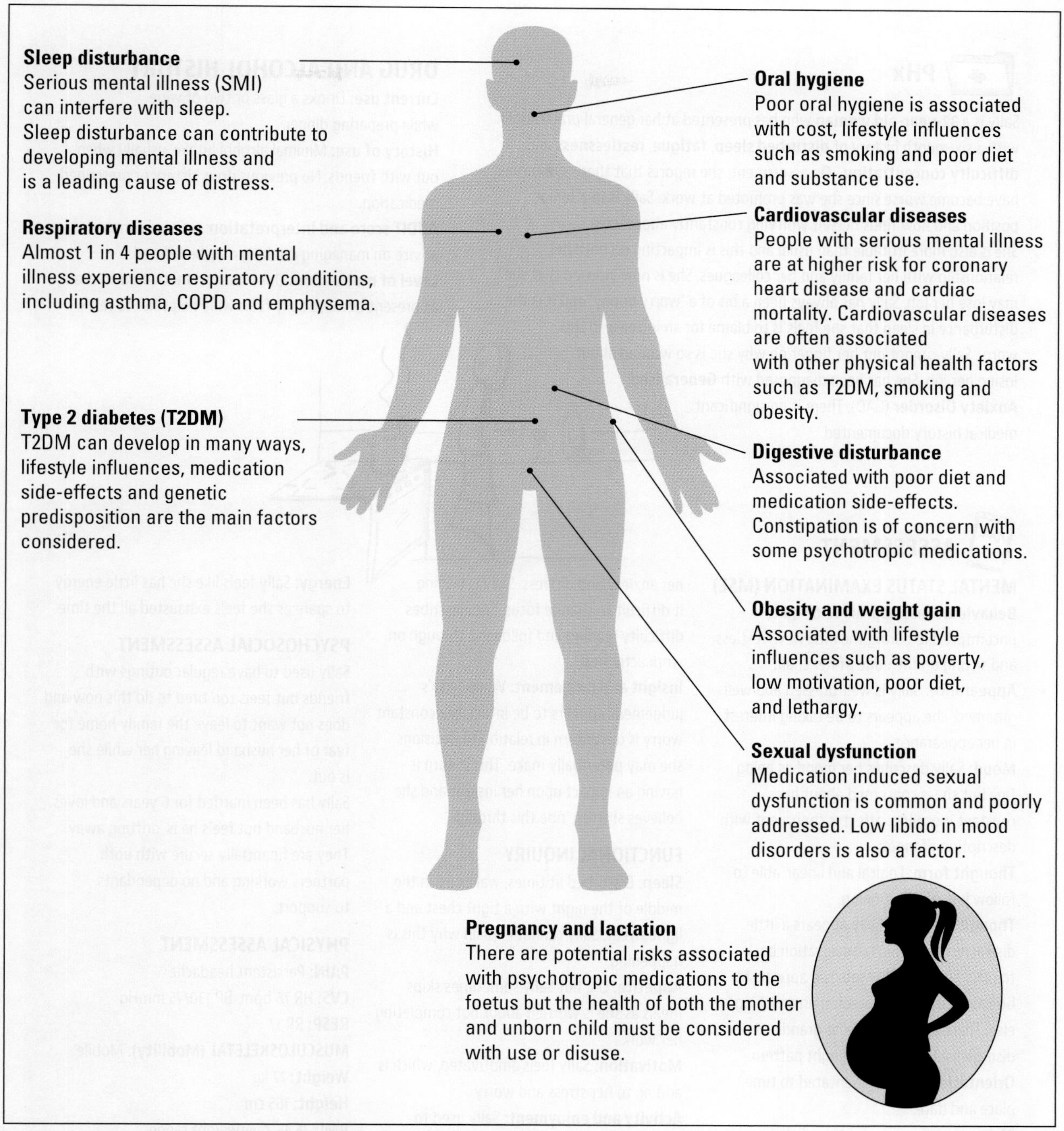

Sleep disturbance
Serious mental illness (SMI) can interfere with sleep. Sleep disturbance can contribute to developing mental illness and is a leading cause of distress.

Respiratory diseases
Almost 1 in 4 people with mental illness experience respiratory conditions, including asthma, COPD and emphysema.

Type 2 diabetes (T2DM)
T2DM can develop in many ways, lifestyle influences, medication side-effects and genetic predisposition are the main factors considered.

Oral hygiene
Poor oral hygiene is associated with cost, lifestyle influences such as smoking and poor diet and substance use.

Cardiovascular diseases
People with serious mental illness are at higher risk for coronary heart disease and cardiac mortality. Cardiovascular diseases are often associated with other physical health factors such as T2DM, smoking and obesity.

Digestive disturbance
Associated with poor diet and medication side-effects. Constipation is of concern with some psychotropic medications.

Obesity and weight gain
Associated with lifestyle influences such as poverty, low motivation, poor diet, and lethargy.

Sexual dysfunction
Medication induced sexual dysfunction is common and poorly addressed. Low libido in mood disorders is also a factor.

Pregnancy and lactation
There are potential risks associated with psychotropic medications to the foetus but the health of both the mother and unborn child must be considered with use or disuse.

FIGURE 11.6 Common physical health problems of people with mental illness

SOURCE: SHUTTERSTOCK.COM/MARTIAL RED (MAIN SILHOUETTE); ISTOCK.COM/MABACI (PREGNANT SILHOUETTE)

- **Personal factors** People with a serious mental illness experience higher rates of smoking, alcohol consumption and other substance use, poor diet, lack of physical exercise and high-risk behaviour.
- **Professional factors** Research suggests that health professionals are less likely to offer preventive health care. This reflects a lack of 'ownership' for the physical health of people with a serious mental illness from both primary care and mental health staff (Jones, 2008). Consumers who have had adverse encounters with health services or health professionals in the past are also less likely to seek help for a physical illness (Hungerford et al., 2021, p. 338).

11.4 ASSESSMENT FOR GENERALISED ANXIETY DISORDER (GAD)

Concept map 11.1 explores the impact of anxiety on Sally's life and strategies to manage these impacts.

PHx

Sally is a **32-year-old woman** who has presented at her general practitioner with a six-month history of **disturbed sleep, fatigue, restlessness** and **difficulty concentrating**. On assessment, she reports that these symptoms have become worse since she was promoted at work. Sally is in a senior position and now finds herself worrying constantly about work. She is also more irritable than usual and this is impacting on both her relationship with her family and her colleagues. She is now worried that she may lose her job. Sally has always been a bit of a 'worry bunny' and it is the disturbance in sleep that she feels is to blame for an increase in this worry. Sally cannot put her finger on why she is so worried about losing her job. She has been diagnosed with **Generalised Anxiety Disorder** (GAD). There is no significant medical history documented.

DRUG AND ALCOHOL HISTORY

Current use: Drinks a glass or two of wine while preparing dinner.
History of use: Minimal alcohol intake, usually when out with friends. No previous drug history or prescribed medication.
AUDIT score and interpretation: 8. Some simple advice on managing drinking may be offered.
Level of motivation: Does not feel motivated to change at present because Sally feels wine helps her to relax.

ASSESSMENT

MENTAL STATUS EXAMINATION (MSE)

Behaviour: Sally appears to be quite uncomfortable during the interview, restless and sitting on the edge of her chair.
Appearance: Sally is well-dressed and well-groomed; she appears to be taking interest in her appearance.
Mood: Sally describes her mood as being fine but she is concerned about her constant worrying; affect is congruent with description of mood.
Thought form: Logical and linear, able to follow line of questioning.
Thought content: Sally appears a little distracted and brings conversation back to concerns about her job. She appears to be having difficulty focusing on anything else. There appears to be no grandiosity or disorganisation to her thought pattern.
Orientation: Sally is orientated to time, place and date.
Memory and concentration: Sally's memory appears to be intact but her concentration appears to be affected by

her anxiety and distress. Sally is finding it difficult to change focus. She describes difficulty reading and following through on work activities.
Insight and judgement: While Sally's judgement appears to be intact, her constant worry is of concern in relation to decisions she may potentially make. This in turn is having an impact upon her insight and she believes she can 'ride this through'.

FUNCTIONAL INQUIRY

Sleep: Disturbed at times, wakes up in the middle of the night with a tight chest and a light sweat; Sally cannot explain why this is happening.
Appetite: OK, but Sally sometimes skips meals as she is worried about not completing her work.
Motivation: Sally feels amotivated, which is adding to her stress and worry.
Activity and enjoyment: Sally used to enjoy swimming and walking but now worries this is a waste of precious time.

Energy: Sally feels like she has little energy to spare as she feels exhausted all the time.

PSYCHOSOCIAL ASSESSMENT

Sally used to have regular outings with friends but feels too tired to do this now and does not want to leave the family home for fear of her husband leaving her while she is out.
Sally has been married for 6 years and loves her husband but feels he is 'drifting away'. They are financially secure with both partners working and no dependants to support.

PHYSICAL ASSESSMENT

PAIN: Persistent headache
CVS: HR 76 bpm, BP 130/75 mmHg
RESP: RR 17
MUSCULOSKELETAL (Mobility): Mobile
Weight: 72 kg
Height: 165 cm
BMI: 26.45, overweight range
GASTROINTESTINAL: Occasional morning diarrhoea

Cues

1. Identify the ways anxiety can impact physical health.
2. Discuss the impact anxiety can have on family relationships.
3. Could alcohol use be contributing to Sally's increased anxiety and sleep disturbance? Why?
4. What is the relationship between anxiety and diarrhoea?
5. What is the relationship between anxiety and sleep disturbance?

CONCEPT MAP 11.1 Nursing assessment for Sally

11.5 PLANNING CARE FOR MANAGING GAD

Planning care for managing generalised anxiety will involve education about the disorder to explain why Sally may be feeling the way she is through a stepped-care approach (**Figure 11.7**) that begins with the therapeutic relationship, assessment and psychoeducation. The nature and intensity of interventions will depend upon evaluation and response to any given stage of treatment. Essentially treatment begins at step 1, the least intrusive, but essentially identifies and understands the problem so psychoeducation can target the areas to change. Treatment options for GAD lean towards psychological and self-help strategies as opposed to hospital care and medication.

Planning for managing Sally's anxiety will have the goals of:

■ reducing the impact anxiety is having on everyday life
■ identifying strategies in partnership with Sally to manage her working environment
■ identifying strategies in partnership with Sally to increase motivation and re-engage with activities she enjoys
■ developing long-term self-help strategies
■ re-stabilising sleep patterns and sleep hygiene
■ examining the use of alcohol as a coping mechanism.

Figure 11.7 introduces the stepped-care model (National Institute for Health and Care Excellence, 2011, p. 12) used in the planning stage of developing long- and short-term strategies.

Areas to be targeted in planning care for a person with GAD are shown in **Box 11.3**.

BOX 11.3 PLANNING CARE FOR A PERSON WITH GAD

➤ Consent
➤ Education
➤ Work arrangements
➤ Activity schedules
➤ Psychotherapy options
➤ Sleep hygiene
➤ Alcohol use
➤ Substance abuse
➤ Medication

Initial planning

➤ Education concerning how anxiety works and the impact this has on mental and physical health.
➤ Write a prioritisation planner with Sally for the next 2 weeks' focus.
➤ Identify and establish 2 short-term goals to achieve in the next 2 weeks.
➤ Discuss realistic potential for lifestyle changes associated with sleep patterns and alcohol use.

Concept map 11.2 illustrates Sally's journey through initial care planning.

FOCUS OF THE INTERVENTION	NATURE OF THE INTERVENTION
Step 1: All known and suspected presentations of GAD	Identification and assessment; education about GAD and treatment options; active monitoring
Step 2: Diagnosed GAD that has not improved after education and active monitoring in primary care	Low-intensity psychological interventions: individual non-facilitated self-help, individual guided self-help and psychoeducational groups
Step 3: GAD with an inadequate response to step 2 interventions or marked functional impairment	Choice of a high-intensity psychological intervention (CBT/applied relaxation) or a drug treatment
Step 4: Complex treatment-refractory GAD and very marked functional impairment, such as self-neglect or a high risk of self-harm	Highly specialist treatment, such as complex drug and/or psychological treatment regimens; input from multi-agency teams, crisis services, day hospitals or inpatient care

FIGURE 11.7 The stepped-care model
SOURCE: NATIONAL INSTITUTE FOR HEALTH AND CARE EXCELLENCE

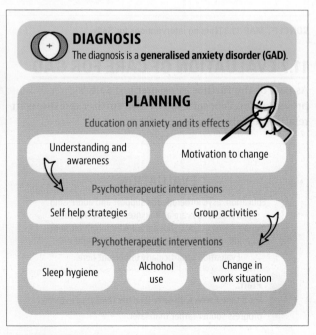

CONCEPT MAP 11.2 Diagnosis and planning for Sally

11.6 NURSING INTERVENTIONS TO SUPPORT HEALTH CARE FOR GAD

Nursing interventions need to be developed in partnership with Sally. Interventions need to be realistic, achievable and, above all, not create more anxiety. Education has been identified as a key aspect of managing GAD since, as the disorder diagnosis itself suggests, there is nothing to actually pinpoint where the anxiety is coming from so trying to timeline intensity and occasions can be very challenging. Sally identified she has recently been promoted and believes this is the cause of the anxiety; that may be the case; it may not. What we do know is that the anxiety is causing

disruption to Sally's life and day-to-day functioning, causing increased anxiety, in rather a vicious circle. It is important to understand that interventions require commitment and are generally long term. A short-term goal would involve education and understanding. This would include the knowledge that these disorders come and go and there may well be a long-term approach to managing vulnerability towards anxiety disorders. In addition, anxiety causes physiological distress due to activation of the autonomic nervous system. Strategies to manage this can include breathing and relaxation techniques, yoga and meditation.

Concept map 11.3 is an illustrated summary of intervention planning focus for Sally.

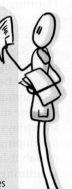

INTERVENTIONS

Education

1 Websites, 1:1 support

2 Family educational support

3 Education on anxiety, its impact, use of alcohol and benefits of being active

4 Substance use/abuse

Psychotherapy

1 Cognitive Behavioural Therapy (CBT)

2 Mindfulness

3 Applied relaxation techniques

4 Support groups

5 Focus on managing one aspect at a time

Lifestyle

1 Explore options to reduce workload

2 Sleep assessment and examination of routine, rumination and management of waking

3 Diet and exercise, identify achievable activities

4 Note alcohol consumption and any substance use/abuse; explore strategies to reduce this.

CONCEPT MAP 11.3 Nursing interventions for Sally

11.7 EVALUATION OF CARE FOR GAD

As part of the further assessment of Sally's presentation, **Concept map 11.4** asks further questions in relation to Sally's management.

EVALUATION

Education, psychotherapeutic support and addressing lifestyle changes are all key interventions for the management of GAD. These require high commitment and may require initial intensive oversight.

Evaluation is particularly important here.

Plan:

Set a time frame with Sally (and her family) to evaluate progress sooner rather than later.

What further assessments should be initiated

CONCEPT MAP 11.4 Evaluation and planning for Sally

REFLECTIVE PRACTICE

1 Why is it important to evaluate planned strategies quickly with Sally?

2 Why might GAD not be recognised in presentations to primary health care?

3 Why is it important to regularly monitor observations and physical health?

11.8 DISCHARGE PLANNING AND COORDINATION OF CARE FOR GAD

Concept map 11.5 explores a plan for Sally's continued care.

11.9 ASSESSMENT FOR DEPRESSION

Concept map 11.6 explores the presentation of Mr Williams.

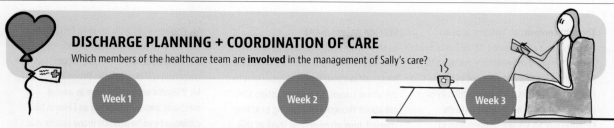

DISCHARGE PLANNING + COORDINATION OF CARE

Which members of the healthcare team are **involved** in the management of Sally's care?

Week 1

Ask Sally to keep a diary of activities and thoughts to bring to a clinical review next week

Ensure Sally has contact details, dates and appointment timesclearly recorded

Offer Sally contact details for support groups in her area or online

Ensure breathing and relaxation techniques are accessible. This could involve apps, websites or local groups

Week 2

Ask if Sally and her family have any further questions about GAD

Review of week one and progress/non-progress, explore any events, emotions, barriers and enablers

Review physiological status and observations

Set goals for week 3

Week 3

As before, evaluate previous week's activities, feelings and events

Revisit plans and goals. What is working /not working?

Set new goals or re-evaluate past goals with a different strategy if needed

Review physiological status and observations

Begin long-term planning or, if required, go back to the start.

CONCEPT MAP 11.5 Discharge planning and coordination of care for Sally

 PHx

Mr Jarrah Williams is a 54-year-old Indigenous Australian male who is being assessed for poor sleep and low mood. This has been developing since Mr Williams received a diagnosis of type 2 diabetes 6 months ago. Mr Williams has been commenced on anti-depressants, but he complained that they were not working so he stopped taking them and now feels that life is not worth living any more. His family do not understand why he is not engaging in community activities any more and are concerned for his wellbeing. Mr Williams has a car but does not like to travel far from his semi-rural community and often loans it out to other community members. Mr Williams is very concerned about his diabetes as he has been instructed to eat a healthy diet and undertake more exercise, something he currently finds very challenging to achieve. Mr Williams missed his last routine diabetic follow-up appointment but has been brought to the clinic by his wife due to recently worsening mood symptoms and disengagement from friends and family. Family are concerned that Mr Williams has been saying that they are better off without him. Mr Williams has not checked his blood glucose level (BGL) for some time as he does not see the point.

 ASSESSMENT

PHYSICAL ASSESSMENT

PAIN: No pain reported

CVS: HR 82 bpm, BP 136/82 mmHg

RESP: RR 18

MUSCULOSKELETAL (Mobility): Mobile, no concerns

Weight: 88 kg

Height: 174 cm

BMI: 29.1, overweight range

Past relevant medical history

Recent diagnosis of type 2 diabetes (previous 6 months). Nil significant medical history, no previous history of mood disturbance. Has been complaining of insomnia for last 4 months, sleeping tablets prescribed with little effect. Diabetes is currently being managed with diet and exercise.

Last HbA1c result 56 mmol/mol (normal range = 48–53 mmol/mol) 5 months ago.

Functional inquiry

Sleep: disturbed at times, wakes up in the middle of the night and cannot get back to sleep.

Appetite: poor at the moment, does not feel like preparing or eating food.

Motivation: Mr Williams does not even want to get out of bed, he only gets up to try and meet family obligations but is finding this increasingly difficult.

Activity and enjoyment: Mr Williams used to enjoy fishing and walking but now can't be bothered. He has not been to work for over 2 weeks.

Energy: Mr Williams reports having little energy to spare and feels exhausted all the time.

Cues: consider the physical impact depression has on overall health. What signs and symptoms of depression (Figure 11.5A) can you see here?

Mental Status Examination

Behaviour: Mr Williams appears quite morose; he is looking down and making minimal eye contact.

Appearance: Mr Williams is casually dressed but admits his wife dressed him this morning.

Mood: Mr Williams reports feeling sad and useless, he feels he is a burden to his family and community.

Thought form: logical and linear, able to follow line of questioning but responses are slow and monosyllabic.

CONCEPT MAP 11.6 Nursing assessment for Mr Williams

Thought content: Mr Williams appears distracted and uninterested. Mr Williams does not see the point of being here and feels he is just being a burden and waste of everyone's time. There appears to be no grandiosity or disorganisation to his thought pattern.

Orientation: Mr Williams is orientated to time, place and date but admits to being more forgetful lately and does not care what day it is.

Memory and concentration: Mr Williams describes difficulty reading and following through on any activities. He is concerned he is forgetting to attend important events in his community.

Insight and judgement: Mr Williams appears to have no understanding of his illness(es) or he is choosing to disengage; difficult to ascertain at the moment. This has resulted in poor judgement as he is not following his treatment routine.

Suicide assessment

As Mr Williams has indicated he feels he is a burden to everyone and they would be better off without him, it is important to ask about suicide. In order to assess this, ask about thoughts of harming or killing yourself, how often do you think of this, how you would do this, what timeframe do you have in mind and does the person have means or access and, importantly, have they tried suicide before (NIMH, 2022).

Mr Williams denies wanting to harm or kill himself despite feeling like he is a burden. He has not made any plans and has not thought about how he would kill himself, and there have been no previous attempts reported.

Psychosocial assessment

Mr Williams lives in a small rural community to which he identifies a strong connection.

Mr Williams lives with his wife, Hattie, their two children and 3 grandchildren.

Mrs Williams describes this as a happy household and they have no financial stressors.

Mr Williams works part time as a local mechanic and is considered an Elder in his community so he attends many ceremonial and traditional occasions.

Mr Williams speaks both language (native tongue) and English.

Mr Williams used to regularly visit friends and family in his community but has not been doing this for some time.

Drug and alcohol assessment

Apart from an occasional beer at the local bar, Mr Williams drinks very little.

Mr Williams has never taken illicit drugs.

AUDIT score = 3

CONCEPT MAP 11.6 Nursing assessment for Mr Williams (continued)

11.10 PLANNING FOR MANAGING DEPRESSION

Box 11.4 illustrates the cultural and social considerations we have to consider in relation to planning and interventions. You can consider this for any person in your care but for this case it is essential.

Planning for managing Mr Williams' depression will have the goals of:

- reducing the impact depression is having on everyday life
- identifying strategies in partnership with Mr Williams and significant others to manage day-to-day activities

- identifying strategies in partnership with Mr Williams and significant others to increase motivation and reengage with activities and commitments.
- developing long-term self-help strategies
- re-stabilising sleep patterns and sleep hygiene
- establishing strategies to manage type 2 diabetes through diet and exercise.

Areas to be targeted when planning for Mr Williams' care are shown in **Box 11.5**.

BOX 11.4 CULTURAL AND SOCIAL CONSIDERATIONS

- Mr Williams' perception of health and wellbeing may differ to yours. Mr Williams may be more concerned about the impact his health is having on his family and community than himself.
- Mr Williams may have cultural obligations associated with Men's Business and lore that he is currently not able to fulfil and this will further fuel feelings of worthlessness as identified in the MSE.
- Mr Williams' understanding of diabetes and depression may be impacted by communication and interpretation of language. Not all terms translate across.
- Mr Williams may not have easy access to services, fresh fruit and vegetables, or exercise opportunities.

BOX 11.5 PLANNING FOR MANAGING DEPRESSION

- Consent
- Management of low mood
- Management of diabetes
- Access to services and support
- Assess level of understanding and interpretation
- Community/ family involvement

Initial planning

- Manage potential suicide risk
- Consultation and establishment of current understanding
- Involve Aboriginal community-controlled health organisation (ACCHO)
- Develop a daily planner with Mr Williams that sets achievable daily goals
- Discuss medication, concerns and benefits
- Discuss and identify meal planning, exercise routines (pre-depression)
- Consult with family and kin

As you can see, planning care for Mr Williams is going to be multifaceted. The way he feels about his physical health is highly likely to be impacted upon by his mental health and as a result, both are being neglected. It is important to understand that there may be a number of complex factors going on here and treatment and intervention considerations are going to be much more than a medical approach. It is important to set realistic and collaboratively developed goals; for example, offering a healthy eating plan may be unattainable without exploring what is currently available and achievable.

Concept map 11.7 illustrates Mr Williams' journey through initial care planning and presents an initial simple visual plan.

11.11 NURSING INTERVENTIONS TO SUPPORT HEALTH CARE FOR DEPRESSION

Nursing interventions, as per any intervention in mental health care, must be developed in partnership with the individual and, in Mr Williams' case, highly likely with the family too. However, never make such an assumption, you must ask Mr and Mrs Williams how they would like to work through this. Looking back on recovery and cultural safety principles, it is really important that connection and identity is maintained and for Mr Williams, as some of this identity has been lost through his disconnection with his cultural and community responsibilities. This in turn impacts upon his mood thus fueling that depressive state of hopelessness and worthlessness. In addition, we are managing the physical health aspect associated with diabetes; poor physical health contributes to poor mental health and vice versa (Collins et al., 2013), so education and interventions need to factor in both along with cultural considerations. Strategies to manage these include education and support, and psychotherapy (talking therapies, Yarning). Yarning is important because it uses stories and anecdotes to share information and minimises risk of misunderstanding through not using jargon while forging connection (Lin et al., 2016).

Concept map 11.8 is an illustrated summary of intervention planning focus for Mr Williams.

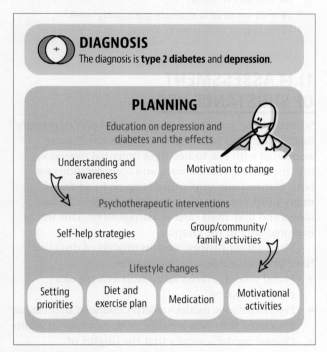

CONCEPT MAP 11.7 Diagnosis and planning for Mr Williams

INTERVENTIONS

Education
1 Indigenous Health Worker, ACCHO, 1:1 support
2 Family educational support
3 Education on depression, its impact, use of medication and benefits of being active
4 Education on diabetes, its impact, use of food as management and benefits of being active

Medication
1 Discuss anti-depressants and how they work, timeframes for how long they take to work and potential side effects.

2 Introduce options around diabetes medication.

Psychotherapy
1 Focus on managing one aspect at a time
2 Cognitive Behavioural Therapy
3 Mindfulness
4 Community-based resources
5 Explore traditional therapies
6 Yarning

Lifestyle
1 Explore options to manage daily routines

2 Sleep assessment and examination of routine, rumination and management of waking
3 Diet and exercise; identify achievable and acceptable activities
4 Identify key community responsibilities and potential strategies to re-engage with these
5 Determine follow-up appointments around Mr Williams' usual routine

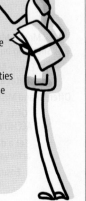

CONCEPT MAP 11.8 Nursing interventions for Mr Williams

11.12 EVALUATION OF CARE FOR DEPRESSION

As part of the further assessment of Mr Williams' presentation, **Concept map 11.9** asks further questions in relation to his management.

EVALUATION

Mr Williams is going to require regular follow-up to monitor both his depression and diabetes which are of equal priority in this case.

Mr Williams really needs to take anti-depressants regularly as prescribed to gain the full effect.

Mr Williams needs to begin to re-engage in his usual activities (at his own pace) and this can be a good measure of improvement.

Education, psychotherapeutic and cultural support are all going to be key to address the long-term changes that are going to be required to manage both diabetes and depression.

Plan:
Having a clear discharge plan and future focused plan is essential and must be evaluated regularly.

Cues

1 Why is it important that any plans are developed and evaluated with Mr Williams?

2 Why is it important to connect with a local ACCHO or Indigenous Health Worker?

3 What barriers can you think of that would impede Mr Williams' engagement with healthcare services?

What further assessments could we consider following evaluation

CONCEPT MAP 11.9 Evaluation and planning for Mr Williams

11.13 DISCHARGE PLANNING AND COORDINATION OF CARE FOR DEPRESSION

Concept map 11.10 is an illustrated view of the discharge planning for Mr Williams.

REFLECTIVE PRACTICE

1 How will undertaking a process of decolonisation assist in your development of a trusting relationship with Mr and Mrs Williams?
2 Why do we need to evaluate goals every week?
3 What targets should we be setting with Mr Williams?

11.14 ASSESSMENT OF SUBSTANCE USE

Substance use assessment is an essential part of primary health care. This type of assessment is much more associated with risk to health of potential overdose, life threatening withdrawals, and considerations for both planned and unplanned surgery. In addition, many intoxicating substances affect judgement and mood and may need careful management. This will be explored later in the chapter.

Throughout history, various models of drug use have been developed, including the:

- Moral model – views **addiction** as a sin or a moral weakness
- Psychodynamic model – asserts childhood traumas are associated with how we cope or do not cope as adults
- Disease model – argues that the origins of addiction lie in the individual him/herself

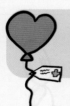

DISCHARGE PLANNING + COORDINATION OF CARE

Which members of the healthcare team are **involved** in the management of Mr Williams care?

Week 1

Ask Mr and Mrs Williams to keep a diary of meals, times and shopping budgets to bring to a clinical review next week

Ensure Mr and Mrs Williams have contact details, dates and appointment times clearly recorded

Offer Mr and Mrs Williams information on depression and diabetes

Offer Mr and Mrs Williams contact details for ACCHO or support groups in their area or online

Set a daily plan with Mr Williams with simple, achievable activities such as attending to ADLs

Ensure BGLs are being done and recorded, offer assistance as required

Week 2

Review of week 1 and progress/non-progress, explore any events, emotions, barriers and enablers

Review physiological status and observations

Align blood glucose levels with diet and exercise, illustrate the connection

Begin discussing the relationship between depression, mood and physical health

Set goals for week 3

Week 3

As before, evaluate previous week's activities, feelings and events

Revisit plans and goals, what is working what is not

Set new goals or re-evaluate past goals with a different strategy if needed

Review physiological status and observations

Begin long-term planning or, if required, go back to the start

CONCEPT MAP 11.10 Discharge planning and coordination of care for Mr Williams

- Social learning model – suggests that **dependence** behaviours are learned, exist on a continuum and consist of a number of behavioural and cognitive (thought) processes
- Public health model – drug use seen as the interaction between the drug, the individual and the environment
- Sociocultural model – argues that substance abuse should be examined in a wider social context and can be linked to inequality (Department of Health and Aged Care, 2004).

It is important for you to reflect on these models because they may influence the way you present support and treatment. It is also important to understand the potential effects that intoxicating substance use can have on general mental health (see **Figure 11.8**) so you can also consider these possible causes and not go straight to a mental health diagnosis (notice the similarities).

Alcohol use and intoxication

Excessive alcohol consumption and **intoxication** is a growing problem and it should be considered a multisystem disease with potentially significant impacts on perioperative morbidity and mortality. Screening should take place at the pre-assessment clinic or on admission to hospital to identify and

treat those at risk of complications. In Australia, the self-reported use of legal substances is much higher than for illegal substances (AIHW, 2017). Legal substances include alcohol, cigarettes and prescribed medications. Summary data from the Coroners Court of Victoria, for example, found that overdose deaths related to prescription medications are more than double those of road accidents (Monheit et al., 2016). The AIHW (2018) reports that 9 per cent of the burden of disease in Australia is attributed to smoking and a further 6.7 per cent to alcohol and substance use. So, in a medical setting we must assess substance use. Many health professionals assume that substance use assessment is the realm of 'specialist' assessors but, as already identified, screening needs to take place on admission. In a 2018 report on screening practices in clinical environments by McNeely et al., they found that participants stated that some patients may never be asked about alcohol or drug use, because screening depends on the provider, the patient's other medical problems, and the amount of time available. As a result, valuable information may not have been gained. McNeely et al. (2018, p. 5) state:

'In addition to providing overall knowledge about the patient's health, providers and patients also talked about specific ways in which

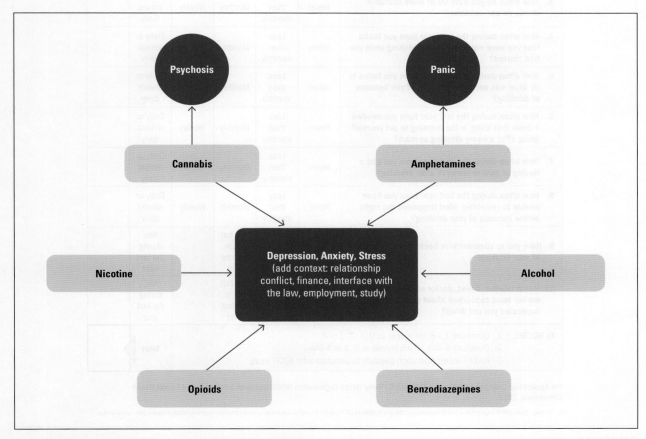

FIGURE 11.8 The impact of alcohol and other drugs on mental health

screening for substance use adds value to the clinical encounter. Screening was felt to be a way of signaling to patients that talking about substance use is permissible, thus opening the door to a conversation that would not otherwise have happened.'

There are many tools health professionals can use. Check with your service which ones they are currently using. Tools that can be used to assess for substance use as recommended by Queensland Health can include:

- AUDIT (Alcohol Use Disorders Identification Test) (WHO, 2001)
- Alcohol, Smoking and Substance Involvement Screening Test (ASSIST) (WHO, 2010)
- Indigenous Risk Impact Screen (IRIS) (Insight, 2023).

The most commonly used tool by nurses is the AUDIT and an example is shown in **Figure 11.9**.

AUDIT Alcohol Screening Tool

The AUDIT (Alcohol Use Disorders Identification Test) is an effective and reliable screening tool for detecting risky and harmful drinking patterns [1].

INSTRUCTIONS: by completing the following questions in the AUDIT Alcohol Screen you will be able to assess whether your drinking is putting you at risk of alcohol-related harm:

1. Answer the following questions about your alcohol use during the **past 12 months**.
2. 'Circle' one box that best describes your answer to each question. Answer as accurately as you can.
3. When you have completed the questions SCORE them and put your total score in the box. Thank you.

Questions	0	1	2	3	4	Score
1. How often do you have a drink containing alcohol?	Never	Monthly or less	2-4 times a month	2-3 times a week	4+ times a week	
2. How many drinks containing alcohol do you have on a typical day when you are drinking?	1 or 2	3 or 4	5 or 6	7 to 9	10 or more	
3. How often do you have six or more standard drinks on one occasion?	Never	Less than monthly	Monthly	Weekly	Daily or almost daily	
4. How often during the last year have you found that you were not able to stop drinking once you had started?	Never	Less than monthly	Monthly	Weekly	Daily or almost daily	
5. How often during the last year have you failed to do what was normally expected of you because of drinking?	Never	Less than monthly	Monthly	Weekly	Daily or almost daily	
6. How often during the last year have you needed a drink first thing in the morning to get yourself going after a heavy drinking session?	Never	Less than monthly	Monthly	Weekly	Daily or almost daily	
7. How often during the last year have you had a feeling of guilt or remorse after drinking?	Never	Less than monthly	Monthly	Weekly	Daily or almost daily	
8. How often during the last year have you been unable to remember what happened the night before because of your drinking?	Never	Less than monthly	Monthly	Weekly	Daily or almost daily	
9. Have you or someone else been injured because of your drinking?	No		Yes, but not in the last year		Yes, during the last year	
10. Has a relative, friend, doctor or other healthcare worker been concerned about your drinking or suggested you cut down?	No		Yes, but not in the last year		Yes, during the last year	

To SCORE:
1. Questions 1 – 8 are scored as 0, 1, 2, 3 or 4
2. Questions 9 and 10 are scored as 0, 2 or 4 only
3. Add all scores from each question to calculate total AUDIT score

Total ▶ [ ]

The Alcohol Use Disorders Identification Test (AUDIT) World Health Organisation (WHO) has been adapted by the Mental Health Commission, 2018.

1. Thomas F. Babor, John C. Higgins-Biddle, John B. Saunders, and Maristela G. Monteiro (2001) AUDIT: The Alcohol Use Disorders Identification Test Guidelines for Use in Primary Care. Second Edition.

FIGURE 11.9 The AUDIT questionnaire

The AUDIT may be completed with the nurse or health professional or independently. Scores indicate levels of drinking and correlate with risk (see **Figure 11.10**).

The AUDIT score here is based upon Australia's standard drinks measure (one standard drink = 10 g of pure alcohol) but this is subject to change, so you need to check. The Department of Health and Aged Care website (www.health.gov.au) has a Standard Drinks Guide that can help a person calculate how many standard drinks they are consuming. **Figure 11.11** shows the 2020 Australian Alcohol Guidelines.

In addition, you may learn about a strategy known as 'harm reduction'. This approach hopes to reassure people that it is okay to talk about substances and to reduce the fear and anxiety that is often associated with limiting use and, most importantly, is non-judgemental.

The National Drug Strategy 2017–2026 (Department of Health and Aged Care, 2017) focuses on reducing harms using three approaches:
1 demand reduction
2 supply reduction
3 harm reduction (see **Figure 11.12**).

Further interventions using this approach can include brief intervention, motivational interviewing and decisional balance charts.

Harm reduction can be assessed through the use of a decisional balance chart (see **Figure 11.13**).

Risk Level	Intervention	AUDIT score*
Zone I	Alcohol Education	0-7
Zone II	Simple Advice	8-15
Zone III	Simple Advice plus Brief Counseling and Continued Monitoring	16-19
Zone IV	Referral to Specialist for Diagnostic Evaluation and Treatment	20-40

*The AUDIT cut-off score may vary slightly depending on the country's drinking patterns, the alcohol content of standard drinks, and the nature of the screening program. Clinical judgment should be exercised in cases where the patient's score is not consistent with other evidence, or if the patient has a prior history of alcohol dependence. It may also be instructive to review the patient's responses to individual questions dealing with dependence symptoms (Questions 4, 5 and 6) and alcohol-related problems (Questions 9 and 10). Provide the next highest level of intervention to patients who score 2 or more on Questions 4, 5 and 6, or 4 on Questions 9 or 10.

FIGURE 11.10 The AUDIT questionnaire scoring

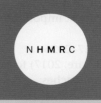

BUILDING
A HEALTHY
AUSTRALIA

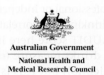

Australian Government
National Health and
Medical Research Council

Alcohol Guidelines

Australian guidelines to reduce
health risks from drinking alcohol

1: HEALTHY ADULTS

Drink no more than
10 standard drinks a week

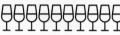

AND
no more than 4 standard drinks
on any one day

to reduce the risk of harm from alcohol.

The less you drink, the lower
your risk of harm.

2: CHILDREN AND PEOPLE UNDER 18 YEARS OF AGE

Should not drink alcohol

to reduce the risk of harm from alcohol.

3: WOMEN WHO ARE PREGNANT OR BREASTFEEDING

Should not drink alcohol

to prevent harm from alcohol
to their unborn child or baby.

www.nhmrc.gov.au/alcohol

FIGURE 11.11 Australian guidelines to reduce health risks from drinking alcohol

SOURCE: NATIONAL HEALTH AND MEDICAL RESEARCH COUNCIL

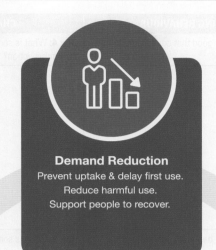

Demand Reduction
Prevent uptake & delay first use.
Reduce harmful use.
Support people to recover.

Harm Minimisation
Building safe, healthy and resillient communities through preventing, responding and reducing alcohol, tobacco and other drugs related health, social and economic harms.

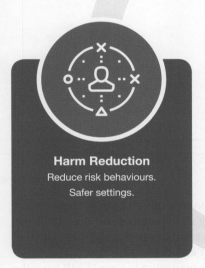

Harm Reduction
Reduce risk behaviours.
Safer settings.

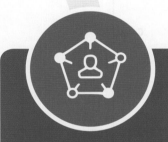

Supply Reduction
Control licit drug and precursor availability.
Reduce illicit drug availability and accessibility.

Strategic Principles

| Partnerships | Coordination & Collaboration | Evidence-informed Responses | National Direction, Jurisdictional Implementation |

FIGURE 11.12 Harm minimisation approach

	NOT CHANGING BEHAVIOUR	CHANGING BEHAVIOUR
Pros	**Box 1:** What is something good that could come from *not* taking this action?	**Box 4:** What is something good that could come from taking this action?
Cons	**Box 2:** What is something bad that could come from *not* taking this action?	**Box 3:** What is something bad that could come from taking this action?

FIGURE 11.13 Example of a decisional balance chart

SOURCE: AGENCY FOR HEALTHCARE RESEARCH AND QUALITY

11.15 ASSESSMENT FOR MANAGING ALCOHOL-INDUCED SLEEP DISTURBANCE

Concept map 11.11 explores the impact of Andrew's persistent insomnia.

11.16 PLANNING CARE FOR MANAGING ALCOHOL-INDUCED SLEEP DISTURBANCE

Planning for managing Andrew's insomnia will have the goals of:

- identifying strategies in partnership with Andrew to manage lifestyle changes
- identifying strategies in partnership with Andrew to reduce alcohol consumption

- developing long-term self-help strategies
- re-stabilising sleep patterns and sleep hygiene
- establishing strategies to manage pre-diabetes through diet and exercise.

Planning for managing insomnia will have the goals of:

- patient education and consent to further investigation and referral
- self-care in relation to diet, exercise and lifestyle changes
- potential management of a continuous positive airway pressure (CPAP) machine.

Andrew is a partner in his care plan and can contribute to his health care by following his plan of care and managing his condition in the home environment. **Box 11.6** indicates the areas that are targeted in the planning stage of developing long- and short-term strategies.

PHx

Andrew Jones is a 42-year-old married man who is seeking support for persistent insomnia which is affecting his day-to-day working life. Following a recent admission for day surgery for tooth extraction, Andrew has been advised to be assessed for a CPAP machine. Andrew requires a full assessment to evaluate and ascertain all possible reasons for his insomnia and disturbed sleep. Andrew's wife complains about his snoring.

DRUG & ALCOHOL HISTORY

Current use: Drinks a 'crate' of beer with friends at the weekend, has the occasional beer during the week at home. Denies any other substance use.

History of use: Since late teens, has never sought help or received treatment.

AUDIT score and interpretation: 12: indicates risky use and requires follow-up.

Level of motivation: Ambivalent, does not link alcohol to insomnia as it gets him off to sleep.

 ## ASSESSMENT

Functional inquiry:

Sleep: Disturbed at present, wakes up around 2–3 a.m. and struggles to get back to sleep. Feels fatigued during the day.

Appetite: Good; no changes.

Energy: Currently low, associates this with poor sleep.

Motivation: Motivated to get insomnia sorted out and go fishing but has been struggling to get up and go to work.

Concentration: Diminished, occasionally forgets things, but able to watch a movie or TV program.

Anxiety: Has been increasingly anxious about increased workload which is becoming stressful. Believes this is contributing to the insomnia.

Mood: Mood is good, just unhappy about impact insomnia is having.

NB. No requirement for an MSE on this occasion

Psychosocial assessment

Andrew has been married to Anne for 15 years. Andrew has 2 children aged 6 and 8. He works as an air traffic controller spending much of his time sitting and working shifts including night shift. Andrew is often tired after work and winds down in the evening with a couple of beers. At the weekend he watches the children playing sport then relaxes by going fishing with friends. This usually ends with 'a few bevvies' with the boys. Andrew has noticed he has become increasingly restless during the night, waking several times. He puts this down to the stress of work and the long shifts he works. He has been advised he may be suffering from sleep apnoea and may need a continuous positive airway pressure (CPAP) machine. He does not know what a CPAP machine is nor how it could help him.

Past medical history:

History of asthma since a child, currently uses Becotide OD and Ventolin PRN. Appendectomy age 12.

No significant previous history reported Last HbA1c result 52 mmol/mol (normal range = 48–53 mmol/mol) 6 months ago as part of routine medical for air traffic controllers.

Physical assessment:

PAIN: Nil

CVS: HR 76 bpm, BP 130/75 mmHg

RESP: RR 17

MUSCULOSKELETAL (Mobility): Mobile

Weight: 102 kg

Height: 171 cm

BMI: 35.3, obese range

BGL: (non-fasting) 7.4 mmol/L

Cues

1 What is the relationship between disturbed sleep and alcohol use?

2 What is the relationship between obesity and sleep apnoea?

3 What is the relationship between pre-diabetes and sleep disturbance?

CONCEPT MAP 11.11 Nursing assessment for Andrew

<table>
<tr><td>

BOX 11.6 PLANNING FOR MANAGING INSOMNIA

» Consent
» Self-care
» Lifestyle modifications
» Dietary changes
» Alcohol consumption
» Physical activity
» Stress management
» Medication
» Sleep study

</td></tr>
</table>

Concept map 11.12 outlines a plan for Andrew's care and illustrates his journey through initial care planning.

11.17 NURSING INTERVENTIONS TO SUPPORT HEALTH CARE FOR ALCOHOL-INDUCED SLEEP DISTURBANCE

Nursing interventions are implemented as part of person-centred care. When considering mental health and/or substance use, this is often divided into short-term, medium-term and long-term goals as

people may need to grasp the concept of differential diagnosis (where one thing may be linked to several other problems). In addition, interventions may include lifestyle changes and it is really important that this is developed in partnership with the patient. Explore what is achievable and set small 'bite-sized' goals where necessary. Sometimes if the goal is too big it becomes unachievable, thereby fuelling a sense of failure and this is often quickly followed by abandonment.

Sleep disturbance is a common sign of risky alcohol use but is often not detected. A significant diagnostic overshadowing risk here could be attributing the insomnia to weight and fitness levels. However, they may all contribute, so a reduction in weight *and* an increase in physical activity *and* a reduction in alcohol use can not only improve sleep but reduce stress as well (Hallgren et al., 2017). So, consider care planning in mental health and substance-related use as a 'journey'. An intervention commonly used in health is a 'brief intervention' or the trans-theoretical model – this is a model that establishes commitment to change (see **Figure 11.14**). It was developed by Prochaska and Diclemente in the 1970s and has gone on to support identification of readiness to change and uses decisional balance to make that change (Prochaska et al., 1994).

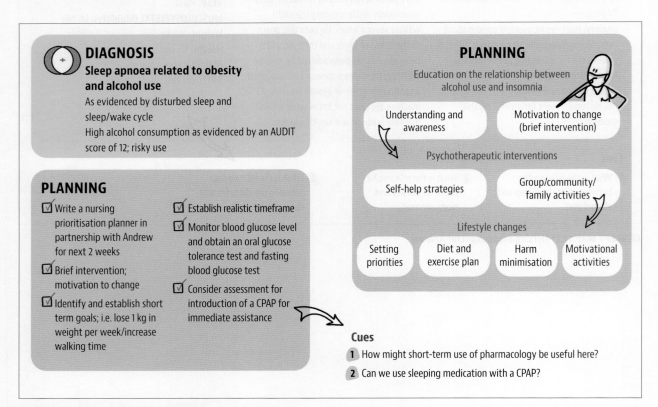

CONCEPT MAP 11.12 Diagnosis and planning for Andrew

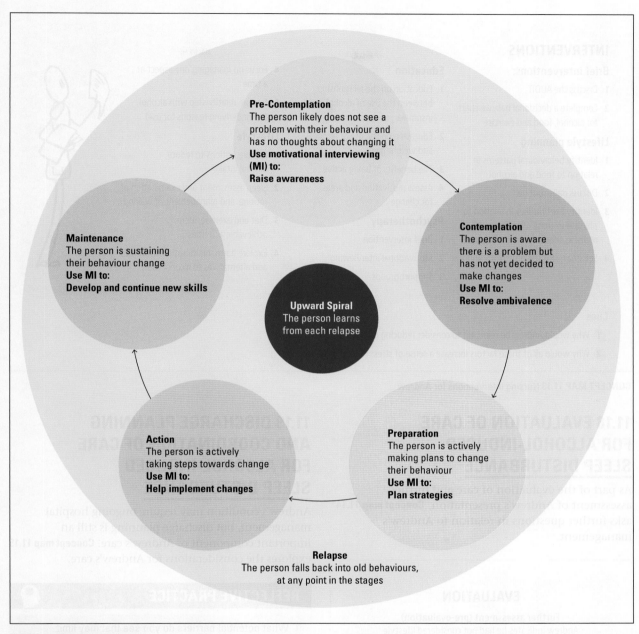

Pre-Contemplation
The person likely does not see a problem with their behaviour and has no thoughts about changing it
Use motivational interviewing (MI) to:
Raise awareness

Contemplation
The person is aware there is a problem but has not yet decided to make changes
Use MI to:
Resolve ambivalence

Maintenance
The person is sustaining their behaviour change
Use MI to:
Develop and continue new skills

Upward Spiral
The person learns from each relapse

Action
The person is actively taking steps towards change
Use MI to:
Help implement changes

Preparation
The person is actively making plans to change their behaviour
Use MI to:
Plan strategies

Relapse
The person falls back into old behaviours, at any point in the stages

FIGURE 11.14 Stages of change

SOURCE: BECKWITH J., BECKWITH V., (S), NASN SCHOOL NURSE, 25 (6), P4, © 2020. REPRINTED BY PERMISSION OF SAGE PUBLICATIONS.

This model is still used today and what it exemplifies is that the change must come from the individual. Health care can advise, educate and direct but if the patient is not ready, change will not happen. Planning, both short and long term, has to reflect this.

The stages of change are ascertained using brief intervention.

There is an example of using brief intervention with Andrew, and an illustrated summary of an intervention planning focus in **Concept map 11.13**.

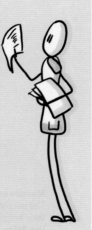

INTERVENTIONS

Brief interventions:

1 Discuss the AUDIT

2 Complete a decisional balance chart for alcohol, food and exercise

Lifestyle planning

1 Identify behavioural patterns in relation to food and alcohol

2 Discuss daily routine

3 Identify likes/dislikes in relation to physical exercise. Planning must be realistic, achievable and affordable

4 Set small, realistic goals with Andrew

Education

1 Education on the relationship between the use of alcohol and insomnia

2 Education on the use of alcohol and weight gain

3 The benefits of being active

4 Assess motivation and areas for change

Psychotherapy

1 Brief intervention

2 Motivational interviewing

3 Support groups

4 Focus on managing one aspect at a time

5 Explore relationship with alcohol (i.e. underlying reasons for use)

Lifestyle

1 Explore options to reduce alcohol intake

2 Sleep assessment and examination of routine, and management of waking

3 Diet and exercise, identify achievable activities

4 Explore harm minimisation strategies and alternatives to alcohol use

Cues

1 Why would Andrew be reluctant to consider reducing drinking at the weekends?

2 Why would all of these factors increase a sense of stress related to work?

CONCEPT MAP 11.13 Nursing interventions for Andrew

11.18 EVALUATION OF CARE FOR ALCOHOL-INDUCED SLEEP DISTURBANCE

As part of the evaluation of care and further assessment of Andrew's presentation, **Concept map 11.14** asks further questions in relation to Andrew's management.

EVALUATION

Further assessment (pre-evaluation)

Andrew indicates he had not considered lifestyle factors as contributing to insomnia.

Andrew finds the decisional balance chart interesting and useful.

Cues

1 How can we use this information to plan further care?

CONCEPT MAP 11.14 Evaluation and planning for Andrew

11.19 DISCHARGE PLANNING AND COORDINATION OF CARE FOR ALCOHOL-INDUCED SLEEP DISTURBANCE

Andrew's condition may require ongoing hospital management, but discharge planning is still an important component of Andrew's care. **Concept map 11.15** explores the considerations for Andrew's care.

REFLECTIVE PRACTICE

1 What potential barriers do you see that may limit Andrew in engagement in management of alcohol use?

2 What about your values and perspectives? Are you at risk of being judgemental?

3 What do you do if Andrew is not interested in changing his habits? How would you approach this?

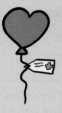

**DISCHARGE PLANNING +
COORDINATION OF CARE**

How do the following areas of healthcare management **relate** to Andrew's presentation? Which members of the healthcare team are **involved** in each area of management?

- Diabetes
- Diet
- Snoring
- Stress management

Week 1

Engage in brief intervention and revisit the AUDIT results to explore goals

Set goals in partnership with Andrew

Ask Andrew to keep a diary of alcohol consumption and occasions

Ask Andrew to jot down sleep disturbances and effects on work, etc.

Begin to explore motivational activities

Week 2

Review of week 1 and progress/non-progress, explore any events, emotions, barriers and enablers

Review physiological status and observations

Continue discussing the relationship between alcohol use, mood and physical health

Set goals for week 3

Week 3

As before, evaluate previous week's activities, feelings and events

Revisit plans and goals; what is working, what is not

Set new goals or re-evaluate past goals with a different strategy if needed

Review physiological status and observations

Begin long-term planning or if required, go back to the start

CONCEPT MAP 11.15 Discharge planning and coordination of care for Andrew

SUMMARY

People with altered mental health and or/substance use problems face the challenges of living within their environment with potentially added stigma and discrimination, increased stress, poor cultural safety and maladaptive coping mechanisms. When providing care for the person who has increased stress, anxiety or other cognitive-related symptoms, the nurse has the additional challenge of providing health education, recognising power differentials and an increased sense of confusion, potential shame or a sense of worthlessness. The individual may present with real or psychosomatic symptoms and diagnostic overshadowing can be (and still is) a real problem for many people. This can result in a reluctance to disclose 'personal' problems. In addition, past history, culture and experience also impact upon engagement to seek help and continue therapy. Nurses must take a person-centred approach to assessment and care planning, and ultimately this can lead to better health outcomes for those seeking assistance.

CLINICAL SKILLS IN MENTAL HEALTH AND SUBSTANCE USE

A broad range of clinical skills are required when managing a person with mental health concerns or substance abuse problems. Consult your Clinical Skills resources, such as Tollefson and Hillman (2022), *Clinical Psychomotor Skills* (8th ed.).

Key skills include:

1 Observation: Nurses must be conscious of their observation skills in relation to picking up cues for distress or discomfort. Many people do not know they have a mental health concern and will often present with a physical health concern. They may feel stigma or fear discrimination. Psychological observation is supported by tools such as the MSE, MMSE or other standardised assessment tools (check in your area) just as observation skills for physiological needs must be augmented by standardised tools and equipment.

2 Assessment: Assessment must be holistic, may be subjective and objective and often involves intuition. Communication is key here, so that is the next clinical skill.

3 Professional communication: An essential skill in nursing, the ability to gain trust, communicate effectively and respectfully are key to developing effective assessments, care planning and delivery. Having a non-judgemental and empathic approach means people are more likely to share concerns with you.

4 Clinical thinking: Are you getting the whole picture? What else could be going on? Understanding complexities associated with co-occurring disorders and diagnostic overshadowing are key attributes in effective and safe care.

5 Person-centred practice, including cultural safety: Cultural safety is not just about culture, creed and ethnicity. Cultural safety is about understanding where you come

from in relation to your perspective, values and potential for affecting practice. Cultural safety recognises the need for reflection, understanding power imbalances and respect.

6   Team work: Nursing is a team effort and in mental health we often see different perspectives, so it is important to share and gain a whole picture. This includes working in partnership with your patients.

PROBLEM-SOLVING SCENARIO

Using a concept map approach, how would you assist Felicity Smith?

Felicity is a 32-year-old female who has developed an infection following constant handwashing that has been interfering with her ability to work and even leave the house. Felicity believes her hands are contaminated and if she touches anyone else or even anything, she will contaminate them. This has been a real challenge as she is a hairdresser. The GP suspects obsessive compulsive disorder (OCD), a disorder that is brought on by extreme anxiety and distorted cognitive thinking, and has referred Felicity to the psychiatric team and to you (as the Practice Nurse) to treat and dress

Felicity's hands. You are asked to establish and implement a long-term plan of care in relation to engagement with the health services and management of the infection.

1   What are the causes of OCD?
2   What are the associated signs and symptoms of OCD?
3   What options are there with regards to treating this condition?
4   What are the lifestyle factors that are also considered in relation to the impact of OCD?
5   Why is working in partnership so important in managing OCD?

PORTFOLIO DEVELOPMENT

Wherever you practise nursing you will need ongoing continuing professional development to ensure that you are delivering current evidence-based nursing care that provides the best possible outcomes for the patient. As mental health- and substance use-related conditions require a specific

knowledge base, the useful websites below will assist in meeting continuing professional development activities to meet the NMBA yearly registration requirements for a Registered Nurse.

USEFUL WEBSITES

Australian Government Aboriginal and Torres Strait Islander mental health program https://www.health.gov.au/initiatives-and-programs/aboriginal-and-torres-strait-islander-mental-health-program
Black Dog Institute https://www.blackdoginstitute.org.au
Diagnostic and Statistical Manual of Mental Disorders, Fifth Edition https://dsm.psychiatryonline.org/doi/book/10.1176/appi.books.9780890425596
Nursing and Midwifery Board of Australia, Decision-making framework for nursing and midwifery (2020) https://www.

nursingmidwiferyboard.gov.au/codes-guidelines-statements/frameworks.aspx
The Royal Children's Hospital Melbourne Clinical Practice Guidelines: MSE https://www.rch.org.au/clinicalguide/guideline_index/Mental_state_examination
WHO: The Alcohol, Smoking and Substance Involvement Screening Test (ASSIST) https://www.who.int/publications/i/item/978924159938-2

REFERENCES AND FURTHER READING

Alexander, V., Ellis, H., & Barrett, B. (2016). Medical–surgical nurses' perceptions of psychiatric patients: A review of the literature with clinical and practice applications. *Archives of Psychiatric Nursing, 30*(2), 262–270. https://doi.org/10.1016/j.apnu.2015.06.018

American Psychiatric Association (APA). (2013) *Diagnostic and Statistical Manual of Mental Disorders,* fifth edition, text revision (DSM-5-TR). https://dsm.psychiatryonline.org/doi/book/10.1176/appi.books.9780890425787

Australian Bureau of Statistics (ABS). 2018. *National health survey: first results, 2017–18.* https://www.abs.gov.au/statistics/health/health-conditions-and-risks/national-health-survey-first-results/latest-release

Australian Institute of Health and Welfare (AIHW). (2017) *National drug strategy household survey 2016: Detailed findings.* https://www.aihw.gov.au/reports/illicit-use-of-drugs/2016-ndshs-detailed/summary.

Australian Institute of Health and Welfare (AIHW). (2018). *Impact of alcohol and illicit drug use on the burden of disease and injury in Australia: Australian Burden of Disease Study 2011.* Canberra: AIHW. https://www.aihw.gov.au/reports/burden-of-disease/impact-alcohol-illicit-drug-use-on-burden-disease/summary

Australian Institute of Health and Welfare (AIHW). (2020, 13 July). *Mental health.* Retrieved from https://www.aihw.gov.au/reports/australias-health/mental-health

Best, O. (2018). The cultural safety journey: An Aboriginal Australian nursing and midwifery context. In O. Best & B. Fredericks (Eds.), *Yatdjuligin: Aboriginal and Torres Strait Islander nursing and midwifery care* (2nd ed., pp. 46–63). Cambridge University Press.

Blincoe, T., & Chamber, D. (2019). Alcohol and anaesthesia. *British Journal of Hospital Medicine, 80*(8). https://doi.org/10.12968/hmed.2019.80.8.485

COAG (Council of Australian Governments) Health Council. (2017). *The fifth national mental health and suicide prevention plan.* Canberra: Department of Health. https://www.mentalhealthcommission.gov.au/getmedia/0209d27b-1873-4245-b6e5-49e770084b81/Fifth-National-Mental-Health-and-Suicide-Prevention-Plan.pdf

Collins, E., Drake, M., Deacon, M. (2013). *The physical care of people with mental health problems, a guide for best practice.* Sage Publications.

Croakey Health Media. (2013, 20 August). *Culture is an important determinant of health: Professor Ngiare Brown at NACCHO Summit.* https://www.croakey.org/culture-is-an-important-determinant-of-health-professor-ngiare-brown-at-naccho-summit

Department of Health and Aged Care. (2004). *Models that help us understand AOD use in society.* https://www1.health.gov.au/internet/publications/publishing.nsf/Content/drugtreat-pubs-front5-wk-toc~drugtreat-pubs-front5-wk-secb~drugtreat-pubs-front5-wk-secb-3~drugtreat-pubs-front5-wk-secb-3-4

Department of Health and Aged Care (2017) *National drug strategy 2017–2026.* Canberra: Commonwealth of Australia. https://www.health.gov.au/resources/publications/national-drug-strategy-2017-2026?language=en

Foye, U., Simpson, A., & Reynolds, L. (2020). 'Somebody else's business': The challenge of caring for patients with mental health problems on medical and surgical wards. *Journal of Psychiatric and Mental Health Nursing, 27*(4), 406–416. https://doi.org/10.1111/jpm.12596

Hallgren, M., Vancampfort, D., Schuch, F., Lundin, A., & Stubbs, B. (2017). More reasons to move: Exercise in the treatment of alcohol use disorders. *Frontiers in Psychiatry, 8*, 160. https://doi.org/10.3389/fpsyt.2017.00160

healthdirect. (2023, March). *Substance abuse.* https://www.healthdirect.gov.au/substance-abuse

Hungerford, C., Hodgson, D., Clancy, R., Murphy, G., & Doyle, K. (2021). *Mental health care: an introduction for health professionals.* John Wiley & Sons.

Insight. (2023). *IRIS screening instrument and risk card (2011 version).* https://insight.qld.edu.au/shop/iris-screening-instrument-and-risk-card

Jones, S., Howard, L., & Thornicroft, G. (2008). Diagnostic overshadowing: worse physical health care for people with mental illness. *Acta Psychiatrica Scandinavica, 118*(3), 169–171. https://doi.org/10.1111/j.1600-0447.2008.01211.x

Leamy, M., Bird, V., Boutillier, C., Williams, J., & Slade, M. (2011). Conceptual framework for personal recovery in mental health: Systematic review and narrative synthesis. *British Journal of Psychiatry, 199*(6), 445–452. https://doi.org/10.1192/bjp.bp.110.083733

Lin, I., Green, C., Bessarab, D. (2016). 'Yarn with me': applying clinical yarning to improve clinician–patient communication in Aboriginal health care. *Australian Journal of Primary Health, 22*, 377–382. https://doi.org/10.1071/PY16051

McNeely, J., Kumar, P. C., Rieckmann, T., Sedlander, E., Farkas, S., Chollak, C., Kannry, J. L., Vega, A., Waite, E. A., Peccoralo, L. A., Rosenthal, R. N., McCarty, D., & Rotrosen, J. (2018). Barriers and facilitators affecting the implementation of substance use screening in primary care clinics: a qualitative study of patients, providers, and staff. *Addiction Science & Clinical Practice, 13*(1), 8. https://doi.org/10.1186/s13722-018-0110-8

Monheit, B., Pietrzak, D., & Hocking, S. (2016). Prescription drug abuse – a timely update. *Australian Family Physician, 45*(12), 862–866. https://search-informit-org.elibrary.jcu.edu.au/doi/10.3316/informit.577080197063309

National Institute for Health and Care Excellence. (2011). *Generalised anxiety disorder and panic disorder in adults: Management.* https://www.nice.org.uk/guidance/cg113

National Institute of Mental Health (NIMH). (2022). *Ask Suicide-Screening Questions (ASQ) toolkit.* https://www.nimh.nih.gov/research/research-conducted-at-nimh/asq-toolkit-materials

O'Hagan, M. (2001). *Recovery competencies for New Zealand mental health workers.* Mental Health Commission (New Zealand).

Prochaska, J. O., Velicer, W. F., Rossi, J. S., Goldstein, M. G., Marcus, B. H., Rakowski, W., Fiore, C., Harlow, L. L., Redding,

C. A., Rosenbloom, D., & Rossi, S. R. (1994). Stages of change and decisional balance for 12 problem behaviors. *Health Psychology, 13*(1), 39–46. https://doi.org/10.1037/0278-6133.13.1.39

Ramsden, I. (2002). Cultural safety and nursing education in Aotearoa and Te Waipounamu. Unpublished doctoral dissertation, Victoria University of Wellington, Wellington, NZ. https://www.nccih.ca/634/Cultural_Safety_and_Nursing_Education_in_Aotearoa_and_Te_Waipounamu.nccih?id=1124

Reeves, E., Henshall, C., Hutchinson, M., & Jackson, D. (2018). Safety of service users with severe mental illness receiving inpatient care on medical and surgical wards: A systematic review. *International Journal of Mental Health Nursing, 27*(1), 46–60. https://doi.org/10.1111/inm.12426

Seligman, M. E. P. (2011). *Flourish: A visionary new understanding of happiness and well-being.* Free Press.

Tyerman, J., Patovirta, A-L., & Celestini, A. (2021). How stigma and discrimination influences nursing care of persons diagnosed with mental illness: A systematic review. *Issues in Mental Health Nursing, 42*(2), 153–163. DOI: 10.1080/01612840.2020.1789788

Webster, L. R, & Webster, R. M. (2005). Predicting aberrant behaviors in opioid-treated patients: Preliminary validation of the opioid risk tool. *Pain Medicine, 6*(6), 432–442. DOI: 10.1111/j.1526-4637.2005.00072.x

World Health Organization (WHO). (2001). Alcohol Use Disorders Identification Test (AUDIT). https://www.who.int/publications/i/item/audit-the-alcohol-use-disorders-identification-test-guidelines-for-use-in-primary-health-care

World Health Organization (WHO). (2010). *The Alcohol, Smoking and Substance Involvement Screening Test (ASSIST): Manual for use in primary care.* http://apps.who.int/iris/bitstream/handle/10665/44320/9789241599382_eng.pdf?sequence=1

World Health Organization (WHO). (2022a). *International classification of diseases,* 11th revision. https://icd.who.int/en

World Health Organization (WHO). (2022b). *Mental health.* https://www.who.int/news-room/fact-sheets/detail/mental-health-strengthening-our-response

World Health Organization (WHO). (2023). *Constitution.* www.who.int/about/accountability/governance/constitution

CHAPTER 12

VISUAL AND AUDITORY SYSTEMS

Visual impairment is a significant health issue for older Australians because it impacts on their physical, functional, emotional and social wellbeing, and in turn reduces their quality of life. Over 13 million people have one or more chronic eye conditions, with glaucoma occurring in 3.5 per cent of males and for females, a 3.8 per cent incidence. For cataracts, females have a higher incidence of 10.6 per cent compared to 7.4 per cent for males (Australian Institute for Health and Welfare [AIHW], 2021). Ear health is important for all age groups, and Aboriginal and Torres Strait Islander children from 0–14 years self-report hearing problems at twice the rate of non-Aboriginal and Torres Strait Islander children (AIHW, 2022).

LEARNING OBJECTIVES

After reading this chapter, you should have an understanding of the:

1 assessment required for a person with a visual condition
2 assessment required for a person with a hearing condition
3 prioritisation of key components in the development of plans of care for people presenting with the conditions of:
   - glaucoma
   - cataracts
   - acute otitis media with effusion
   - tinnitus
4 prioritised and targeted nursing interventions required to promote recovery or prevent further deterioration of people presenting with visual and hearing conditions
5 evaluation phase and how the prioritised and targeted nursing interventions inform further assessment of the person, planning of care and collaboration with the healthcare team
6 discharge planning and coordination of care required in preparing the person for discharge and subsequent continuity of care between the person and their healthcare providers.

INTRODUCTION

Our senses connect us to each other and the environment. When there is a disruption to one or more of the senses, such as sight and hearing, the ability to pick up stimuli and cues from other people and the environment are diminished and interfere with the quality of life for the person. Not being able to pick up all the stimuli from others and the environment can place the individual at risk for injury and depression.

The visual system includes the external and internal structure of the eyes, along with the visual pathway through the optic nerves to the visual cortex of the occipital lobe in the brain.

The auditory system includes the three parts of the ear: the external ear, middle ear and inner ear.

Whether a condition of the visual or auditory systems is newly diagnosed or is long term and considered chronic in presentation, the concepts of person-centred care are the same, with the goal of maintaining the sensory systems so the individual can interact at the best level possible with their environment and others.

12.1 ASSESSMENT OF VISUAL PROBLEMS

A health assessment entails the collection of patient data, both subjective and objective. In **Box 12.1**, the subjective health assessment components are applied to all patients, but the emphasis on each of the components is influenced by the person's presentation in seeking health care.

BOX 12.1   SUBJECTIVE ASSESSMENT

- ➤ History of illness
- ➤ Past health history
- ➤ Medications
- ➤ Surgery
- **Functional health patterns:**
  - – Health perception and management
  - – Nutritional and metabolic
  - – Elimination
  - – Activity and exercise
  - – Sleep and rest
  - – Cognitive and perceptual
  - – Self-perception and concept
  - – Role relationship
  - – Sexuality and reproductive
  - – Coping and stress
  - – Values and beliefs
- ➤ Risk calculation

The collection of objective data is informed by the subjective data and is highlighted in the physical assessment and diagnostic studies results for the person. Objective data is collected via the systems approach, and as the topic of eyes is presented in the first part of this chapter, the focus of **Box 12.2** is the eyes, and the remaining physical assessment will be guided by the person's health history that was obtained in **Box 12.1**.

BOX 12.2   OBJECTIVE ASSESSMENT

- ➤ Visual fields
- ➤ Visual acuity – Snellen and Rosenbaum charts
- ➤ Extraocular muscle function
- ➤ Diagnostic tests – tonometry, fundoscopy, gonioscopy, red reflex
- ➤ Inspection of internal structures
- ➤ Other body systems as appropriate

12.2 ASSESSMENT FOR OPEN-ANGLE GLAUCOMA

Open-angle is the most common type of glaucoma and the outflow (reabsorption) of aqueous humour in the trabecular meshwork is decreased. It develops slowly and there are no symptoms of pain. Visual field loss is not noted until peripheral vision has been affected. In the collection of subjective data (**Box 12.1**), previous and current person-reported information is important in the determination of visual symptoms.

Presentation

Elizabeth Richardson is a 58-year-old married woman who is admitted for day surgery to reduce left eye intraocular pressure due to open-angle glaucoma. Elizabeth is scheduled for trabeculectomy filtration surgery to the left eye.

See **Concept map 12.1** to further explore Elizabeth's initial care in the day surgery unit.

12.3 PLANNING CARE FOR OPEN-ANGLE GLAUCOMA

Planning for glaucoma will have the goals of:
- informed consent to surgery
- patient education for self-care in relation to the application of an eye pad
- ocular antiglaucoma drops (Broyles et al., 2023)
- reducing physical activity for the first week
- ensuring a safe home environment
- adverse effects of therapy.

Elizabeth is a partner in her care plan and is able to contribute to her health care by being able to follow her plan of care and manage her condition in the home environment. **Box 12.3** indicates the areas that are targeted in the planning stage of glaucoma and trabeculectomy filtration surgery.

BOX 12.3   PLANNING FOR EYE SURGERY

- ➤ Surgery and consent
- ➤ Self-care
- ➤ Lifestyle modifications
- ➤ Physical activity
- ➤ Medication

Concept map 12.2 outlines a plan for Elizabeth's care.

PHx

Elizabeth, a **58-year-old female** with bilateral open-angle glaucoma (that was diagnosed 8 years ago), has now become **less responsive to antiglaucoma medication**, with increasing intraocular eye pressures, and the left eye least responsive to medication.

Elizabeth has had three changes in the types of antiglaucoma medication, due to **intraocular pressures rising to high levels**, which necessitates a change of antiglaucoma medication.

Her **older brother has also been diagnosed with bilateral glaucoma**, and has had laser surgery to control right eye pressure, and is prescribed antiglaucoma eye drops to reduce intraocular pressures.

Cues

1. What is the relationship between acute angle glaucoma and family history?

2. Why do intraocular pressures rise even though a patient is prescribed a specific antiglaucoma medication?

CONCEPT MAP 12.1 Nursing assessment for Elizabeth

 ASSESSMENT

Primary survey

A: Patent
B: RR 14
C: Warm, intact
D: Alert
E: T 36.5 °C
F: Fasting, HNPU
G: BGL 4.8 mmol/L

Secondary survey

CNS (Cognition): Alert and orientated

PAIN: Nil
CVS: HR 72 bpm, BP 130/75 mmHg
RESP: RR 14
GIT (Input): Fasting since 7 a.m. for food, and for the last 2 hours for water.
MUSCULOSKELETAL (Mobility): Mobile

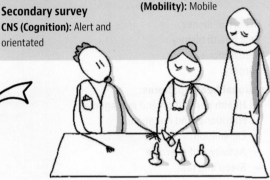

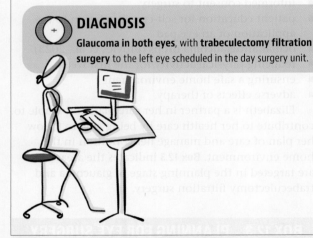 **DIAGNOSIS**

Glaucoma in both eyes, with **trabeculectomy filtration surgery** to the left eye scheduled in the day surgery unit.

CONCEPT MAP 12.2 Diagnosis and planning for Elizabeth

PLANNING

☑ Anaesthesia, surgery and post-anaesthesia

☑ Write a Nursing Prioritisation Planner

Health education and home care:

☑ Eye dressing at night

☑ Not to touch or rub eye

☑ Pain medication – anti-inflammatory eye drops and oral paracetamol

☑ Antiglaucoma medication

☑ Avoid lifting, strenuous activity, coughing, sneezing and constipation for two weeks

☑ Avoid driving and operating heavy machinery

☑ Report eye pain, changes in vision, red eye, headache

☑ Postoperative appointment

12.4 NURSING INTERVENTIONS TO SUPPORT HEALTH CARE FOR OPEN-ANGLE GLAUCOMA

Nursing interventions are implemented as part of person-centred care, with the aim of controlling the signs and symptoms that represent the pathophysiology of glaucoma.

Concept map 12.3 explores Elizabeth's journey in the day surgery unit.

12.5 EVALUATION OF CARE FOR OPEN-ANGLE GLAUCOMA

As part of the further assessment of Elizabeth's presentation, **Concept map 12.4** asks further questions in relation to Elizabeth's management.

EVIDENCE-BASED PRACTICE

To reduce the systemic absorption of eye medication, apply nasolacrimal occlusion for five minutes.

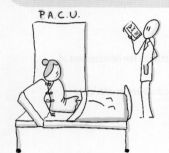

INTERVENTIONS

1 Patient health education

2 Check for valid consent

3 Accompany to anaesthetic area

4 Undertake postoperative assessments in the post-anaesthetic care unit (PACU)

5 Position with head elevated

Cues

1 Why does Elizabeth state that the corner of her eye feels gritty?

What further assessments should be initiated

CONCEPT MAP 12.3 Nursing interventions for Elizabeth

12.6 DISCHARGE PLANNING AND COORDINATION OF CARE FOR OPEN-ANGLE GLAUCOMA

Elizabeth's glaucoma in both eyes and trabeculectomy filtration surgery requires discharge planning and further management at home and a post-surgical review with the ophthalmologist.

In planning for Elizabeth's discharge, **Concept map 12.5** explores the considerations for her care.

12.7 ASSESSMENT FOR CATARACT SURGERY

A cataract is age-related degeneration of the eye, where metabolic processes are less effective and water is accumulated with subsequent alterations in lens fibre structure. The transparency of the lens is reduced and there are changes in the person's vision with decreased vision, abnormal colour perception and sensitivity to glare.

Presentation

Daphne Ferrier is an 85-year-old female who has bilateral cataracts. Daphne's visual acuity of both eyes has been decreasing, and throughout the day whatever the intensity of light is, it appears always to be glaring. At her last optometrist appointment, she was referred to an ophthalmologist for assessment. She has noticed that her dog Gemma who is white and black in colour has become shades of grey.

Please refer to **Box 12.1** and **Box 12.2** for the subjective and objective components that are addressed in a health history.

See **Concept map 12.6** to further explore Daphne's initial care in the day surgery unit.

EVALUATION

Whilst Elizabeth was being monitored in PACU, the ophthalmologist discussed the outcome of the surgery and reminded Elizabeth about her **post-surgical appointment for review and eye pressure measurement**. Elizabeth's left eye dressing was dry and intact and vital signs were within normal limits.

Plan:
Elizabeth's husband is to collect her for the journey home once postoperative observations are completed.

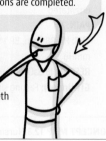

Cues **1** Why is it important that Elizabeth continues to apply antiglaucoma medication to both eyes?

2 What lifestyle changes can Elizabeth adopt to reduce the likelihood of intraocularpressures rising?

CONCEPT MAP 12.4 Evaluation and planning for Elizabeth

DISCHARGE PLANNING + COORDINATION OF CARE

How do the following areas of healthcare management **relate** to Elizabeth's presentation? Which members of the healthcare team are **involved** in each area of management?

Written postoperative instructions

Wear protective eye shield at night to protect the eye when sleeping

Postoperative medication

Anti-inflammatory eye drops and oral paracetamol

Post-surgical review

Optical prescription

Sunglasses

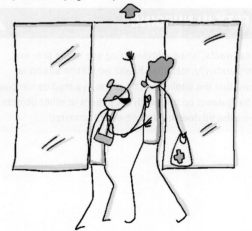

CONCEPT MAP 12.5 Discharge planning and coordination of care for Elizabeth

PHx

Daphne is an **85-year-old female** who is admitted for day surgery to remove a cataract from the right eye. Visual acuity of both eyes has been decreasing, with the right eye having the most mature cataract. The right eye cataract surgical removal will involve extracapsular extraction and intraocular lens insertion.

 ASSESSMENT

CNS (Cognition): Alert and orientated
PAIN: Nil
CVS: HR 88 bpm, BP 145/80 mmHg
RESP: RR 18, SaO$_2$ 98% on room air
GIT (Input): Fasting since 8 p.m. last evening for food, and for the last 2 hours for water. Bowel sounds present.
SKIN/INTEG: Warm feet with slight oedema
MUSCULOSKELETAL (Mobility): Mobile

Cues

1 What is the relationship between the development of cataracts and ageing?

2 What lifestyle factors are considered in relation to cataracts?

CONCEPT MAP 12.6 Nursing assessment for Daphne

12.8 PLANNING CARE FOR CATARACT SURGERY

Planning for cataract removal will have the goals of:
- informed consent to surgery
- patient education for self-care in relation to eye pad application
- eye drops (antibiotic and anti-inflammatory)
- paracetamol for pain (Broyles et al., 2023)
- reducing physical activity for the first week
- knowledge of the adverse effects of therapy
- promotion of a safe home environment.

Daphne is a partner in her care with the nurse and is able to contribute by discussing the plan of care and the subsequent management of her condition at home. Please refer to **Box 12.3** for the areas that are targeted in the planning stage of cataract surgery.

SAFETY IN NURSING ⚠

For cataracts, when administering eye drops pre- and postoperatively, including health education sessions, ensure that the application tip of the eye medication does not have direct contact with the patient or other objects to ensure the tip does not become contaminated.

Concept map 12.7 outlines a plan for Daphne's care.

 DIAGNOSIS

Bilateral cataracts, with the removal of the right eye cataract as a day surgery procedure.

PLANNING

☑ Preoperative medication eye drops

☑ Anaesthesia, surgery and post-anaesthesia

☑ Write a Nursing Prioritisation Planner

Health education and home care:

☑ Clean eye and dressing

☑ Not to touch or rub eye dressing

☑ Antibiotic eye drops

☑ Pain medication – anti-inflammatory eye drops and oral paracetamol

☑ Avoid reading and pressure to face for two days, avoid strenuous activity, bending over, lifting, coughing and sneezing for two weeks

☑ Report eye pain, changes in vision, red eye, headache

☑ Postoperative appointment

☑ Avoid driving or operating a vehicle

☑ Wear eye cover at night to protect eye

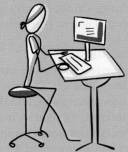

CONCEPT MAP 12.7 Diagnosis and planning for Daphne

12.9 NURSING INTERVENTIONS TO SUPPORT HEALTH CARE FOR CATARACT SURGERY

Nursing interventions are implemented as part of person-centred care, and to remove the cataract that has reduced Daphne's vision.

Concept map 12.8 explores Daphne's journey in the day surgery unit.

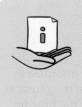

INTERVENTIONS

1 Patient health education
2 Check for valid consent
3 Preoperative topical anaesthetic drops and mydriatic eye drops
4 Accompany to anaesthetic area
5 Undertake postoperative assessments in the post-anaesthetic care unit (PACU)

What further assessments should be initiated ?

Cues ① Why does Daphne state that her eye feels full?

CONCEPT MAP 12.8 Nursing interventions for Daphne

12.10 EVALUATION OF CARE FOR CATARACT SURGERY

As part of the further assessment of Daphne's presentation, **Concept map 12.9** asks further questions in relation to Daphne's management.

EVALUATION

The ophthalmologist visited Daphne in the PACU. He was happy with the surgery and will see Daphne when she has her follow-up appointment for review. Daphne's vital signs were within normal limits and the right eye dressing was dry and intact.

Plan:
Discharge Daphne in the care of a family member for the journey home once postoperative observations are completed.

Cues

① What criteria should Daphne use to measure whether her vision has improved? Would Gemma the dog return to her original colour of black and white?

CONCEPT MAP 12.9 Evaluation and planning for Daphne

12.11 DISCHARGE PLANNING AND COORDINATION OF CARE FOR CATARACT SURGERY

The removal of the cataract from Daphne's right eye requires discharge planning and further management at home and a post-surgical review with the ophthalmologist. **Concept Map 12.10** explores the considerations for Daphne's care.

DISCHARGE PLANNING + COORDINATION OF CARE

How do the following areas of healthcare management **relate** to Daphne's presentation? Which members of the healthcare team are **involved** in each area of management?

Written postoperative instructions	Postoperative medication	Post-surgical review
Wear protective eye shield at night to protect the eye when sleeping	Antibiotic eye drops, anti-inflammatory eye drops and oral paracetamol	Optical prescription Sunglasses

CONCEPT MAP 12.10 Discharge planning and coordination of care for Daphne

12.12 ASSESSMENT OF HEARING PROBLEMS

In the collection of subjective data, previous and current person-reported information is important in the determination of hearing symptoms. See **Box 12.4** for the health assessment data collection areas.

BOX 12.4   SUBJECTIVE ASSESSMENT

➤ History of illness
➤ Past health history
➤ Medications
➤ Family history
➤ Recent air travel
➤ Recent deep sea diving
➤ Recent or ongoing industrial exposure
➤ Surgery

Functional health patterns:
  - Health perception and management
  - Nutritional and metabolic
  - Elimination
  - Activity and exercise
  - Sleep and rest
  - Cognitive and perceptual
  - Self perception and concept
  - Role relationship
  - Sexuality and reproductive
  - Coping and stress
  - Values and beliefs
➤ Risk calculation

The collection of objective data is informed by the subjective data and highlighted in the physical assessment and diagnostic studies for the hearing system (see **Box 12.5**).

BOX 12.5   OBJECTIVE ASSESSMENT

➤ Inspection of external structures
➤ Hearing acuity
➤ Inspection of auditory canal and tympanic membrane
➤ Diagnostic tests:
➤ Audiometry
➤ Weber test
➤ Rinne test
➤ Whisper test
➤ Other body systems as appropriate

12.13 ASSESSMENT FOR OTITIS MEDIA WITH EFFUSION

Otitis media with effusion occurs when the middle ear is inflamed with fluid and mucus and does not drain effectively via the auditory tube. As this is a more chronic presentation, there is a feeling of fullness, popping sensation and decreased hearing in the ear. The presentation of pain and fever is not present as in an acute episode of otitis media. As part of the health assessment please refer to **Box 12.4** and **Box 12.5**.

Presentation

Katie Namatjira is an Aboriginal 7-year-old girl who is admitted for day surgery for bilateral myringotomy with grommets. Katie has had recurring middle ear infections for the last six months which have recurred after antibiotic treatment has been completed. Katie and her mother have come from an Aboriginal community located in far north Queensland.

See **Concept map 12.11** to further explore Katie's initial care in the day surgery unit.

PHx

Katie is a 7-year-old girl who has had recurring middle ear infections for the last six months, that have not responded to antibiotics. Katie's hearing levels have decreased significantly in the last 2 months.

ASSESSMENT

Primary survey	Secondary survey
A: Patent	**CNS (Cognition):** Alert and orientated
B: RR 16	
C: Warm	**PAIN:** Both ears feel full
D: Alert	**CVS:** HR 88 bpm, BP 90/60 mmHg
E: T 35.8 °C	
F: Fasting, HNPU	**RESP:** RR 16
G: BGL 4.2 mmol/L	**GIT (Input):** Fasting since 8 p.m. the previous evening for food, last 2 hours for water

Cues

1. What is the relationship between acute otitis media and upper respiratory tract infections?
2. Why does Katie have hearing loss?

CONCEPT MAP 12.11 Nursing assessment for Katie

REFLECTIVE PRACTICE

Cultural considerations
Aboriginal and Torres Strait Islander children have the highest incidence of persistent otitis media in Australia, and it is characterised by development at a young age with a long duration of the disease. Hearing loss from the disease impacts on verbal and written communication, which leads to impaired school performance (language, reading, attention levels, anxiety and depression) and lower employment prospects in adulthood (Menzies School of Health Research, 2020).

12.14 PLANNING CARE FOR OTITIS MEDIA SURGERY

The planning for bilateral myringotomy with ventilation tubes (grommet) insertions (tympanostomy) will have the goals of:
■ relieving increased middle ear pressures and preventing spontaneous rupturing of the eardrum

- enabling ventilation and drainage of the middle ear during the postoperative phase.

Both Katie and her mother are partners in culturally competent care that is required in the day surgery unit and for appropriate health education for the home environment. **Box 12.6** indicates the areas that are targeted in the planning stage of otitis media surgery.

BOX 12.6   PLANNING FOR OTITIS MEDIA SURGERY

- ➤ Surgery and consent
- ➤ Self-care
- ➤ Use of age-appropriate language
- ➤ Medication
- ➤ Diet

Concept map 12.12 outlines a plan for Katie's care.

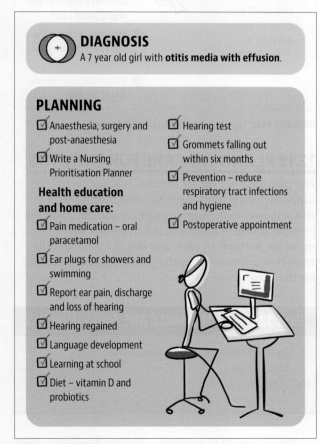

DIAGNOSIS

A 7 year old girl with **otitis media with effusion**.

PLANNING

- ☑ Anaesthesia, surgery and post-anaesthesia
- ☑ Write a Nursing Prioritisation Planner

Health education and home care:

- ☑ Pain medication – oral paracetamol
- ☑ Ear plugs for showers and swimming
- ☑ Report ear pain, discharge and loss of hearing
- ☑ Hearing regained
- ☑ Language development
- ☑ Learning at school
- ☑ Diet – vitamin D and probiotics

- ☑ Hearing test
- ☑ Grommets falling out within six months
- ☑ Prevention – reduce respiratory tract infections and hygiene
- ☑ Postoperative appointment

CONCEPT MAP 12.12 Diagnosis and planning for Katie

12.15 NURSING INTERVENTIONS TO SUPPORT HEALTH CARE FOR OTITIS MEDIA SURGERY

Nursing interventions are implemented as part of person-centred care, and Katie's surgical procedure has the aim to reverse the signs and symptoms and the associated pathophysiology of otitis media.

Concept map 12.13 explores Katie's journey in the day surgery unit.

INTERVENTIONS

1 Child and mother health education

2 Check for valid consent

3 Accompany to anaesthetic area

4 Undertake postoperative assessments in the post-anaesthetic care unit (PACU)

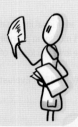

What further assessments should be initiated

Cues   **1** Katie states that everyone is very loud in PACU. What is your response?

CONCEPT MAP 12.13 Nursing interventions for Katie

12.16 EVALUATION OF CARE FOR OTITIS MEDIA SURGERY

As part of the further assessment of Katie's presentation, **Concept map 12.14** asks further questions in relation to the support for Katie and her mother in returning to their remotely located community.

12.17 DISCHARGE PLANNING AND COORDINATION OF CARE FOR OTITIS MEDIA SURGERY

Katie's otitis media surgery requires discharge planning and further management at home and a post-surgical review with the local health clinic and Royal Flying Doctor Service. **Concept Map 12.15** explores the considerations for Katie's care.

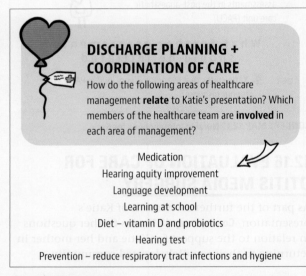

EVALUATION

While Katie and her mother are in PACU, the surgeon visits and part of the discussion is to encourage attendance to the local healthcare clinic and to attend a Royal Flying Doctor Service visit that includes a review of Katie's ears.

Plan:
Discharge Katie and her mother for the journey home to far north Queensland.

Cues

1. What additional information can be provided to assist Katie's mother in providing an environment where there will be lower incidence of ear infection?

CONCEPT MAP 12.14 Evaluation and planning for Katie

DISCHARGE PLANNING + COORDINATION OF CARE

How do the following areas of healthcare management **relate** to Katie's presentation? Which members of the healthcare team are **involved** in each area of management?

Medication
Hearing aquity improvement
Language development
Learning at school
Diet – vitamin D and probiotics
Hearing test
Prevention – reduce respiratory tract infections and hygiene

CONCEPT MAP 12.15 Discharge planning and coordination of care for Katie

12.18 ASSESSMENT FOR TINNITUS

Tinnitus is often the first symptom of hearing loss for older adults. Hearing loss occurs due to inner ear nerve damage where the organ of Corti hair cells are damaged. This damage produces hearing loss and sounds that vary from soft to loud and can be low to high pitched. Please Refer to **Box 12.4** and **Box 12.5** when conducting a health assessment.

Presentation

Francoise Cole is 37-year-old woman who is attending the general practitioner (GP) with ringing in the right ear. The ringing has been ongoing for the last three weeks, and started with a head cold but has not resolved. The ringing in the right ear has prevented the placement of her mobile telephone to the right ear.

See **Concept map 12.16** to further explore Francoise's initial care.

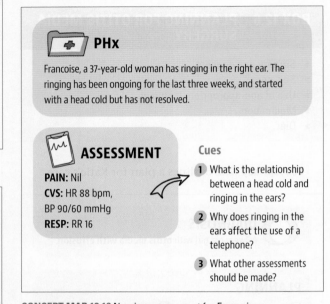

PHx

Francoise, a 37-year-old woman has ringing in the right ear. The ringing has been ongoing for the last three weeks, and started with a head cold but has not resolved.

ASSESSMENT

PAIN: Nil
CVS: HR 88 bpm, BP 90/60 mmHg
RESP: RR 16

Cues

1. What is the relationship between a head cold and ringing in the ears?

2. Why does ringing in the ears affect the use of a telephone?

3. What other assessments should be made?

CONCEPT MAP 12.16 Nursing assessment for Francoise

12.19 PLANNING CARE FOR TINNITUS

The planning of care for tinnitus is based on supportive interventions of focused hearing tests and self-care, including medication and diet, and the possible fitting of a hearing aid. Francoise and the nurse are partners in care, and **Box 12.7** indicates the areas that are targeted in the planning stage of caring for the person with tinnitus.

BOX 12.7 PLANNING CARE FOR TINNITUS
➤ Further assessment and potential hearing aid
➤ Medication
➤ Diet
➤ Self-care

Concept map 12.17 outlines a plan for Francoise's care.

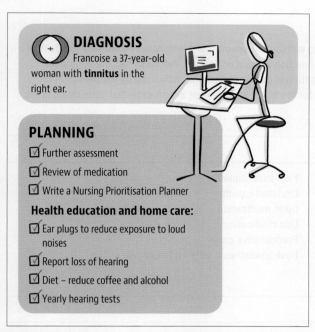

DIAGNOSIS

Francoise a 37-year-old woman with **tinnitus** in the right ear.

PLANNING

☑ Further assessment

☑ Review of medication

☑ Write a Nursing Prioritisation Planner

Health education and home care:

☑ Ear plugs to reduce exposure to loud noises

☑ Report loss of hearing

☑ Diet – reduce coffee and alcohol

☑ Yearly hearing tests

CONCEPT MAP 12.17 Diagnosis and planning for Francoise

12.20 NURSING INTERVENTIONS TO SUPPORT HEALTH CARE FOR TINNITUS

Nursing interventions are implemented as part of person-centred care, and to manage the symptoms of tinnitus.

Concept map 12.18 explores the management of Francoise's tinnitus.

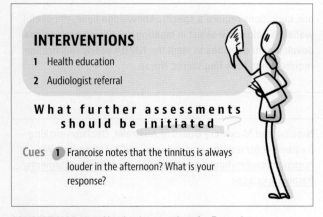

INTERVENTIONS

1 Health education

2 Audiologist referral

What further assessments should be initiated?

Cues 1 Francoise notes that the tinnitus is always louder in the afternoon? What is your response?

CONCEPT MAP 12.18 Nursing interventions for Francoise

12.21 EVALUATION OF CARE FOR TINNITUS

As part of the further assessment of Francoise's tinnitus, **Concept map 12.19** asks further questions in relation to supporting Francoise with living with tinnitus.

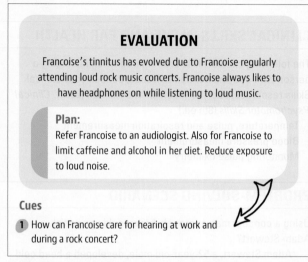

EVALUATION

Francoise's tinnitus has evolved due to Francoise regularly attending loud rock music concerts. Francoise always likes to have headphones on while listening to loud music.

Plan:
Refer Francoise to an audiologist. Also for Francoise to limit caffeine and alcohol in her diet. Reduce exposure to loud noise.

Cues

1 How can Francoise care for hearing at work and during a rock concert?

CONCEPT MAP 12.19 Evaluation and planning for Francoise

12.22 DISCHARGE PLANNING AND COORDINATION OF CARE FOR TINNITUS

Francoise's tinnitus requires management at home and an annual review by the audiologist. **Concept Map 12.20** explores the considerations for Francoise's care

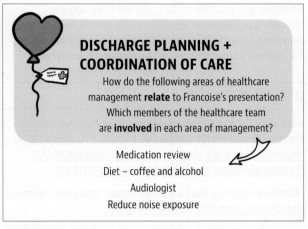

DISCHARGE PLANNING + COORDINATION OF CARE

How do the following areas of healthcare management **relate** to Francoise's presentation? Which members of the healthcare team are **involved** in each area of management?

Medication review

Diet – coffee and alcohol

Audiologist

Reduce noise exposure

CONCEPT MAP 12.20 Discharge planning and coordination of care for Francoise

SUMMARY

People with eye and hearing disorders have the challenges of living within their environment with reduced sensory input while remaining safe. When providing care for a person with decreased function of sight or hearing, the nurse has the additional challenge of providing health education when either eyesight or hearing is decreased and not fully used by the person in the education session. Hence, written instructions (often in large font) for the home environment are an essential component in the health education process.

CLINICAL SKILLS IN EYE AND EAR HEALTH

The following clinical skills are required when managing a person with eye and ear health issues; consult your Clinical Skills resources, such as Tollefson and Hillman (2022), *Clinical Psychomotor Skills* (8th ed.).

- Temperature, pulse and respiration measurement
- Blood pressure measurement
- Monitoring pulse oximetry
- Pain assessment
- Oral medication
- Optic medication
- Otic medication
- Preoperative care
- Post-anaesthesia care and handover

PROBLEM-SOLVING SCENARIO

Using a concept map approach, how would you assist Adam Stewart?

Adam Stewart, a 52-year-old male, developed a head cold one week ago. He recovered quickly, but tinnitus started in his left ear. The tinnitus was then heard in his right ear and two incidences of dizziness occurred in the last 24 hours. Adam now reports that he finds it difficult to hear. The general practitioner (GP) suspects Meniere's disease. The GP orders tests and refers Adam to you (as the Practice Nurse) to establish and implement a long-term plan of care.

1 What are the causes of Meniere's disease?
2 What are the associated signs and symptoms of Meniere's disease?
3 How is medication management used in treating the condition?
4 What are the lifestyle factors that are also considered in controlling Meniere's disease?
5 How does self-care assist in reducing the severity of Meniere's disease?

PORTFOLIO DEVELOPMENT

Wherever you practise nursing you will need ongoing continuing professional development to ensure that you are delivering current evidence-based nursing care that provides the best possible outcomes for the patient. As ocular and otic conditions require a specific knowledge base, the useful websites below will assist in meeting continuing professional development activities to meet the NMBA yearly registration requirements for a Registered Nurse.

USEFUL WEBSITES

Australian Ophthalmic Nurses Association National Council, Practice Standards for Ophthalmic Nurses in Australia (2018) http://www.aonanc.com.au/images/Documents/AONANC-Practice-standards-for-Ophthalmic-Nurses-2018.pdf

Otorhinolaryngology, Head and Neck Nurses Group Inc, Podcasts https://ohnng.com.au/category/podcasts

Nursing and Midwifery Board of Australia, Decision-making framework for nursing and midwifery (2020) https://www.nursingmidwiferyboard.gov.au/codes-guidelines-statements/frameworks.aspx

REFERENCES AND FURTHER READING

Australian Institute of Health and Welfare (AIHW). (2021). *Eye health*. https://www.aihw.gov.au/reports-data/health-conditions-disability-deaths/eye-health/overview

Australian Institute of Health and Welfare (AIHW). (2022). *Ear health*. https://www.indigenoushpf.gov.au/measures/1-15-ear-health

Awad Abid, D., Ahmed Hassanin, A., Abubakr Salama H, & Salama, M., H. (2018). Effect of implementing nursing guideline on nurses' performance regarding patients undergoing cataract or glaucoma surgery. *International Journal of Nursing Didactics*, *8*(8), 10–21.

Bauer, C. A. (2018). Tinnitus. *The New England Journal of Medicine*, *378*(13), 1224–1231. DOI: 10.1056/NEJMcp1506631

Broyles, B., Reiss, B., Evans, M., Pleunik, S., Page, R., & Badoer, E. (2023). *Pharmacology in nursing* (4th ANZ ed.). Cengage Learning Australia.

Choi, A. R., & Greenburg, P. B. (2018). Patient education strategies in cataract surgery: a systematic review. *Journal of Evidence-based Medicine*, *11*(2), 71–82. https://doi.org/10.1111/jebm.12297

Daley, M., & Howe, R. (2021). Myringotomy and insertion of grommets as day surgery: a case study. *British Journal of Nursing*, *30*(3), 142–147. https://doi.org/10.12968/bjon.2021.30.3.142

DeLaune S., Ladner, P., McTier, L., Tollefson, J., & Lawrence, J. (2024). *Fundamentals of nursing* (3rd ed.). Cengage Learning Australia.

Menzies School of Health Research. (2020). *2020 Otitis media guidelines for Aboriginal and Torres Strait Islander children*. https://otitismediaguidelines.com/wpcontent/uploads/2021/07/OtitisMedia_Guideline_2020.pdf

Mohamed Taha, N., & Ahmed Abd Elaziz, N. (2015). Effect of nursing intervention guidelines on nurses' role, patients' needs, and visual problems post cataract surgery.

American Journal of Nursing Science, *4*(5), 261–269. DOI: 10.11648/j.ajns.20150405.13

Neighbors, M., & Tannehill-Jones, R. (2023). *Human diseases* (6th ed.). Cengage.

Obuchowska, I., Lugowska, D., Mariak, Z., & Konopinska, J. (2021). Subjective opinions of patients about step-by-step cataract surgery preparation. *Clinical Ophthalmology*, *15*, 713–721. DOI: 10.2147?OPTH.S298876

Sowka, J. W., & Kabat, A. G. (2017). A pop fly straight to the eye: a refresher on hyphema management, just in time for wiffleball season. *Review of Optometry*, *154*(6), 98–100.

Tollefson, J., & Hillman, E. (2022). *Clinical psychomotor skills: Assessment tools for nurses* (8th ed.). Cengage Learning Australia.

Watkinson, S., & Seewoodhary, M. (2015). Cataract management: effect on patients' quality of life. *Nursing Standard*, *29*(21), 42–48. https://doi.org/10.7748/ns.29.21.42.e9222

CHAPTER 13

GASTROINTESTINAL SYSTEM

Gastrointestinal illnesses – such as gastroenteritis, abdominal and pelvic pain, and nausea and vomiting – make up a very large percentage of emergency department presentations annually within Australia. Abdominal and pelvic pain is the most frequently occurring principal diagnosis, with more than 355 000 people presenting annually for investigations and treatment around this pain. Gastroenteritis is seventh in the presentations annually, with over 110 000 people of all ages presenting with symptoms. Nausea and vomiting see more than 85 000 people present annually. These figures highlight that ages of patients presenting with symptoms are spread evenly across the lifespan; therefore, regardless of what area or specialty your nursing career is in, you will need specific assessment skills for the abdomen, and head-to-toe assessment for your patient (Australian Institute of Health and Welfare [AIHW], 2018).

LEARNING OBJECTIVES

After reading this chapter, you should have an understanding of the:
1 assessment required for a person with gastrointestinal conditions
2 prioritisation of key components in the development of a plan of care for people presenting with the conditions of:
   – diverticulitis
   – pancreatitis
3 prioritised and targeted nursing interventions required to promote recovery or prevent further deterioration of people presenting with the conditions of diverticulitis and pancreatitis
4 evaluation phase and how the prioritised and targeted nursing interventions inform further assessment, planning and collaboration with the healthcare team
5 discharge planning and coordination of care required in preparing the person for discharge and subsequent continuity of care between the person and their healthcare providers.

INTRODUCTION

The gastrointestinal (GI) system is also referred to as the digestive system. The GI system contains the mouth, oesophagus, stomach, small intestines, large intestines, rectum, anus, liver, pancreas and the gallbladder (Brown et al., 2019; Rizzo, 2015). As you can see, these organs and this system contain many factors that can be impacted by ill health, injury and chronic illness. Factors outside the GI system can also contribute or influence functioning and these include emotional and psychological factors, such as stress, anxiety and some other nervous disorders. The impact or the manifestation of stress or anxiety is different for every person, and can be seen through such symptoms as abdominal pain, diarrhoea, constipation, or even anorexia (Brown et al., 2019). Some chronic conditions or diseases of the GI system, such as ulcerative colitis or peptic ulcer disease, can be directly impacted by stress and, generally, stress worsens the symptoms of the conditions for the person. Other considerations in GI tract 'health' are nutrition, activity, medications and injury.

There are many common GI conditions, including:
- gastritis
- peptic ulcer
- irritable bowel syndrome
- coeliac disease
- inflammatory bowel disease
- Crohn's disease
- ulcerative colitis
- diverticulitis

- cholecystitis
- hepatitis
- pancreatitis
- cancer/tumours/malignancies

- gastroenteritis
- norovirus
- abdominal pain – unspecified.

You will need to rely upon your foundation anatomy and physiology and the application of this to your patient's condition. Some conditions will contain a variety of different presenting symptoms or care progression, and you will need to ensure that your care is always patient specific. Patients will also respond differently to treatment, intervention and management of their condition. With each variable of GI conditions, there are a number of factors that can directly impact the patient's condition such as age, medications, previous history and treatment, and emotional or physiological stressors (Brown et al., 2019; DeLaune et al., 2024).

Abdominal pain

Abdominal pain is the most common cause for presentation to emergency departments in Australia (AIHW, 2018). Abdominal pain can mask underlying serious conditions, and it should not be assumed that someone with abdominal pain is constipated or has gastroenteritis; rather, everything should be excluded prior to coming to this conclusion.

There have been 'red flags' identified in abdominal pain that require close assessment and review of the patient regardless of their presentation or situation in a hospital environment. These are shown in **Figure 13.1**.

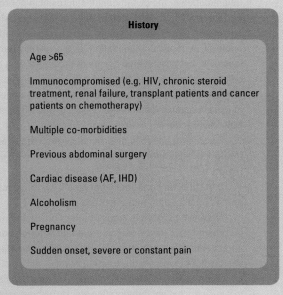
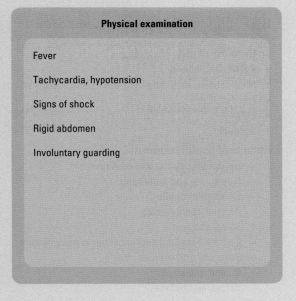

History	Physical examination
Age >65	Fever
Immunocompromised (e.g. HIV, chronic steroid treatment, renal failure, transplant patients and cancer patients on chemotherapy)	Tachycardia, hypotension
Multiple co-morbidities	Signs of shock
Previous abdominal surgery	Rigid abdomen
Cardiac disease (AF, IHD)	Involuntary guarding
Alcoholism	
Pregnancy	
Sudden onset, severe or constant pain	

FIGURE 13.1 Abdominal emergencies

SOURCE: AGENCY FOR CLINICAL INNOVATION

13.1 ASSESSMENT OF GASTROINTESTINAL CONDITIONS

Abdominal assessment or GI assessment is a focused assessment that requires inspection, auscultation, percussion and palpation as with any other body system. Inspection should be undertaken with the patient laying supine to review bloating, presence of a mass, or even blood from the anus. Auscultation requires listening for the presence of bowel sounds in the four quadrants. Percussion can be used to determine liver edges, and palpation can also identify a mass, pain on palpation, rebound tenderness, guarding and rigidity. All aspects or components of these findings will contribute to your patient care and interventions (Brown et al., 2019; DeLaune et al., 2024).

Due to the complexity of the GI system, patients can present with a myriad of symptoms. For example, a patient presenting with irritable bowel syndrome (IBS) can present with incredibly varied symptoms compared to other patients with IBS. The 'umbrella' of symptoms includes abdominal pain, constipation, diarrhoea, bloating and anorexia. So, your assessment will need to be abdominally focused, but patient specific, as no two patients will have the exact same symptoms for any GI condition.

In the collection of subjective data, previous and current person-reported information is important in the determination of symptoms that are related directly to the GI system and its associated organs. See **Box 13.1** for the health assessment data collection areas.

BOX 13.1   SUBJECTIVE ASSESSMENT

- ➤ History of illness, or symptoms
- ➤ Past health history
- ➤ Medications, including over-the-counter medications
- ➤ Family history
- ➤ Pain
- ➤ Surgery

Functional health patterns:
- – Health perception and management
- – Nutritional and metabolic
- – Elimination habits
- – Activity and exercise
- – Sleep and rest
- – Cognitive and perceptual aspects of symptoms
- – Sexuality and reproductive
- – Coping and stress
- – Values and beliefs

The collection of objective data is informed by the subjective data. The data collected can be impacted by other systems; for example, if the person has nausea, vomiting and diarrhoea, you may see a decline in blood pressure and fluid volume status and this will impact their vital signs. Other considerations are shown in **Box 13.2**.

BOX 13.2   PHYSICAL ASSESSMENT

- ➤ Vital signs
- ➤ Head-to-toe physical assessment
- ➤ Diagnostic – bloods, electrolytes, glucose, renal function, clotting profile, cholesterol
- ➤ Chest x-ray – abdomen
- ➤ Computed tomography – abdomen

13.2 ASSESSMENT FOR DIVERTICULITIS

Presentation

Ruby is a 38-year-old woman who has been hospitalised for diverticulitis. Diverticulitis is inflammation of the diverticulum that can result in peritonitis, perforation, fistula formation or even an abscess (Craft & Gordon, 2019). **Concept map 13.1** further explores Ruby's status.

SAFETY IN NURSING

DIVERTICULITIS

Inflammation of the diveriticulum can result in peritonitis, perforation, fistula formation or even an abscess. Micro and macro perforation develops, which releases intestinal bacteria, leading to inflammation. This generally remains localised, but will develop as one of the above with the inflammatory response. Patients will present with pain, tenderness in the lower left quadrant of the abdomen, fever, nausea, vomiting, distention or bloating, and PR bleeding. Most diverticula occur in the sigmoid colon.

If a patient has mild diverticulitis, often they can be treated as an outpatient, but it requires follow-up and review with a GP within 48–72 hours.

Diverticulitis can rapdily become a systemic infection and be a cascading factor in sepsis.

Assessing systemic signs of infection, including increasing pain, fever, tachycardia and hypotension is an escalation in care and requires a thorough patient assessment to inform the treating team.

Diverticulitis is a chronic condition, but one that can lead to significant patient deterioration quickly without appropriate observations and ongoing assessments.

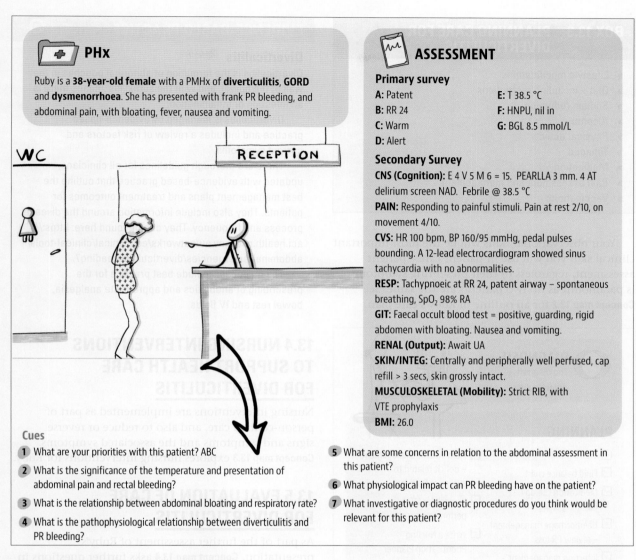

PHx

Ruby is a **38-year-old female** with a PMHx of **diverticulitis**, **GORD** and **dysmenorrhoea**. She has presented with frank PR bleeding, and abdominal pain, with bloating, fever, nausea and vomiting.

WC

RECEPTION

ASSESSMENT

Primary survey

A: Patent

B: RR 24

C: Warm

D: Alert

E: T 38.5 °C

F: HNPU, nil in

G: BGL 8.5 mmol/L

Secondary Survey

CNS (Cognition): E 4 V 5 M 6 = 15. PEARLLA 3 mm. 4 AT delirium screen NAD. Febrile @ 38.5 °C

PAIN: Responding to painful stimuli. Pain at rest 2/10, on movement 4/10.

CVS: HR 100 bpm, BP 160/95 mmHg, pedal pulses bounding. A 12-lead electrocardiogram showed sinus tachycardia with no abnormalities.

RESP: Tachypnoeic at RR 24, patent airway – spontaneous breathing, SpO$_2$ 98% RA

GIT: Faecal occult blood test = positive, guarding, rigid abdomen with bloating. Nausea and vomiting.

RENAL (Output): Await UA

SKIN/INTEG: Centrally and peripherally well perfused, cap refill > 3 secs, skin grossly intact.

MUSCULOSKELETAL (Mobility): Strict RIB, with VTE prophylaxis

BMI: 26.0

Cues

1 What are your priorities with this patient? ABC

2 What is the significance of the temperature and presentation of abdominal pain and rectal bleeding?

3 What is the relationship between abdominal bloating and respiratory rate?

4 What is the pathophysiological relationship between diverticulitis and PR bleeding?

5 What are some concerns in relation to the abdominal assessment in this patient?

6 What physiological impact can PR bleeding have on the patient?

7 What investigative or diagnostic procedures do you think would be relevant for this patient?

CONCEPT MAP 13.1 Nursing assessment for Ruby

13.3 PLANNING CARE FOR DIVERTICULITIS

Planning for the patient with diverticulitis will involve the nurse having an understanding of what diverticulitis 'is' and how it is diagnosed. Abdominal and chest x-rays will rule out other causes of acute abdominal pain, and a CT with a contrast (oral) is the preferred test to determine a diagnosis of diverticulitis. There are many other conditions that may be misdiagnosed as diverticulitis because the symptoms mimic those of diverticulitis. These include appendicitis, bowel obstruction, gastroenteritis, pelvic inflammatory disease, perforated gastric ulcer, peritonitis or an ectopic pregnancy. For example, in Ruby's case, blood tests such as full blood count, white cell count, haemoglobin, C-reactive protein, estimated glomerular filtration rate, creatinine, urea and electrolytes, liver function tests, blood cultures

(temperature 38.5 °C), group and hold (in case of surgery) and a pregnancy test to rule out ectopic pregnancy will be required.

There are multiple reasons for abdominal pain and GI dysfunction. For example, bloating could be related to an obstruction or a paralytic ileus. A mass on palpation could be a tumour or a cyst. Rebound tenderness can be peritonitis secondary to appendicitis. Malaena can be indicative of cancer or bleeding in the upper GI tract from ulcers or varices. And finally, constipation with pain can be due to inflammatory bowel disease, IBS or an infection. For Ruby's care, appropriate investigations would be to rule out other conditions and to identify the cause of her symptoms and pain (Brown et al., 2019; Craft & Gordon, 2019).

Box 13.3 indicates the areas that are targeted in the planning stage of Ruby's care for both abdominal pain and PR bleeding.

BOX 13.3 PLANNING CARE FOR DIVERTICULITIS

- ❯ Lifestyle modifications
- ❯ Diet – including restrictions
- ❯ Sodium reduction
- ❯ Alcohol
- ❯ Physical activity
- ❯ Tobacco
- ❯ Medication
- ❯ Pain assessment and management
- ❯ Vaccinations

Your observational skills will be the most important clinical skill you will use in patient care – patient assessment, regardless of their presenting symptoms, is paramount as no two patients are the same. See **Concept map 13.2** for an outline of Ruby's care plan.

EVIDENCE-BASED PRACTICE 🔍

Diverticulitis

Diverticulitis is the formation of abnormal pouches in the wall of the bowel, and with the suffix 'itis' means there is an infection or inflammation.

Diverticulitis is managed by evidence-based practice and includes a review of risk factors and current symptoms.

There are thorough guidelines for all clinicians, updated with evidence-based practice that outline the best management plans and treatment outcomes for patients. They also include information around the disease process and frequency. They can be found here: https://aci.health.nsw.gov.au/networks/eci/clinical/clinical-tools/abdominal-emergencies/diverticulitis#heading7.

The guidelines include best practice for the prescribing of antibiotics and appropriate analgesia, bowel rest and IV fluids.

13.4 NURSING INTERVENTIONS TO SUPPORT HEALTH CARE FOR DIVERTICULITIS

Nursing interventions are implemented as part of person-centred care, and also to reduce or reverse signs and symptoms and the associated symptoms. **Concept map 13.3** explores nursing interventions for Ruby.

13.5 EVALUATION OF CARE FOR DIVERTICULITIS

As part of the further assessment of Ruby's presentation, **Concept map 13.4** asks further questions in relation to Ruby's management.

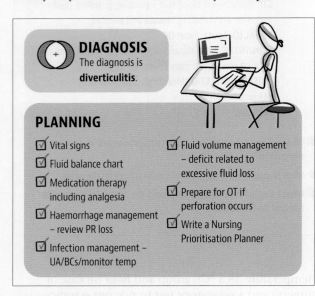

DIAGNOSIS
The diagnosis is **diverticulitis**.

PLANNING

- ☑ Vital signs
- ☑ Fluid balance chart
- ☑ Medication therapy including analgesia
- ☑ Haemorrhage management – review PR loss
- ☑ Infection management – UA/BCs/monitor temp
- ☑ Fluid volume management – deficit related to excessive fluid loss
- ☑ Prepare for OT if perforation occurs
- ☑ Write a Nursing Prioritisation Planner

CONCEPT MAP 13.2 Diagnosis and planning for Ruby

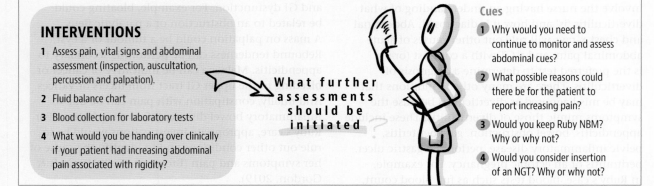

INTERVENTIONS

1 Assess pain, vital signs and abdominal assessment (inspection, auscultation, percussion and palpation).
2 Fluid balance chart
3 Blood collection for laboratory tests
4 What would you be handing over clinically if your patient had increasing abdominal pain associated with rigidity?

What further assessments should be initiated?

Cues

1 Why would you need to continue to monitor and assess abdominal cues?
2 What possible reasons could there be for the patient to report increasing pain?
3 Would you keep Ruby NBM? Why or why not?
4 Would you consider insertion of an NGT? Why or why not?

CONCEPT MAP 13.3 Nursing interventions for Ruby

EVALUATION

The medical team have been notified of Ruby's increasing abdominal pain (despite analgesia) and increased rigidity.

Plan:
Whilst Ruby was being prepared to have a repeat CT abdomen for the alterations in condition, she becomes hypotensive and tachycardic.

Cues

1. What interventions need to be considered now for Ruby? Prioritise these interventions in order of urgency.

2. Does this deterioration in her condition relate to the reason for presentation?

3. What do the deteriorations in vital signs indicate pathophysiologically?

CONCEPT MAP 13.4 Evaluation and planning for Ruby

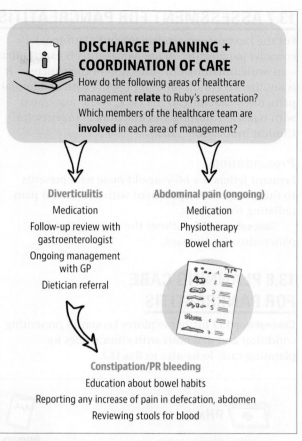

DISCHARGE PLANNING + COORDINATION OF CARE

How do the following areas of healthcare management **relate** to Ruby's presentation? Which members of the healthcare team are **involved** in each area of management?

Diverticulitis
Medication
Follow-up review with gastroenterologist
Ongoing management with GP
Dietician referral

Abdominal pain (ongoing)
Medication
Physiotherapy
Bowel chart

Constipation/PR bleeding
Education about bowel habits
Reporting any increase of pain in defecation, abdomen
Reviewing stools for blood

CONCEPT MAP 13.5 Discharge planning and coordination of care for Ruby

13.6 DISCHARGE PLANNING AND COORDINATION OF CARE FOR DIVERTICULITIS

The nature of GI conditions is diverse, and this generally means that the patient and their family will not be prepared for the impact or the outcome of their hospitalisation and treatment. Your role will include discussing the processes and planned care with the patient alongside the medical and allied healthcare team.

Ruby has presented with three (3) specific conditions that require discharge planning and further management at home and with assistance from the general practice. How do the management of the three conditions intersect? Review the findings in **Concept map 13.5**.

REFLECTIVE PRACTICE

Gastrointestinal nursing – Diverticulitis

Nutrition plays a very large role in the management of diverticulitis. The increase in consumption of processed foods and low-fibre foods has seen an increase in presentations of people developing diverticulitis. The risk factors for diverticulitis increase with age, and it generally occurs from the pressure on the colon which forms pouches. Diverticulitis can be caused by seeds or pieces of food becoming stuck in the pouch, or even faeces from constipation or diarrhoea. Infection is the result of something being lodged in these pouches.

In Australia, the United States and England there is a higher incidence of diverticulosis – which is an ongoing condition where more than one bulging pouch exists and it is thought to be directly related to a diet high in processed foods. It is often referred to as 'diverticulosis of the colon'.

As with any chronic condition there is often new research, new suggestions or practices, and new information to review (Craft & Gordon, 2019).

Questions

1. How would you determine the most appropriate material to source to provide health information to your patient who has diverticulitis?
2. How would you support your patient in sourcing accurate information for their condition?
3. What other allied health professionals would be relevant in the health education and promotion of a patient with diverticulitis?

13.7 ASSESSMENT FOR PANCREATITIS

For the next patient assessment and planning, let's consider pancreatitis. Acute pancreatitis is exactly that – an acute inflammation/infection of the pancreas. It is another GI condition that presents with abdominal pain, often radiating to the back, and is associated with nausea, vomiting and diaphoresis (Agency for Clinical Innovation, 2022).

Presentation

Leonard Jeffers is a 66-year-old male who presents to the emergency department with abdominal pain radiating to the back.

Concept map 13.6 outlines the nursing care for pancreatitis for Leonard.

13.8 PLANNING CARE FOR PANCREATITIS

Concept map 13.7 further explores Leonard's presenting condition and diagnosis with clinical cues for planning care. Refer also to **Box 13.3**.

13.9 NURSING INTERVENTIONS TO SUPPORT HEALTH CARE FOR PANCREATITIS

Concept map 13.8 outlines the interventions for Leonard's nursing care.

13.10 EVALUATION OF CARE FOR PANCREATITIS

Concept map 13.9 outlines the evaluation process for Leonard's care.

 PHx

Leonard is a 68-year-old male who presents with a 2-day history of **abdominal pain**, radiating to his back. Associated with nausea and vomiting.
PMHx: Alcoholism, smoking (nicotine) 20/day, CAD, HTN, NIDDM, truncal obesity.

Cues

1. What are your priorities with this patient?
2. What is the significance of the pain severity?
3. What is the significance of VTE prophylaxis ?
4. What is the pathophysiological relationship between pancreatitis and NIDDM?
5. What are some concerns in relationship to the patient's cardiovascular presentation?
6. What investigative or diagnostic procedures would you think would be relevant for this patient?

 ASSESSMENT

Primary survey
A: Patent, clear
B: RR 22 no increased WOB
C: Tachy @ 115, regular
D: 7/10
E: T 38.6 °C
F: Dry mucous membranes, IVF to be inserted
G: BGL 10.6 mmol/L

Secondary survey
CNS: E4 V5 M6 = 15 PEARLA 4 mm.
T 38.8 °C
PAIN: C/o pain to abdomen, and radiating to the back – rated as 7/10, pain unchanged on movement. Diaphoretic, generalised.
CVS: HR 115 bpm, regular. BP 110/70 mmHg. Centrally warm, peripherally cooler. cap refill <3 secs

RESP: RR 22, no increased WOB, related to pain? Chest on auscultation clear throughout R = L with decreased AE bibasally. Nil cough. SpO$_2$ 98% RA. Clubbing.
GIT: BS Audible in all quadrants. Pain to RUQ/epigastric region, radiating to back. BGL 12.5 mmol/L. Nausea, reports vomiting prior to presentation.
RENAL (output): HNPU for past 6 hours.
SKIN/INTEG: Poor integrity, dry skin, grossly intact. Nil skin tears.
MUSCULOSKELETAL (mobility): Strict RIB, with VTE prophylaxis. Tremor present.
BMI: 28.0

CONCEPT MAP 13.6 Nursing assessment for Leonard

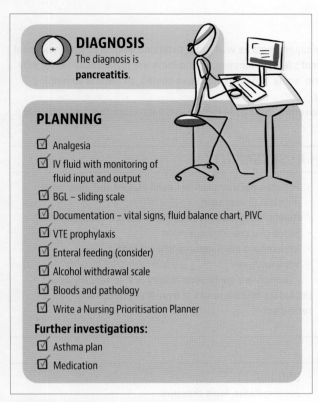

DIAGNOSIS

The diagnosis is **pancreatitis**.

PLANNING

- ☑ Analgesia
- ☑ IV fluid with monitoring of fluid input and output
- ☑ BGL – sliding scale
- ☑ Documentation – vital signs, fluid balance chart, PIVC
- ☑ VTE prophylaxis
- ☑ Enteral feeding (consider)
- ☑ Alcohol withdrawal scale
- ☑ Bloods and pathology
- ☑ Write a Nursing Prioritisation Planner

Further investigations:

- ☑ Asthma plan
- ☑ Medication

CONCEPT MAP 13.7 Diagnosis and planning for Leonard

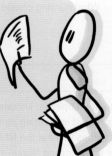

INTERVENTIONS

1 Assess pain, BGLs and vital signs.

2 Assess alcohol withdrawal scale hourly or more frequently if required.

3 ISBAR handover preparation for end-of-shift handover – what would you be handing over if your patient has increasing pain?

What further assessments should be initiated?

Cues

1 What further questions or information would you like to know from the patient?

2 What is the deterioration or change in patient status here?

3 What could be the pathophysiological reason for the increase in pain?

CONCEPT MAP 13.8 Nursing interventions for Leonard

EVALUATION

The medical team have been notified of the increase in your patient's pain. It is now rated as 9/10.

Plan:
Medical officer has requested further analgesia, and a repeat in vital signs, including BGL.

Cues

1 What interventions need to be considered now for your patient? What is your priority here?

2 The patient has been prescribed 5 mg subcutaneous morphine. What are the considerations for administration of this medication?

3 What do you think is the reason for the increase in pain?

CONCEPT MAP 13.9 Evaluation and planning for Leonard

13.11 DISCHARGE PLANNING AND COORDINATION OF CARE FOR PANCREATITIS

Concept map 13.10 introduces the key concepts relevant for Leonard's discharge and coordination of care.

DISCHARGE PLANNING + COORDINATION OF CARE

How do the following areas of healthcare management **relate** to Leonard's presentation? Which members of the healthcare team are **involved** in each area of management?

Pancreatitis

Medication

Diet review

Pain management plan

Follow-up with GP for repeat lipase and other indices

Smoking and alcohol use – cessation or minimisation of nicotine and alcohol

Medication

Referral (with consent) to AOD team

QUIT

NIDDM

Patient education and health promotion on BGL management

Diet review

Alcohol and impact on NIDDM – follow up with Diabetic Educator

CONCEPT MAP 13.10 Discharge planning and coordination of care for Leonard

SUMMARY

Abdominal pain is a frequent cause for presentation to emergency departments as well as for extended lengths of stay in hospital post-procedure. Abdominal pain has significant impact on the patient's level of functioning and there are myriad reasons for why someone could experience abdominal pain. It is in part why the term 'acute abdomen' has been coined, as there is something 'acutely' wrong, but it is not always immediately clear what or why.

Your nursing assessment should follow the systematic approach and focus on the patient and their subjective and objective data findings.

CLINICAL SKILLS IN GASTROINTESTINAL HEALTH ASSESSMENT

The following clinical skills are required when managing a person with GI issues; consult your Clinical Skills resources, such as Tollefson and Hillman (2022), *Clinical Psychomotor Skills* (8th ed.).

- Temperature, pulse and respiration measurement
- Blood pressure measurement
- Monitoring pulse oximetry
- Pain assessment

- Focused gastrointestinal health history and abdominal physical assessment
- Height, weight and waist circumference measurement
- Blood glucose measurement
- Intravenous medication administration
- Venipuncture

Obtaining a medication history is also very important (including an awareness of over-the-counter and herbal remedies).

PROBLEM-SOLVING SCENARIO

Using a concept map approach, how would you assist Tiffany Fredericks?

Tiffany Fredericks is a 90-year-old woman who has been in hospital for the past 7 days, post a mechanical fall. Tiffany has not had her bowels open for 10 days. She is currently on abdominal assessment, and has:

- abdominal pain, upper right and left quadrants with diminished bowel sounds

- BNO 10/7
- passing flatus, feels pressure.
1   With these symptoms and observations what are some pathophysiological processes in place that are impacting Tiffany's pain?
2   What nursing considerations would you have for Tiffany?

PORTFOLIO DEVELOPMENT

Wherever you practise nursing you will need ongoing continuing professional development to ensure that you are delivering current evidence-based nursing care that provides the best possible outcomes for the patient. As GI conditions require a specific knowledge base, the useful websites below will assist in meeting continuing professional development activities to meet the NMBA yearly registration requirements for a Registered Nurse.

USEFUL WEBSITES

Registered Nurse Standards for Practice
The Registered Nurse Standards for Practice consist of seven crucial standards that all nurses must follow. Download and review the standards at the following link. https://www.nursingmidwiferyboard.gov.au/Codes-Guidelines-Statements/Professional-standards/registered-nurse-standards-for-practice.aspx

Emergency Care Institute – NSW Health
Clinical guidelines for all clinicians in the treatment, management, and diagnosis of diverticulitis.
https://aci.health.nsw.gov.au/networks/eci/clinical/clinical-tools/abdominal-emergencies/diverticulitis#heading7

Clinical guidelines for all clinicians in the treatment, management, and diagnosis of abdominal emergencies.
https://aci.health.nsw.gov.au/networks/eci/clinical/clinical-tools/abdominal-emergencies

Gastroenterological Nurses College of Australia
Provides resources and specialised education for gastroenterological nursing. https://www.genca.org

Gastroenterological Society of Australia
Provides ongoing education and resources specific to gastroenterological nursing. https://www.gesa.org.au

REFERENCES AND FURTHER READING

Agency for Clinical Innovation. (2022). *Acute pancreatitis*. https://aci.health.nsw. gov.au/networks/eci/clinical/clinical-tools/abdominal-emergencies/acute-pancreatitis

Australian Institute of Health and Welfare (AIHW). (2018). *Emergency department care 2017–2018. Australian hospital statistics.* Canberra: Australian Government

Brown, D., Edwards, H., Buckley, T., Aitken, R. L., Lewis, S. L., Bucher, L., McLean Heitkemper, M., Harding, M. M., Kwong, J., & Roberts, D. (2019). *Lewis's medical-surgical nursing ANZ* (5th ed.). Elsevier.

Craft, J., & Gordon, C. (2019). *Understanding pathophysiology* (3rd ed.). Elsevier Australia.

DeLaune, S., Ladner, P., McTier, L., Tollefson, J., & Lawrence, J. (2024). *Fundamentals of nursing* (3rd ed.). Cengage Learning Australia.

Rizzo, D. C. (2015). *Fundamentals of anatomy and physiology* (4th ed.). Cengage Learning.

Tollefson, J., & Hillman, E. (2022). *Clinical psychomotor skills: Assessment tools for nurses* (8th ed.). Cengage Learning Australia.

CHAPTER 14

LIVER, PANCREAS AND BILIARY TRACT

Liver disease is one of the leading causes of premature death in Australia. In the premature death statistics, males predominate and were aged 50 years and over. Aboriginal and Torres Strait Islander peoples' mortality rates are higher than non-Aboriginal and Torres Strait Islander people; males have a three times higher rate of death and females a five times higher rate of death (Australian Institute of Health and Welfare, 2016).

LEARNING OBJECTIVES

After reading this chapter, you should have an understanding of the:
1 assessment required for a person with a liver, pancreas and biliary condition
2 prioritisation of key components in the development of plans of care for a person with the liver, pancreas and biliary conditions of:
   – hepatitis
   – cirrhosis
   – gallstones (cholelithiasis)
3 prioritised and targeted nursing interventions required to promote recovery or prevent further deterioration of people presenting with the liver, pancreas and biliary conditions of hepatitis, cirrhosis and gallstones
4 evaluation phase and how the prioritised and targeted nursing interventions inform further assessment of the person, planning of care and collaboration with the healthcare team
5 discharge planning and coordination of care required in preparing the person for discharge and subsequent continuity of care between the person and their healthcare providers.

INTRODUCTION

The liver, gallbladder and pancreas all play a role in facilitating digestion. The liver has the diverse roles of metabolising proteins, carbohydrates and fats, and detoxification and filtration of steroids, hormones and drugs. It also synthesises plasma proteins, fibrogen, clotting factors and antibodies. Then, importantly, it stores carbohydrates, amino acids, vitamins, minerals and blood. The liver's secretion of bile is stored in the gallbladder, and the gallbladder releases the bile via the common bile duct into the duodenum to increase fat digestion and absorption. The pancreas releases enzymes and fluids into the pancreatic duct, which then joins the common bile duct and breaks down proteins, starch and fats in the small intestine. The pancreas also has a hormonal function for carbohydrate, protein and fat metabolism.

People with disorders of the liver, pancreas and biliary system (or biliary tract), experience disruption in activity levels and decreased sense of wellbeing. Whether the condition is newly diagnosed or is long term and considered chronic in presentation, the concepts of person-centred care are the same, with the goal of maintaining digestive and metabolic processes so the individual can maintain wellbeing.

It is important to consider that the liver, gallbladder and pancreas influence each other's functions. The liver may experience fibrosis and scarring, portal hypertension and impeded excretion of bile. The liver can experience hepatitis, fatty liver disease, liver cancer and obstruction of bile flow due to gallstones (cholelithiasis). Gallstones may lodge at the end of the common bile duct and impede the flow of pancreatic digestive enzymes as well to produce pancreatitis.

14.1 ASSESSMENT OF LIVER, PANCREAS AND BILIARY PROBLEMS

In the collection of subjective data, previous and current person-reported information is important in the determination of liver, pancreas and biliary symptoms. See **Box 14.1** for the health assessment data collection areas.

BOX 14.1 SUBJECTIVE ASSESSMENT

- ➤ History of illness
- ➤ Past health history
- ➤ Medications
- ➤ Family history
- ➤ Surgery

Functional health patterns:
- – Health perception and management
- – Nutritional and metabolic
- – Elimination
- – Activity and exercise
- – Sleep and rest
- – Cognitive and perceptual
- – Self-perception and concept
- – Role relationship
- – Sexuality and reproductive
- – Coping and stress
- – Values and beliefs
- ➤ Risk calculation

The collection of objective data is informed by the subjective data and is highlighted in the physical assessment of the person and results of diagnostic studies. **Box 14.2** lists the objective assessment components for the liver, pancreas and biliary tract, and as required, other body systems will also be assessed for data.

BOX 14.2 OBJECTIVE ASSESSMENT

- ➤ Abdomen
- ➤ Inspection
- ➤ Auscultation
- ➤ Percussion
- ➤ Palpation
- ➤ Diagnostic tests – endoscopy, oesophageal studies, liver biopsy, liver function studies, x-ray, ultrasound, tomography, magnetic resonance imaging, cholangiography, endoscopic retrograde cholangiopancreatography, liver biopsy, serum amylase, serum lipase, liver function tests
- ➤ Other body systems as appropriate

14.2 ASSESSMENT FOR HEPATITIS

As part of the health assessment for an individual, the components of **Box 14.1** and **Box 14.22** are incorporated for a person-centred approach to the assessment of hepatitis.

Presentation

Ngoc Bui is a 28-year-old information technology developer and has been admitted to the emergency department with nausea and vomiting for the last week, and now a rash has appeared on his body. His mother noted that the white part of his eyes has a tinge of yellow colour, and he was told to go to the emergency department straight away.

See **Concept map 14.1** to further explore Ngoc's initial care in the emergency department.

📁➕ PHx

Ngoc had **hepatitis** when he was 5 years old, but does not know which type. Ngoc has had no recent overseas travel nor been in contact with people with hepatitis. He does not take medication and has no known allergies. Ngoc denies illicit drug use. His **nausea** and **vomiting** has **increased** in the last 2 days. He does not have a significant family history.

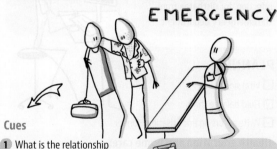

EMERGENCY

Cues

1. What is the relationship between yellow sclera and hepatitis?

2. Is there a relationship between the bout of hepatitis that Ngoc had as a child and the current presentation?

3. What systems would be of note during the secondary survey?

4. Does the liver change in size due to an infection?

📈 ASSESSMENT

Primary survey

A: Patent

B: RR 18, SpO$_2$ 99%. Clear breath sounds.

C: HR 89 bpm, BP 125/80 mmHg

D: Alert

E: 37.2 °C

CONCEPT MAP 14.1 Nursing assessment for Ngoc

14.3 PLANNING CARE FOR HEPATITIS

Planning for the nursing care for acute hepatitis has the goals of:

- increasing nutrition and activity
- maintaining liver function.

Ngoc is a partner in his care plan and contributes to his health care by following his plan of care and managing his condition in the home environment. **Box 14.3** lists the areas that are targeted in the planning stage of acute hepatitis management.

BOX 14.3   PLANNING FOR HEPATITIS
> Nutrition > Activity > Liver function > Tests > Medication > Self-care

Concept map 14.2 outlines a plan for Ngoc's care.

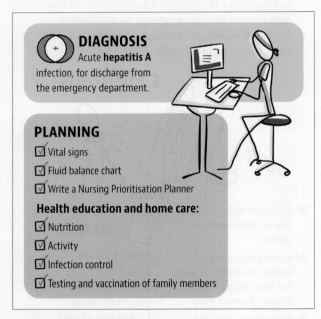

CONCEPT MAP 14.2 Diagnosis and planning for Ngoc

14.4 NURSING INTERVENTIONS TO SUPPORT HEALTH CARE FOR HEPATITIS

Nursing interventions are implemented as part of person-centred care and reverse the signs and symptoms and the associated pathophysiology of hepatitis.

Concept map 14.3 explores Ngoc's journey in the emergency department, before discharge to home.

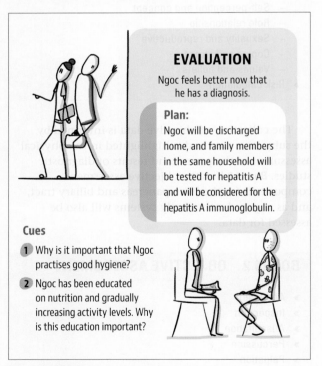

CONCEPT MAP 14.3 Nursing interventions for Ngoc

14.5 EVALUATION OF CARE FOR HEPATITIS

As part of the further assessment of Ngoc's presentation, **Concept map 14.4** asks further questions in relation to Ngoc's management.

CONCEPT MAP 14.4 Evaluation and planning for Ngoc

14.6 DISCHARGE PLANNING AND COORDINATION OF CARE FOR HEPATITIS

Ngoc's hepatitis requires discharge planning and further management at home (see **Concept map 14.5**).

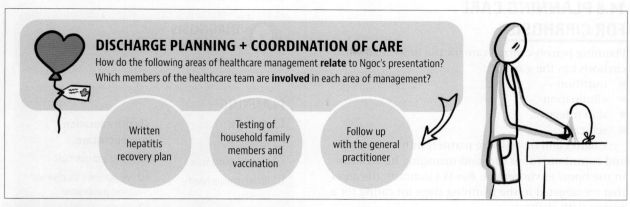

DISCHARGE PLANNING + COORDINATION OF CARE

How do the following areas of healthcare management **relate** to Ngoc's presentation? Which members of the healthcare team are **involved** in each area of management?

- Written hepatitis recovery plan
- Testing of household family members and vaccination
- Follow up with the general practitioner

CONCEPT MAP 14.5 Discharge planning and coordination of care for Ngoc

14.7 ASSESSMENT FOR CIRRHOSIS

As cirrhosis is part of the liver disease trajectory, **Box 14.1** and **Box 14.2** subjective and objective assessment foci are incorporated into Charles' health assessment.

Presentation

Charles Wilson is a 62-year-old man who was brought into the emergency department by ambulance. Charles' wife states that he has had ongoing problems with alcohol abuse for the last 25 years. He is thin in build and has a florid face.

Charles states that he has no appetite and is only an occasional drinker.

See **Concept map 14.6** to further explore Charles' initial care in the emergency department, before transfer to the medical ward for further care.

SAFETY IN NURSING

Paracetamol, as an over-the-counter medication, is present in pain medication, fever relievers and cough medications. A person can unintentionally overdose on paracetamol.

 PHx

Charles had a **bleeding gastric ulcer** 3 years ago, which was treated. He now has had significant weight loss, and nausea and vomiting for the last 3 weeks. Charles states that he does not have an alcohol problem, and the gastric ulcer was not caused by alcohol.

 ASSESSMENT

Primary survey
A: Clear
B: RR 28, pulse oximetry 96% on room air, breath sounds reveal lower lobe bilateral fine crackles on auscultation.
C: HR 102 bpm, BP 150/90 mmHg, spider angiomas on cheeks and nose
D: Orientated but does not always follow statements and questions
E: 38.3 °C
F: IVF to be commenced, urine dark
G: BGL 7.2 mmol/L

Secondary survey
CNS: E 4 V 4 M 5 = 13/15 PEARL 3mm. Does not always follow statements and questions. Denies alcohol abuse.
CVS: HR 104 bpm, BP 155/90 mmHg, T 38.6 °C, peripherally perfused
Resp: RR 30, SaO$_2$ 96%
GIT: Bowel sounds present. Left upper quadrant tender. Enlarged liver. Haemorrhoids. Poor appetite for the last 3 weeks, so eating very little. So has regular constipation.

Renal: Urine concentrated and dark
Metabolic: BGL 7.2 mmol/L
Integumentary: Warm dry skin, spider angiomas.
Musculoskeletal: Equal limb strength with limbs showing muscle wastage.
Blood drawn for liver function, protein metabolism, and lipid metabolism.
Chest x-ray to be reviewed.

CONCEPT MAP 14.6 Nursing assessment for Charles

14.8 PLANNING CARE FOR CIRRHOSIS

Planning person-centred care for the individual with cirrhosis has the goals of:

- nutrition
- elimination
- skin integrity
- self-care.

Charles and his wife are partners in his care plan and contribute to his care and managing his health in the home environment. **Box 14.4** indicates the areas that are targeted in the planning stage for caring for a person with cirrhosis.

BOX 14.4   PLANNING FOR CIRRHOSIS

- ➤ Respond to severity of symptoms
- ➤ Nutrition
- ➤ Elimination
- ➤ Alcohol withdrawal scale
- ➤ Skin integrity
- ➤ Health education and home care:
  - – self-care
  - – physical activity
  - – alcohol cessation

SAFETY IN NURSING ⚠

Cirrhosis

Older adults are more susceptible to central nervous system adverse effects of antiemetic drugs. The adverse effects are exemplified by confusion and an increased risk of patient falls.

Concept map 14.7 outlines a plan for Charles' care.

DIAGNOSIS

Alcohol-induced cirrhosis, with admission to the medical ward

PLANNING

- ☑ Vital signs
- ☑ Pulse oximetry
- ☑ Glasgow Coma Scale
- ☑ Breath sounds, heart sounds
- ☑ IV therapy 0.9% sodium chloride
- ☑ Fluid balance chart
- ☑ Medication – lactulose, proton pump inhibitor
- ☑ Nutrition
- ☑ Oral hygiene
- ☑ Skin care
- ☑ Falls risk
- ☑ Write a Nursing Prioritisation Planner

Health education and home care:

- ☑ Fluids and nutrition
- ☑ Medication – laxative and avoid paracetamol
- ☑ Alcohol cessation

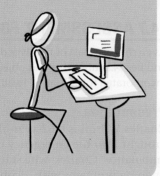

CONCEPT MAP 14.7 Diagnosis and planning for Charles

14.9 NURSING INTERVENTIONS TO SUPPORT HEALTH CARE FOR CIRRHOSIS

Nursing interventions are implemented as part of person-centred care, and to address the signs and symptoms associated with progressive cirrhosis.

Concept map 14.8 explores Charles' journey from the emergency department to the medical ward.

INTERVENTIONS

1 Vital signs 4 hourly
2 Pulse oximetry 4 hourly
3 Glasgow Coma Scale 4 hourly
4 Breath sounds and heart sounds daily
5 Hourly alcohol withdrawal scale
6 IV therapy 0.9% sodium chloride 8/24
7 Fluid balance chart
8 Lactulose 6 hourly, Esomeprazole daily
9 High protein diet

10 Oral care after meals and snacks
11 Skin care 2 hourly
12 Falls risk 8 hourly

Health education and home care:

- Nutrition – small regular meals and increased fluid intake
- Medication – lactulose, esomeprazole
- Alcohol cessation program

What further assessments should be initiated ?

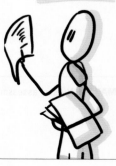

CONCEPT MAP 14.8 Nursing interventions for Charles

14.10 EVALUATION OF CARE FOR CIRRHOSIS

As part of the further assessment of Charles' presentation, **Concept map 14.9** asks further questions in relation to Charles' management.

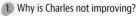

EVALUATION

Still not able to have full conversations, aware that he is in hospital

Constipation still evident

Urine less concentrated

Plan:
Continue planned care

Cues
1. Why is Charles not improving?
2. What is the rationale for the Glasgow Coma Scale observations, increased fluid intake and a laxative?

CONCEPT MAP 14.9 Evaluation and planning for Charles

14.11 DISCHARGE PLANNING AND COORDINATION OF CARE FOR CIRRHOSIS

The discharge planning for Charles' cirrhosis has the foci of further management at home and a follow-up appointment with his general practitioner (see **Concept map 14.10**).

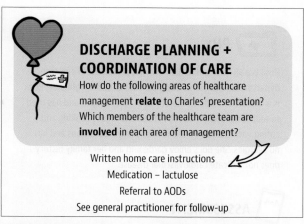

DISCHARGE PLANNING + COORDINATION OF CARE

How do the following areas of healthcare management **relate** to Charles' presentation? Which members of the healthcare team are **involved** in each area of management?

Written home care instructions

Medication – lactulose

Referral to AODs

See general practitioner for follow-up

CONCEPT MAP 14.10 Discharge planning and coordination of care for Charles

14.12 ASSESSMENT FOR GALLSTONES (CHOLELITHIASIS)

Presentation

Rosa Futura is a 56-year-old woman who was brought to the emergency department by her husband. Rosa was making pasta sauce for dinner, when suddenly she felt excruciating pain on her upper right side and bent over with pain. Rosa's face is quite sweaty.

Rosa's presentation requires a person-centred health assessment, which includes the components of **Box 14.1** and **Box 14.2** for conducting a health assessment.

See **Concept map 14.11** to further explore Rosa's initial care in the emergency department.

14.13 PLANNING CARE FOR CHOLELITHIASIS

The planning of person-centred care for a patient with cholelithiasis will have the goals of:
- relieving pain
- removing gallstones
- nutrition.

Rosa is a partner in the planning of her care.
Box 14.5 indicates the areas that are targeted in the planning stage of gallstones care.

BOX 14.5 PLANNING CARE FOR CHOLELITHIASIS

- Medication
- Fluids
- Endoscopic retrograde cholangiopancreatography (ERCP)
- Pain assessment and management
- Health education and home care

PHx

Rosa is a 58-year-old female. She has presented to emergency department with excruciating pain in her upper right side. Rosa is a mother of 3 adult children. She is overweight, and has tried to reduce her weight but she states she enjoys cooking and eating with the family. She is not taking medications and has no allergies. She does enjoy gardening and her family history does not indicate cardiovascular disease.

ASSESSMENT

Primary survey

A: Clear

B: RR 25. Breath sounds clear

C: HR 100 bpm, BP 160/90 mmHg

D: Alert and orientated, pain scale 8/10

E: 36.9 °C

F: HNPU, NBM

G: BGL 11.2 mmol/L

Cues

1 As part of the secondary survey

What is the relationship between the upper right abdominal pain and biliary function?

2 What are the indicators in Rosa's past history for gall bladder disease?

3 What tests should be obtained to confirm a diagnosis of gallstones (cholelithiasis)?

CONCEPT MAP 14.11 Nursing assessment for Rosa

Concept map 14.12 outlines a plan for Rosa's care.

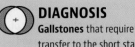

DIAGNOSIS

Gallstones that require transfer to the short stay unit attached to the emergency department.

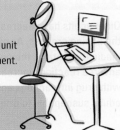

PLANNING

☑ Position: high Fowlers

☑ Vital signs

☑ Pain assessment and management

☑ IV fluid

☑ Fluid balance chart

☑ NBM

☑ Medication – antiemetic, analgesics, antispasmodics

☑ Endoscopic retrograde cholangiopancreatography (ERCP)

☑ Write a Nursing Prioritisation Planner

Health education and home care:

☑ Weight loss and small meals

CONCEPT MAP 14.12 Diagnosis and planning for Rosa

14.14 NURSING INTERVENTIONS TO SUPPORT HEALTH CARE FOR CHOLELITHIASIS

Nursing interventions are implemented as part of person-centred care to address the signs and symptoms of gallstones. Medication therapy is an essential component of the interventions required for Rosa, and the medications include an antiemetic, analgesic and an antispasmodic (Broyles et al., 2023).

Concept map 14.13 explores Rosa's journey in the emergency department and the attached short stay unit.

What further assessments should be initiated

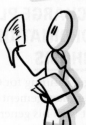

INTERVENTIONS

1 Positioning – high Fowlers

2 Vital signs – every 2 hours, then 4 hourly overnight

3 Pain scale hourly

4 IV therapy

5 Fluid balance chart

6 NBM and mouth care

7 Medication – ondansetron, morphine and atropine

8 Prepare for ERCP next day.

Health education and home care:

• Weight loss

• Low fat small meals

CONCEPT MAP 14.13 Nursing interventions for Rosa

14.15 EVALUATION OF CARE FOR CHOLELITHIASIS

As part of the further assessment of Rosa's presentation, **Concept map 14.14** asks further questions in relation to Rosa's care.

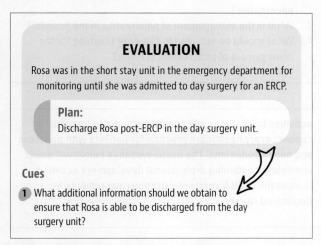

EVALUATION

Rosa was in the short stay unit in the emergency department for monitoring until she was admitted to day surgery for an ERCP.

Plan:
Discharge Rosa post-ERCP in the day surgery unit.

Cues

1 What additional information should we obtain to ensure that Rosa is able to be discharged from the day surgery unit?

CONCEPT MAP 14.14 Evaluation and planning for Rosa

14.16 DISCHARGE PLANNING AND COORDINATION OF CARE FOR CHOLELITHIASIS

Rosa's ongoing short inpatient stay and discharge planning are important components of the care trajectory (see **Concept map 14.15**).

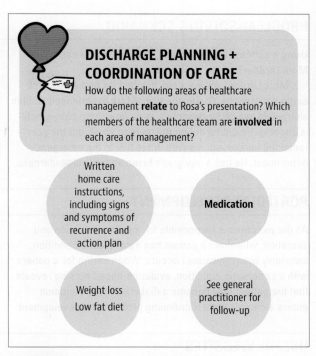

DISCHARGE PLANNING + COORDINATION OF CARE

How do the following areas of healthcare management **relate** to Rosa's presentation? Which members of the healthcare team are **involved** in each area of management?

Written home care instructions, including signs and symptoms of recurrence and action plan

Medication

Weight loss
Low fat diet

See general practitioner for follow-up

CONCEPT MAP 14.15 Discharge planning and coordination of care for Rosa

SUMMARY

The liver, pancreas and biliary tract are essential organs that enable individuals to provide themselves with self-care. When providing care to a person who has decreased liver, pancreas and biliary function, the nurse has the additional challenge of providing care to an individual whose activity levels are curtailed and self-care is challenged due to digestion dysfunction.

CLINICAL SKILLS IN LIVER, PANCREAS AND BILIARY HEALTH

The following clinical skills are required when managing a person with liver, pancreas and biliary conditions; consult your Clinical Skills resources, such as Tollefson and Hillman (2022), *Clinical Psychomotor Skills* (8th ed.).

- Temperature, pulse and respiration measurement
- Blood pressure measurement
- Monitoring pulse oximetry
- Pain assessment

- Focused gastrointestinal health history and abdominal physical assessment
- Height, weight and waist circumference measurements
- Nasogastric tube insertion
- Oral medication
- Intravenous medication administration
- Oxygen therapy via nasal cannula or various masks

PROBLEM-SOLVING SCENARIO

Using a concept map approach, how would you assist Mark Lardner?

Mark Lardner, 45 years old, has had his first episode of acute pancreatitis. During the night Mark experienced sudden sharp pain, which he describes as severe sharp pain which is ongoing. He got up during the night to vomit, but the pain remained unrelieved. His wife drove him to the emergency department. He has a low grade fever, abdominal tenderness with muscle guarding, and decreased bowel sounds. Serum amylase was high and abdominal CT confirmed pancreatitis.

1   What are the causes of pancreatitis?
2   What are the associated signs and symptoms of pancreatitis?
3   What is the management of pancreatitis in the hospital?
4   What should be included in self-care teaching for the management of pancreatitis at home?

PORTFOLIO DEVELOPMENT

As the pancreas is responsible for insulin production and secretion, whenever a patient has a pancreatic condition, invariably hyperglycaemia occurs. When caring for a patient with a pancreatic condition, evidence-based nursing reveals that the patient may become a diabetic if their condition enters a chronic state. Continuing professional development activities for diabetes will enable the nurse to provide contemporary healthcare practice for patients with pancreas and biliary conditions. The useful websites below will assist in meeting continuing professional development activities to meet the NMBA yearly registration requirements for a Registered Nurse.

USEFUL WEBSITES

The Registered Nurse Standards for Practice consist of seven crucial standards that all nurses must follow. Download and review the standards at the following link. https://www.nursingmidwiferyboard.gov.au/Codes-Guidelines-Statements/Professional-standards/registered-nurse-standards-for-practice.aspx

Australian Diabetes Society https://www.diabetessociety.com.au/

Gastroenterology Society of Australia https://www.gesa.org.au

Nursing and Midwifery Board of Australia, Decision-making framework for nursing and midwifery (2020) https://www.nursingmidwiferyboard.gov.au/codes-guidelines-statements/frameworks.aspx

REFERENCES AND FURTHER READING

Australian Institute of Health and Welfare (AIHW). (2015). *Leading cause of premature mortality in Australia fact sheet: liver disease.* Cat. no. PHE 199. Canberra: AIHW.

Broyles, B., Reiss, B., Evans, M., Pleunik, S., Page, R., & Badoer, E. (2023). *Pharmacology in nursing* (4th ANZ ed.). Cengage Learning Australia.

Bufton, S. (2016). The treatment of hepatitis. *Nursing in Practice.* https://www.nursinginpractice.com/clinical/vaccinations-and-infections/travel-health/the-treatment-of-hepatitis

Chaney, A. (2019). Caring for patients with chronic hepatitis C infection. *Nursing, 49*(3), 36–42. DOI: 10.1097/01.NURSE.0000553271.39804.a4

Clements, A., & Greenslade, L. (2014). Nursing care for end-stage liver disease. *Nursing Times, 10*(29), 16–19.

DeLaune, S., Ladner, P., McTier, L., Tollefson, J., & Lawrence, J. (2024). *Fundamentals of nursing* (3rd ed.). Cengage Learning Australia.

Fabrellas, N., Carol, M., Palacio, E., Aban, M., Lanzilliotti, T., Nicolao, G., Chiappa, M. T., Esnault, V., Graf-Dirmeier, S., Helder, J., Gossard, A., Lopez, M., Cervera, M., & Dols, L. (2020). Nursing care of patients with cirrhosis: The LiverHope nursing project. *Hepatology, 71*(3), 1106–1116. DOI: 10.1002/hep.31117

Johnstone, C. (2018). Pathophysiology and nursing management of acute pancreatitis. *Nursing Standard, 33*(4). DOI: 10.7748/ns.2018.e11179

Krenzer, M. (2016). Understanding acute pancreatitis. *Nursing, 46*(8), 34–40. DOI: 10.1097/01.NURSE.0000484959.78110.98

Lindseth, G., & Denny, D. (2014). Patients' experiences with cholecystitis and a cholecystectomy. *Gastroenterology Nursing, 37*(6), 407–414. DOI:10.1097/SGA.0000000000000072

Neighbors, M., & Tannehill-Jones, R. (2023). *Human diseases* (6th ed.). Cengage.

Tollefson, J., & Hillman, E. (2022). *Clinical psychomotor skills: Assessment tools for nurses* (8th ed.). Cengage Learning Australia.

15.1 ASSESSMENT OF
MUSCULOSKELETAL PROBLEMS
15.2 ASSESSMENT FOR FRACTURE

CHAPTER 15

MUSCULOSKELETAL SYSTEM

Musculoskeletal conditions are conditions that affect the bones, muscles and/or connective tissues. The most common condition in Australia is arthritis – with around 7 million people reporting arthritis in 2017–2018.

The impacting factor of arthritis is that one in five Australians report very high or high levels of psychological distress associated with severe to moderate pain. The impact of musculoskeletal conditions is not just the joint itself or ability to move, but many facets of daily life. Another significant impact, both financially and psychologically, for Australians is that of back pain. Many Australians report ongoing distress and pain associated with chronic back pain and subsequent impact on quality of life (Australian Institute of Health and Welfare [AIHW], 2022).

LEARNING OBJECTIVES

After reading this chapter, you should have an understanding of the:
1. assessment required for a person with a musculoskeletal condition
2. prioritisation of key components in the development of plans of care for people presenting with the musculoskeletal injuries of:
   – fracture
   – back pain
3. prioritised and targeted nursing interventions required to promote recovery or prevent further deterioration of people presenting with fractures or back pain
4. evaluation phase and how the prioritised and targeted nursing interventions inform further assessment, planning and collaboration with the healthcare team
5. discharge planning and coordination of care required in preparing the person for discharge and subsequent continuity of care between the person and their healthcare providers.

INTRODUCTION

Musculoskeletal conditions or problems are an incredibly common occurrence and they are also a common source of both disability and pain. Not all conditions are related to trauma, and many are degenerative conditions such as osteoporosis, bone cancer, metabolic bone diseases and muscular dystrophy. The nursing care and management of any person with an acute or chronic (or a mixture of both) musculoskeletal conditions is absolutely individual and reliant upon their response to any interventions (AIHW, 2022; Brown et al., 2019; Craft & Gordon, 2019; Waugh & Grant, 2023).

The main function of our musculoskeletal system is to support, protect and ensure movement. Other factors it is responsible for are the storage of minerals and blood cell production (in the bone marrow). Bones are our 'framework' and provide protection to vital organs; for example, the skull encases our brain and the sternum covers the heart and is one of the most difficult bones to break (Waugh & Grant, 2023). Our bones lead to joints and connective tissue such as cartilage, ligaments, tendons, fascia, bursae and muscle. As we age, there is degeneration of joints and loss of strength, leading to the increased risk of falling, and slower recovery to any such fall or injury (Brown et al., 2019).

The most common cause of injury to the musculoskeletal system is trauma/traumatic injury. Potential injuries are:
- fracture
- dislocation
- soft-tissue injury.

The impact of traumatic events is not just the initial pain, but the ongoing disability, loss of income and ability to live well. In all age groups in Australia and New Zealand, accidents are the fourth highest causative factor in death – with heart disease, cancer and strokes being the top three. Falls are one of the leading causes of hospitalisation in Australia, with falls occurring in hospital also contributing to this statistic (AIHW, 2022; Brown et al., 2019).

15.1 ASSESSMENT OF MUSCULOSKELETAL PROBLEMS

See **Box 15.1** for health assessment data collection areas.

BOX 15.1   SUBJECTIVE ASSESSMENT

- ➤ Past history of illness and injury
- ➤ Family history
- ➤ Medications
- ➤ Surgery

Functional health patterns
  - – Health perception and management
  - – Nutritional and metabolic
  - – Elimination
  - – Activity and exercise
  - – Sleep and rest
  - – Cognitive and perceptual
  - – Self-perception and concept
  - – Role relationship
  - – Sexuality and reproductive
  - – Coping and stress
  - – Values and beliefs
- ➤ Risk calculation

Box 15.2 assists the nurse in the physical assessment for musculoskeletal problems.

BOX 15.2   PHYSICAL ASSESSMENT

- ➤ Glasgow Coma Scale (GCS), including pupillary assessment
- ➤ Vital signs
- ➤ Perfusion to limbs (or any limbs in casts from fracture)
- ➤ Diagnostic investigations such as x-ray or CT
- ➤ Blood tests such as full blood count
- ➤ Blood glucose level (BGL)
- ➤ Electrocardiogram
- ➤ Pain assessment
- ➤ Neurovascular assessment

15.2 ASSESSMENT FOR FRACTURE

Presentation

Michael, a 15-year-old male, was admitted to the surgical short stay unit after a fall from an electric scooter at approx. 20 km/hr. Michael sustained a FOOSH (fall on outstretched hand) resulting in a distal radial fracture to his right arm. He has been hospitalised overnight for monitoring post-sedation to a closed reduction. Post-sedation, Michael will have a POP cast put in place.

Concept map 15.1 further explores Michael's admission.

EVIDENCE-BASED PRACTICE

Pain control/management in the emergency presentation

There are over 7 million reported presentations to emergency departments (EDs) annually, with more than 75 per cent of these presentations related to pain. Pain management is not always adequatly addressed within the ED, and as such, the National Health and Medical Research Council (NHMRC) has developed acute pain guidelines for presentations (common) to EDs. The guidelines aim to improve pain management based on best practice, formulate recommendations to ensure consistency across Australia and to evaluate and inform future ED care improvements.

The goals for analgesia in fractures and dislocation are:

1 immobilisation of the affected site, ice and elevation (these are all effective in provision of analgesia)

2 anticipation of procedures where movement is required such as x-ray and ensure adequate analgesic cover is given.

For less severe pain, commence with paracetamol 1 g orally 4 hourly PRN with or without oxycodone 5 mg immediate release 4–6 hourly PRN (National Institute of Clinical Studies, 2011).

The manual provides an excellent insight into many presenting conditions for musculoskeletal causes, and can be accessed here: https://www.cesphn.org.au/images/Emergency_acute_pain_management_manual-1.pdf

PHx

Michael, a **15-year-old male** was admitted via the emergency department with a **distal radial fracture** following a fall at speed (20 km/hr).
NKDA
Nil previous medical or surgical history
Nil medications
Weight: 65 kg

 ASSESSMENT

Primary survey
A: Patent
B: RR 14
C: CRT <3 sec to affected limb
D: Alert
E: T 36.9 °C
F: IVF 65 ml/hr, HPU
G: BGL 6.9 mmol/L

Secondary survey
CNS: E 4 V 5 M 6 = 15
PEARLA 3 mm

PAIN: C/o to right wrist, 4/10 (easing)
CVS: HR 90 bpm, BP 110/65 mmHg, cap refill, < 3 sec to affected limb. Emergency/Ambulance trauma splint in situ
T: 36.9 °C
RESP: RR 14, patent airway – spontaneous breathing, SpO$_2$ 99%
GIT (Input): IVF 65 mL/hr

RENAL (Output): Voided via bottle – no sediment, straw coloured
SKIN/INTEG: Centrally and peripherally well perfused. Pulses present to right radial and brachial. Deformity to right wrist.
MUSCULOSKELETAL (Mobility): RIB – has been administered methoxyflurane by QAS

Cues

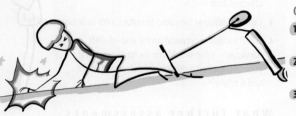

1 What are your priorities with this patient?
2 What is the significance of the deformity?
3 What is the relationship between the FOOSH and the distal fracture?
4 What are some concerns in mobility related to the medication administered by QAS?
5 How frequently would you assess pain levels?
6 What investigative or diagnostic procedures do you think would be relevant for this patient?

CONCEPT MAP 15.1 Nursing assessment for Michael

15.3 PLANNING CARE FOR A FRACTURE

Planning for any musculoskeletal injury or condition will have the goals of:
- ensuring adequate analgesia
- assessing safety for mobilisation regardless of the mechanism of injury or pain.

Box 15.3 indicates the areas that are targeted in the planning stage of musculoskeletal assessment and nursing care.

BOX 15.3 PLANNING CARE FOR MUSCULOSKELETAL INJURY

- Physical activity
- Pain assessment and management
- Medication
- Monitor vital signs
- Neurovascular observations – paraesthesia, absence of sensation
- Reduced or absent pulses to affected extremity
- Restricted function – attending to ADLs as dominant hand is right
- Management of cast/splint or assistive devices

Musculoskeletal injuries can cause changes or alterations to the neurovascular status of the affected/injured extremity. In planning any care for your patient, ensure you are assessing the pulses relevant to the affected limb, in comparison to the other side, for strength, and then assess for colour, warmth, movement and sensation. All aspects here relate directly to the blood flow to the affected limb and are crucial in ensuring you are not 'missing' a significant deterioration in the patient's condition (Brown et al., 2019; Crisp & Taylor, 2021; DeLaune et al., 2024).

See **Concept Map 15.2** for an outline of Michael's care plan.

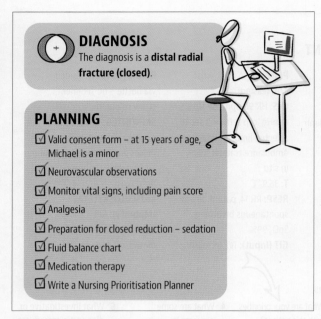

DIAGNOSIS
The diagnosis is a **distal radial fracture (closed)**.

PLANNING
- ☑ Valid consent form – at 15 years of age, Michael is a minor
- ☑ Neurovascular observations
- ☑ Monitor vital signs, including pain score
- ☑ Analgesia
- ☑ Preparation for closed reduction – sedation
- ☑ Fluid balance chart
- ☑ Medication therapy
- ☑ Write a Nursing Prioritisation Planner

CONCEPT MAP 15.2 Diagnosis and planning for Michael

15.4 NURSING INTERVENTIONS TO SUPPORT HEALTH CARE FOR A FRACTURE

Nursing interventions are implemented as part of person-centred care and ensure the safest care for the patient is undertaken. Interventions in musculoskeletal care will focus on the affected extremity or location and ensuring that pulses are assessed on both the affected and unaffected side for their strength (see example neurovascular observation chart in **Figure 15.1**). Pulses are documented or described as:

- strong
- diminished

- audible by Doppler only
- absent.

An absent or diminished pulse indicates vascular dysfunction – meaning that swelling from the injury is impacting upon the arterial flow to the affected limb. This is an urgent escalation or intervention in the patient's care (Brown et al., 2019). Nursing interventions for Michael are explored in **Concept map 15.3**.

INTERVENTIONS

1 Assess pain, neurovascular observations, level of consciousness and vital signs regularly

2 Neurovascular assessment of POP cast and affected limb

3 Limb elevation as tolerated to reduce limb oedema

4 ISBAR handover preparation for end-of-shift handover – what would you be handing over if your patient had a diminished pulse to his right radial artery?

What further assessments should be initiated

Cues

1 Why are neurovascular observations crucial to fractures?

2 What possible reasons could there be for the patient to report pain?

3 What has likely occurred for Michael's pulse to be diminished in the right radial artery?

CONCEPT MAP 15.3 Nursing interventions for Michael

SAFETY IN NURSING ⚠

NEUROVASCULAR OBSERVATIONS – POST-FRACTURE

The affected limb's colour (pink, pale, cyanotic) and temperature (hot, warm, cool, cold) is important and needs to be assessed regularly and compared to the unaffected limb to determine 'normal' or baseline for the person. Unexpected findings such as coolness or paleness can indicate arterial insufficiency potentially related to the fracture causing pressure or damage to the artery. Another assessment that the nurse will need to perform is

a capiliary refill test (CRT). This needs to be performed on the nailbed of both the affected and unaffected side, and colour should return to normal/original colour within three seconds – to yield a 'normal' finding, both sides should have the same capillary refill time.

Any concerns or alterations should be escalated through the appropriate measures in your facility. It is crucial to prioritise circulation in any injury, as the impact of loss of circulation can be irreversible. Refer to **Figure 15.1**.

TRAINING ONLY

Queensland Government

Neurovascular Observation Chart – Lower Limb

Facility: Couni Hospital

✓ Left | Right

Affix patient identification label here

URN: 45678

Family Name: Richards

Given Names: Jo

Address:

Date of Birth: 01 JAN 1970   Sex: ☐M ☐F ☐I

Date: xx/xx/xx

Time: 0800

Pain Score (Please tick: ☑ Numerical ☐ Faces Pain Scale – Revised ☐ FLACC) — scale 10, 9, 8, 7, 6, 5, 4, 3, 2, 1 — recorded: 4

Sensation
Peroneal Nerve (dorsal surface) · Tibial Nerve (plantar surface)

A = Absent
P = Pins and needles / fuzzy / numb
M = Moves to touch
N = Normal

Peroneal: A, P, M, N — recorded: N
Tibial: A, P, M, N — recorded: N

Movement
Peroneal Nerve (dorsiflexion) · Tibial Nerve (plantarflexion)

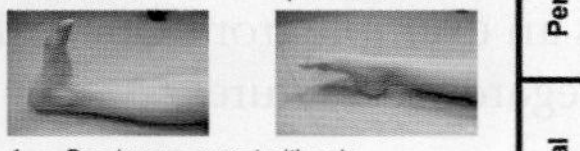

4 = Passive movement with pain
3 = Active movement with pain
2 = Passive movement without pain
1 = Active movement without pain

Peroneal: 4, 3, 2, 1 — recorded: 2
Tibial: 4, 3, 2, 1 — recorded: 2

Pulses
A = Absent
W = Weak
S = Strong

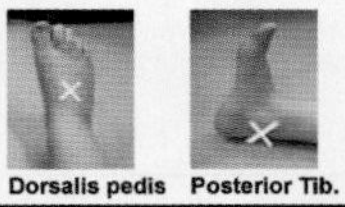
Dorsalis pedis
Posterior Tib.

D.P: A, W, S — recorded: S
P.T: A, W, S — recorded: S

Capillary Refill — 4 = 4+ sec; 3 = 3 sec; 2 = < 2 sec — recorded: 2

Warmth — Cold, Cool, Hot, Warm — recorded: Warm

Colour — Dusky, Pale, Pink — recorded: Pink

Swelling — L = Large; M = Moderate; S = Small; N = Nil — recorded: S

Ooze — L = Large; M = Moderate; S = Small; N = Nil — recorded: N

Date	Time	Prescribed alteration to parameters	Signature	Designation
xx/xx/xx	0800hrs	Nil	Mlie	MO

INSTRUCTIONS FOR USE: Refer to CHS NS 00253 Considerations for Paediatric Observations for instructions.

Source: All images property of Lady Cilento Children's Hospital, Queensland Health.

Page 1 of 2

DO NOT WRITE IN THIS BINDING MARGIN

v1.00 - 06/2015 Mat. No.: 10317311

SW376

NEUROVASCULAR OBSERVATION CHART – LOWER LIMB

FIGURE 15.1 Example of a neurovascular observation chart

SOURCE: STATE OF QUEENSLAND (QUEENSLAND HEALTH)

15.5 EVALUATION OF CARE FOR A FRACTURE

As part of the further assessment of Michael's presentation, **Concept map 15.4** asks further questions in relation to his management.

Priorities of care for the patient with a fracture or injury relate to pain management and neurovascular compromise due to oedema, swelling and ongoing insufficiency from the trauma (Brown et al., 2019).

15.6 DISCHARGE PLANNING AND COORDINATION OF CARE FOR A FRACTURE

The nature of any musculoskeletal injury, condition or 'illness' is going to differ depending upon the person. The impact of the condition will vary – and this is due to the very nature of the traumatic event or fall. Nurses are the conduit at the bedside between the patient and all the allied and multidisciplinary healthcare staff. If the patient has injured their dominant hand, for instance, nurses will work with the patient and other healthcare staff to ensure they can attend to their ADLs even using modified conditions. To put it bluntly, nurses will make sure that the person can wipe their bum.

See further information for Michael's discharge planning in **Concept map 15.5**.

Figure 15.2 is an example from Queensland Health of a factsheet regarding fractures.

EVALUATION

The medical team have been notified of Michael's **decreased sensation** and **increased pain** to his right wrist.

Plan:
Michael is to have a closed reduction, under sedation, and then a plaster of paris (POP) applied in the ED. He will be admitted to the short stay surgical unit overnight due to age and sedation.

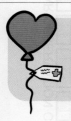

Cues

1. What interventions need to be considered now for Michael?

2. What would your assessment entail post sedation for Michael?

3. Michael is prescribed ketamine for the sedation (one medication of many) but you have not administered this before. What would you need to ensure and understand prior to administration?

CONCEPT MAP 15.4 Evaluation and planning for Michael

DISCHARGE PLANNING + COORDINATION OF CARE

How do the following areas of healthcare management **relate** to Michael's presentation? Which members of the healthcare team are **involved** in each area of management?

   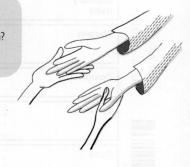

Fractured distal radius

Medication/analgesia

Follow-up review with fracture clinic (appointment made prior to discharge)

Education handout for fractures

Report any increase in pain

Report any decrease in sensation to affected limb

Occupational therapist referral for aids for dominant hand

Post sedation observation

Instructions to parents/care giver for any side effects (ketamine-induced nightmares)

Superficial bruising and abrasions

Keeping site clean

Education about signs of localised infection

Reporting any increase in pain

CONCEPT MAP 15.5 Discharge planning and coordination of care for Michael

Clinical Excellence Division

Queensland Health

Fracture
Emergency Department factsheets

What is a fracture?

A fracture is a medical term for a broken bone. A bone usually breaks when too much force is exerted against it, often during a fall or common activities such as sport. Given time and the right care, the bone heals itself.

Treatment

In the emergency department, you may have had x-rays to check for a fracture. In most instances, a plaster (cast) will be applied to hold the broken bone/s in place while the bone heals. It is important for your recovery that you keep the plaster in good condition.

Injured limbs often swell 24-48 hours after the injury and a normal plaster may become too tight and need to be 'split' or cut off. Sometimes a half plaster or 'back slab' is applied. This requires extra care as it only goes halfway around the affected limb, and does not offer as much protection as a full plaster.

What to expect

- Fractures can be painful. The pain can be extreme at the beginning but it will ease once the plaster is on and the fractured limb is supported and rested. The pain will settle even further over the next few weeks.
- Simple painkillers, such as paracetamol, are often needed. Follow the instructions on the packet. You may be prescribed stronger painkillers. Take them as needed and follow the instructions on the packet. Some medications may make you drowsy; if so do not drive or operate machinery.
- The plaster may be itchy for a few days, but this should ease.
- After the plaster is removed, there may be some stiffness and weakness in the limb. This should improve as you go about your normal activities.

- Sometimes physiotherapy is needed to help recovery.
- The bone will continue to recover, even after the plaster is removed. You need to take extra care and precautions to not re-injure the recovering bone, especially for the next month.
- You may feel a lump at the site of the fracture. This is the new bone, which will eventually take on the shape of your original bone.

Caring for the fracture

The plaster will support and protect the bone while the fracture heals. It can sometimes cause problems with blood flow, especially in the first couple of days. The following advice may help to avoid problems.

- Frequently move or wiggle the fingers (in the case of an upper limb plaster) or toes (for lower limb plaster).
- Keep the plaster raised to prevent swelling, especially for the first 48 hours (for example, use a sling to keep an arm raised or place pillows under your leg).

Caring for the plaster

It is important that you look after your plaster cast.

- Rest for a couple of days after the plaster is applied to allow it to set completely. Don't rest the plaster on anything immediately after having it applied.
- Keep the plaster dry. When having a shower or bath, put a plastic bag over the plaster and seal it with a rubber band. Try to keep the limb away from water, to prevent any leaking in. Keep the plaster out of the rain.
- Do not stick objects down the plaster, as this may damage the skin and cause infection.
- Do not cut or interfere with the cast.

Queensland
Government

FIGURE 15.2 Fracture factsheet

- Do not walk on a plaster. Use crutches as directed.
- Do not lift anything or drive until the fracture is healed.
- Do not smoke as this slows the healing process.

Follow-up

You may be asked to visit a specialist fracture clinic about one week after your injury so the fracture can be checked (with x-rays). If this happens, make sure you attend this appointment.

If there are any problems with the fracture or the way it is healing, you may be referred to an orthopaedic surgeon (specialist bone doctor). It is important that you keep this appointment and take your x-rays with you if possible.

On average, a plaster stays on for about six weeks. This may be longer or shorter, depending on your age, general health and the type of fracture.

You may need to see a physiotherapist for exercises to help with muscle strength, joint mobility and balance. These exercises will help you return safely to normal activities.

Report immediately to GP or local hospital in the below situations:

- marked swelling
- marked color change to fingers/ toes
- numbness, pins and needles or altered sensation
- inability to move fingers/ toes
- continuous pressure at one point beneath the cast
- if cast gets wet.

Seeking help

In a medical emergency, go to the nearest hospital emergency department or call an ambulance (dial 000).

For other medical problems see your local doctor or health-care professional.

13 HEALTH (13 43 25 84) provides health information, referral and teletriage services to the public in all parts of Queensland and is available 24 hours a day, 7 days a week, 365 days a year for the cost of a local call*.

*Calls from mobile phones may be charged at a higher rate. Please check with your telephone service provider

Disclaimer: This health information is for general education purposes only. Please consult with your doctor or other health professional to make sure this information is right for you.

The design and general content of this factsheet are reproduced with the permission of the Victorian Minister for Health, from factsheets that are Copyright © the State of Victoria. Unauthorised reproduction and other uses comprised in the copyright are prohibited without permission.

Fracture - 2-

FIGURE 15.2 Fracture factsheet (continued)

15.7 ASSESSMENT FOR BACK PAIN

Back problems or pain are a range of conditions related to the bones, joints and connective tissue (including muscles and nerves) of the back. These conditions include pain in the lower, middle and upper back, tingling, numbness and weakness in legs, degeneration of spine from wear and tear on the joints, neck pain or stiff neck from disc degeneration. A host of symptoms can result from a range of injuries or conditions and have significant impact upon the person. It is reported that pain is the most common symptom, with 16 per cent of Australians reporting back problems. It is further estimated that 70–90 per cent of the population will suffer from lower back pain at some point in their life (AIHW, 2019).

Presentation

Rebecca Ferguson is a 59-year-old-female who has presented post a fall, with a background of chronic back pain. She has fallen onto her left side and is complaining of pain in her lower back and shoulder.

Concept map 15.6 further explores Rebecca's admission.

 PHx

Rebecca, a 59-year-old female, has **chronic back pain** and has fallen in the garden today on a slippery tile. She has fallen onto her left side and is complaining of pain to her lower back, and shoulder. Her 'normal' back pain is in her cervical and thoracic region from a motor vehicle accident 25 years ago.

PMHx, #T9–11 – MVA 25 years ago.

Meds – amitriptyline 25 mg, targin 40/10 BD, telmisarten 40 mg, aspirin 100 mg. NKDA.

Smokes 15 cigs/day

ETOH – 2 wines/day

 ASSESSMENT

Primary survey

A: Patent
B: RR 20
C: Warm
D: Alert
E: T 36.2 °C
F: HNPU nil in
G: BGL 6.5 mmol/L

Secondary survey

CNS: E 4 V 5 M 6 = 15 PEARL 4 mm
PAIN: C/o pain to mid lower back, centralised, pain also in her right shoulder from fall. Rating pain as 7/10.

Has taken her a.m. dose of targin (it is now 1400 hours)

CVS: HR 82 bpm, regular. BP 140/65 mmHg. Centrally and peripherally warm, cap refill <3 sec. T 36.2 °C

RESP: RR 20, chest on auscultation clear throughout R=L. Nil cough. SpO$_2$ 98% RA

GIT: BS audible in all quadrants. BGL 6.5 mmol/L

RENAL (output): HNPU as yet

SKIN/INTEG: Abrasions to right shoulder, nil other breaks in integument

MUSCULOSKELETAL (mobility): Await physio review due to pain

Cues

1. What are your priorities with this patient?

2. What is the concern regarding analgesia here?

3. What does targin do? Will it be safe to administer this patient further analgesia?

4. What are the concerns for this patient with acute on chronic pain?

5. How could you assess her right shoulder for pain? Would you also perform neurovascular observations?

6. What investigative or diagnostic procedures do you think would be relevant for this patient?

CONCEPT MAP 15.6 Nursing assessment for Rebecca

15.8 PLANNING CARE FOR BACK PAIN

Planning for any musculoskeletal injury or condition, including back pain, will have the goals of:

■ ensuring adequate analgesia
■ assessing safety for mobilisation regardless of the mechanism of injury or pain.

Refer back to **Box 15.3** for the areas that are targeted in the planning stage of musculoskeletal assessment and nursing care.

See **Concept map 15.7** for an outline of Rebecca's care plan.

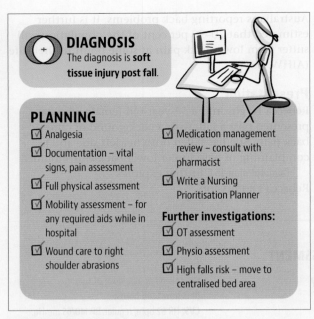

DIAGNOSIS
The diagnosis is **soft tissue injury post fall**.

PLANNING
- ☑ Analgesia
- ☑ Documentation – vital signs, pain assessment
- ☑ Full physical assessment
- ☑ Mobility assessment – for any required aids while in hospital
- ☑ Wound care to right shoulder abrasions
- ☑ Medication management review – consult with pharmacist
- ☑ Write a Nursing Prioritisation Planner

Further investigations:
- ☑ OT assessment
- ☑ Physio assessment
- ☑ High falls risk – move to centralised bed area

CONCEPT MAP 15.7 Diagnosis and planning for Rebecca

15.9 NURSING INTERVENTIONS TO SUPPORT HEALTH CARE FOR BACK PAIN

Nursing interventions for Rebecca are explored in Concept map 15.8.

INTERVENTIONS
1. Assess pain, abrasions and neurovascular observations to affected limb. Assess for falls risk in hospital.
2. Referral to pain specialist
3. Establish acute on chronic pain management in collaboration with healthcare team
4. ISBAR handover preparation for end-of-shift handover – what would you be handing over if your patient was a high falls risk?

What further assessments should be initiated

Cues
1. What further questions or information would you like to know from the patient?
2. What is the potential impact on the patient's mobility if she already has chronic back pain in her upper back, and now has pain in her lower back?
3. What frequency would you assess her pain?

CONCEPT MAP 15.8 Nursing interventions for Rebecca

15.10 EVALUATION OF CARE FOR BACK PAIN

As part of the further assessment of Rebecca's presentation, **Concept map 15.9** asks further questions in relation to her management.

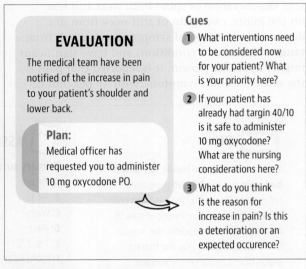

EVALUATION
The medical team have been notified of the increase in pain to your patient's shoulder and lower back.

Plan:
Medical officer has requested you to administer 10 mg oxycodone PO.

Cues
1. What interventions need to be considered now for your patient? What is your priority here?
2. If your patient has already had targin 40/10 is it safe to administer 10 mg oxycodone? What are the nursing considerations here?
3. What do you think is the reason for increase in pain? Is this a deterioration or an expected occurence?

CONCEPT MAP 15.9 Evaluation and planning for Rebecca

15.11 DISCHARGE PLANNING AND COORDINATION OF CARE FOR BACK PAIN

See further information for Rebecca's discharge planning in **Concept Map 15.10**.

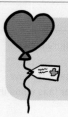

DISCHARGE PLANNING + COORDINATION OF CARE

How do the following areas of healthcare management **relate** to the patient presentation? Which members of the healthcare team are **involved** in each area of management?

Soft tissue injury – right shoulder and lumbar spine	Mobility post-fall and wound care	Pain management
Management and education to patient on non-pharmaceutical analgesia such as change of position, movement, etc.	Gait assessment – physiotherapist	Patient education and health promotion regarding pain management and activity
Ongoing review of chronic pain management with current pain medication	Management of wound – keep abrasions clean and dry, for review by GP in one week	Review by chronic pain team to establish analgesia for old injury
Follow up with GP in one week		Review by physiotherapist for ongoing management of acute pain

CONCEPT MAP 15.10 Discharge planning and coordination of care for Rebecca

REFLECTIVE PRACTICE

Pain assessment

Jenson is a 30-year-old male who has chronic back pain. He has been hospitalised for the same condition several times this year and has been admitted to the medical ward for analgesia and further investigation. Jenson describes the pain as constant, burning and radiating down his spine to his lower back. He initially injured his back in an accident at work six years ago. He has been unable to work since this time and is considerably less able to attend to his ADLs and function due to 'the intense pain that never goes away even when I sleep'.

You have just commenced your shift and have received bedside handover for Jenson. As you return to the nurses' station, the nurse who has just handed over states 'he is just a bloody whinger, he needs to just get over it, it happened six years ago, look at all the meds he is on and he is still whinging about pain! I don't believe he has pain at all, he is just seeking now'.

Questions

1 Is this comment appropriate for patient care? Is this in accordance with NMBA standards?
2 What could you do to educate this nurse on chronic pain?

SUMMARY

The musculoskeletal system is often an underrated one until it is injured. Fractures, trauma and chronic conditions significantly alter the ability to mobilise, protect and function. The impact on ADLs for back pain is significant, and the impact on quality of life for chronic back pain even more so.

Nursing assessment will vary for each patient and their specific needs and impact of the condition. Recovery also will differ and is reliant upon underlying conditions, past trauma/fractures and response to treatment.

CLINICAL SKILLS IN MUSCULOSKELETAL HEALTH

The following clinical skills are required when managing a person with musculoskeletal conditions; consult your Clinical Skills resources, such as Tollefson and Hillman (2022), *Clinical Psychomotor Skills* (8th ed.).

- Pain assessment
- Physical assessment
- Height, weight and waist circumference
- Focused musculoskeletal health history and physical assessment and range-of-motion exercises

PROBLEM-SOLVING SCENARIO

Using a concept map approach, how would you assist Tiffany?

Tiffany is a 78-year-old female who is hospitalised for a surgical procedure. Tiffany has dementia and has been admitted from a residential aged care facility (RACF). Tiffany normally wanders safely around her RACF, but in hospital is unable to do so due to the surgery. How could you mitigate

risk factors for Tiffany in relation to a fall or an injury while in hospital?

1   With Tiffany's dementia and wandering behaviours, how can you ensure her safety and reduce risk for falls while in hospital? What role would you play here?

2   What nursing considerations would you have for Tiffany?

PORTFOLIO DEVELOPMENT

The useful websites below will assist in meeting continuing professional development activities to meet the NMBA yearly registration requirements for a Registered Nurse.

Musculoskeletal Australia is an organisation that caters to patients and their families. There is a great deal of information on their website that will increase your awareness and understanding of the impact of these conditions on a person. https://msk.org.au

The Musculoskeletal Network is an initiative of the New South Wales government and brings together clinicians, health managers and consumers to review the healthcare experiences and outcomes for people with musculoskeletal conditions. https://aci.health.nsw.gov.au/networks/musculoskeletal/about

USEFUL WEBSITES

The Registered Nurse Standards for Practice consist of seven crucial standards that all nurses must follow. Download and review the standards at the following link. https://www.nursingmidwiferyboard.gov.au/Codes-Guidelines-Statements/Professional-standards/registered-nurse-standards-for-practice.aspx

Emergency Care Acute Pain Management Manual
Compiled by the NHMRC, Australian College of Emergency Medicine and College of Emergency Nurses Australia this is a manual to address pain management in the ED. https://www.cesphn.org.au/images/Emergency_acute_pain_management_manual-1.pdf

Pain Australia
Pain Australia is Australia's leading pain advocacy body working to improve patient quality of life for people living with pain, their family, and carers, and to minimise the social and economic burden of pain. https://www.painaustralia.org.au

Australia and New Zealand Orthopaedic Nurses Association
AONA is a network for communication and education for orthopaedic nurses across Australia and New Zealand. http://www.connmo.org.au/index.php/9-members/22-australian-new-zealand-orthopaedic-nurses-association

REFERENCES AND FURTHER READING

Australian Institute of Health and Welfare (AIHW). (2019). *Back problems*. https://www.aihw.gov.au/getmedia/0d9f8959-2a1c-4c99-8c7e-0c8a878f4d6c/Back%20problems.pdf.aspx?inline=true

Australian Institute of Health and Welfare (AIHW). (2022). *Chronic musculoskeletal conditions*. https://www.aihw.gov.au/reports-data/health-conditions-disability-deaths/chronic-musculoskeletal-conditions/overview

Brown, D., Edwards, H., Buckley, T., Aitken, R. L., Lewis, S. L., Bucher, L., McLean Heitkemper, M., Harding, M. M., Kwong, J., & Roberts, D. (2019). *Lewis's medical-surgical nursing ANZ* (5th ed.). Elsevier.

Craft, J., & Gordon, C. (2019). *Understanding pathophysiology* (3rd ed.). Elsevier Australia.

Crisp, J., & Taylor, C. (2021). *Potter and Perry's fundamentals of nursing* (4th ed.). Elsevier.

DeLaune, S., Ladner, P., McTier, L., Tollefson, J., & Lawrence, J. (2024). *Fundamentals of nursing* (3rd ed.). Cengage Learning Australia.

National Institute of Clinical Studies. (2011). *Emergency care – Acute pain management manual*.

Waugh, A., & Grant, A. (2023). *Ross & Wilson anatomy and physiology in health and illness* (14th ed.). Elsevier.

CHAPTER 16

FEMALE REPRODUCTIVE SYSTEM

Chlamydia is a sexually transmitted disease, and it is a notifiable communicable disease. Women in the 20–24 age group have the highest rate of chlamydia in Australia (Australian Institute of Health and Welfare [AIHW], 2023).

LEARNING OBJECTIVES

After reading this chapter, you should have an understanding of the:

1 assessment required for a woman with a female reproductive condition
2 prioritisation of key components in the development of plans of care for a woman with the female reproductive conditions of:
   – endometriosis
   – polycystic ovary syndrome
   – chlamydia
3 prioritised and targeted nursing interventions required to promote recovery or prevent further deterioration of people presenting with the female reproductive conditions of endometriosis, polycystic ovary syndrome and chlamydia
4 evaluation phase and how the prioritised and targeted nursing interventions inform further assessment of the person, planning of care and collaboration with the healthcare team
5 discharge planning and coordination of care required in preparing the person for discharge and subsequent continuity of care between the person and their healthcare providers.

INTRODUCTION

The female reproductive system includes external and internal structures. The genitalia consists of the mons pubis, labia, clitoris, urethral opening, vaginal opening and glands. Internally, there is the vagina, cervix, uterus, fallopian tubes and ovaries. Women with disorders of the female reproductive system experience disruption in their activity levels and decreased sense of wellbeing. Whether the condition is newly diagnosed or is long term and considered chronic in presentation, the concepts of woman-centred care is the same, with the goal of improving reproductive health so the woman can achieve the best possible quality of life that represents their situation.

Common problems include menstrual disorders, fistulas, reproductive tissue disorders (cysts, polyps, **endometriosis**, cervical cancer, ovarian cancer) and menopause.

16.1 ASSESSMENT OF FEMALE REPRODUCTIVE SYSTEM PROBLEMS

In the collecting of subjective data, previous and current person-reported information is important in the determination of female reproductive symptoms. See **Box 16.1** for the health assessment data collection areas.

BOX 16.1   SUBJECTIVE ASSESSMENT

- ➤ History of illness
- ➤ Past health history
- ➤ Family history
- ➤ Medications
- ➤ Surgery
- **Functional health patterns:**
  - – Health perception and management
  - – Nutritional and metabolic
  - – Elimination
  - – Activity and exercise
  - – Sleep and rest
  - – Cognitive and perceptual
  - – Self-perception and concept
  - – Role relationship
  - – Sexuality and reproductive
  - – Coping and stress
  - – Values and beliefs
- ➤ Risk calculation

The collection of objective data is informed by the subjective data and is highlighted in the physical assessment and results of diagnostic studies of the person (see **Box 16.2**). While a reproductive system assessment is the focus of the patient presentations in this chapter, other systems will also be assessed from the information collected in the health history.

BOX 16.2   OBJECTIVE ASSESSMENT

- ➤ Inspect and palpate breasts
- ➤ Inspect and palpate external genitalia
- ➤ Diagnostic tests – hormone studies – urine and blood, cultures and smears, cytological studies, mammography, ultrasound, biopsy, and computed tomography, magnetic resonance imaging, hysteroscopy, hysterosalpingogram, colposcopy, conisation, laparoscopy, dilation and curettage
- ➤ Other body systems as appropriate

16.2 ASSESSMENT FOR ENDOMETRIOSIS

The components of **Box 16.1** and **Box 16.2** are included in the assessment of a woman presenting with a reproductive system problem.

Presentation

Lee Jones is a 28-year-old receptionist who has attended the general practice clinic to work out why she has painful periods. The painful periods started when she was 17 years old, and the period pain has recently become so debilitating that she now needs to take time off from work.

Concept map 16.1 further explores Lee's initial care with the general practice nurse.

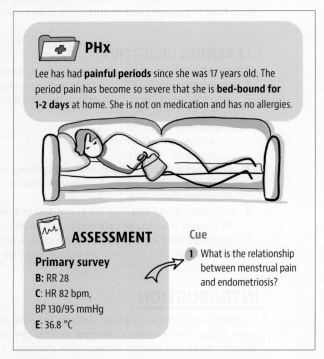

PHx

Lee has had **painful periods** since she was 17 years old. The period pain has become so severe that she is **bed-bound for 1-2 days** at home. She is not on medication and has no allergies.

ASSESSMENT

Primary survey
B: RR 28
C: HR 82 bpm,
BP 130/95 mmHg
E: 36.8 °C

Cue
1 What is the relationship between menstrual pain and endometriosis?

CONCEPT MAP 16.1 Nursing assessment for Lee

16.3 PLANNING CARE FOR ENDOMETRIOSIS

Planning for the nursing care for acute endometriosis has the goals of:
- pain management
- psychological support.

Lee is a partner in her care plan and contributes to her health care by following her plan of care and managing her condition in the home environment. **Box 16.3** lists the areas that are targeted in the planning stage of acute endometriosis management.

BOX 16.3   PLANNING CARE FOR ENDOMETRIOSIS

➤ Pain management
➤ Psychological support
➤ Tests
➤ Medication
➤ Self-care

Concept map 16.2 outlines a plan for Lee's care.

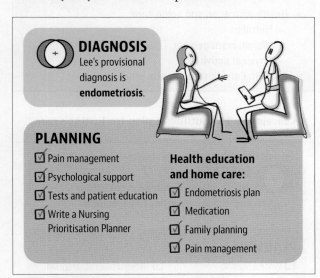

DIAGNOSIS

Lee's provisional diagnosis is **endometriosis**.

PLANNING

☑ Pain management
☑ Psychological support
☑ Tests and patient education
☑ Write a Nursing Prioritisation Planner

Health education and home care:

☑ Endometriosis plan
☑ Medication
☑ Family planning
☑ Pain management

CONCEPT MAP 16.2 Diagnosis and planning for Lee

16.4 NURSING INTERVENTIONS TO SUPPORT HEALTH CARE FOR ENDOMETRIOSIS

Nursing interventions are implemented as part of woman-centred care to reduce the presenting signs and symptoms of endometriosis.

Concept map 16.3 explores Lee's journey in the general practice before returning to her home.

INTERVENTIONS

Health education and home care:

Endometriosis plan – NSAIDs

What further assessments should be initiated

CONCEPT MAP 16.3 Nursing interventions for Lee

16.5 EVALUATION OF CARE FOR ENDOMETRIOSIS

As part of the further assessment of Lee's presentation, Concept map 16.4 asks further questions in relation to Lee's management.

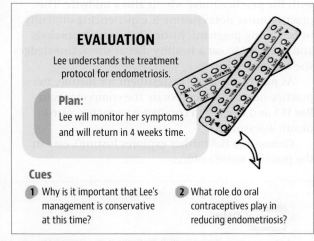

EVALUATION

Lee understands the treatment protocol for endometriosis.

Plan:
Lee will monitor her symptoms and will return in 4 weeks time.

Cues

1 Why is it important that Lee's management is conservative at this time?

2 What role do oral contraceptives play in reducing endometriosis?

CONCEPT MAP 16.4 Evaluation and planning for Lee

16.6 DISCHARGE PLANNING AND COORDINATION OF CARE FOR ENDOMETRIOSIS

Lee's endometriosis requires further management at home. Concept map 16.5 explores discharge planning and coordination of care for Lee.

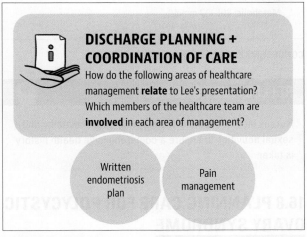

DISCHARGE PLANNING + COORDINATION OF CARE

How do the following areas of healthcare management **relate** to Lee's presentation? Which members of the healthcare team are **involved** in each area of management?

Written endometriosis plan

Pain management

CONCEPT MAP 16.5 Discharge planning and coordination of care for Lee

16.7 ASSESSMENT FOR POLYCYSTIC OVARY SYNDROME

Presentation

Justine Rebeiro is a 32-year-old woman who has presented to her general practice for an appointment with the practice nurse who is also a midwife. The practice nurse notes Justine is experiencing difficulty in becoming pregnant. Justine has irregular periods and has tried to eat a healthy diet as she acknowledges she is overweight.

As part of the health assessment for Justine, the practice nurse will incorporate the components in **Box 16.1** and **Box 16.2** to conduct a woman-centred health assessment.

Concept map 16.6 further explores Justine's care in the practice nurse's office.

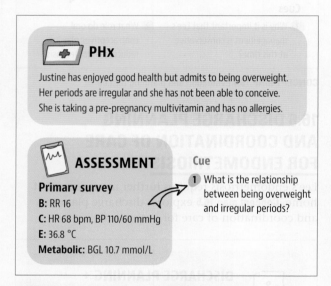

PHx

Justine has enjoyed good health but admits to being overweight. Her periods are irregular and she has not been able to conceive. She is taking a pre-pregnancy multivitamin and has no allergies.

ASSESSMENT

Primary survey
B: RR 16
C: HR 68 bpm, BP 110/60 mmHg
E: 36.8 °C
Metabolic: BGL 10.7 mmol/L

Cue

1 What is the relationship between being overweight and irregular periods?

CONCEPT MAP 16.6 Nursing assessment for Justine

REFLECTIVE PRACTICE

Nurses must feel comfortable asking about sexuality and sexual activities to ensure a comprehensive health history is taken.

16.8 PLANNING CARE FOR POLYCYSTIC OVARY SYNDROME

Planning person-centred care for a woman with polycystic ovary syndrome has the goals of:

- nutrition
- weight management
- exercise
- controlling blood glucose levels.

Justine is a partner in her care plan and contributes to her health care by following her plan of care and managing her condition in the home environment. **Box 16.4** lists the areas that are targeted in the planning stage for caring for a woman with polycystic ovary syndrome.

BOX 16.4   PLANNING CARE FOR POLYCYSTIC OVARY SYNDROME

» Health education and home care:
  – Nutrition
  – Weight management
  – Physical activity
» Consultation with the general practitioner

Concept map 16.7 outlines a plan for Justine's care.

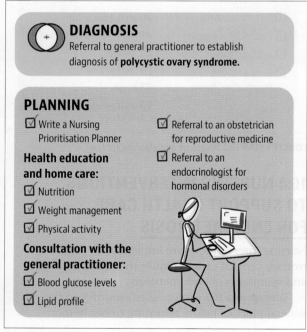

DIAGNOSIS
Referral to general practitioner to establish diagnosis of **polycystic ovary syndrome.**

PLANNING
☑ Write a Nursing Prioritisation Planner

Health education and home care:
☑ Nutrition
☑ Weight management
☑ Physical activity

Consultation with the general practitioner:
☑ Blood glucose levels
☑ Lipid profile

☑ Referral to an obstetrician for reproductive medicine
☑ Referral to an endocrinologist for hormonal disorders

CONCEPT MAP 16.7 Diagnosis and planning for Justine

16.9 NURSING INTERVENTIONS TO SUPPORT HEALTH CARE FOR POLYCYSTIC OVARY SYNDROME

Nursing interventions are implemented as part of woman-centred care to promote reproductive health and pregnancy.

Concept map 16.8 explores Justine's journey in the general practice.

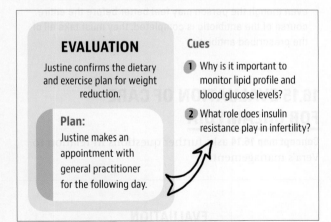

INTERVENTIONS

What further assessments should be initiated

1 Referred to general practitioner for follow up:
- blood glucose level
- lipid profile
- referrals to obstetrician and endocrinologist as needed

Health education and home care:
- Nutrition – moderate carbohydrate and fat intake
- Physical activity
- Weight measurement

CONCEPT MAP 16.8 Nursing interventions for Justine

16.10 EVALUATION OF CARE FOR POLYCYSTIC OVARY SYNDROME

As part of the further assessment of Justine's presentation, **Concept map 16.9** asks further questions in relation to Justine's management.

EVALUATION

Justine confirms the dietary and exercise plan for weight reduction.

Plan:
Justine makes an appointment with general practitioner for the following day.

Cues

① Why is it important to monitor lipid profile and blood glucose levels?

② What role does insulin resistance play in infertility?

CONCEPT MAP 16.9 Evaluation and planning for Justine

16.11 DISCHARGE PLANNING AND COORDINATION OF CARE FOR POLYCYSTIC OVARY SYNDROME

The discharge planning for Justine's polycystic ovary syndrome is a follow-up appointment with her general practitioner. **Concept map 16.10** explores discharge planning and coordination of care for Justine.

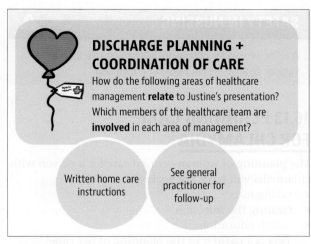

DISCHARGE PLANNING + COORDINATION OF CARE

How do the following areas of healthcare management **relate** to Justine's presentation? Which members of the healthcare team are **involved** in each area of management?

Written home care instructions

See general practitioner for follow-up

CONCEPT MAP 16.10 Discharge planning and coordination of care for Justine

16.12 ASSESSMENT FOR CHLAMYDIA

Presentation

Vera Voroski is a 22-year-old university student who has experienced painful urination for the last three days. She has made an appointment with the practice nurse at her general practitioner's office.

As part of the health assessment for Vera, the practice nurse will incorporate the components in **Box 16.1** and **Box 16.2** to conduct a woman-centred health assessment.

Concept map 16.11 further explores Vera's care in the practice nurse's office.

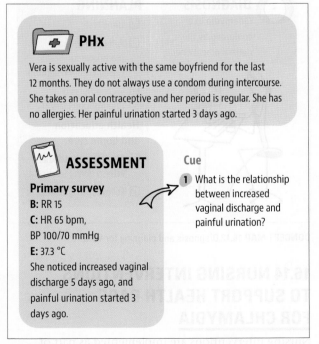

PHx

Vera is sexually active with the same boyfriend for the last 12 months. They do not always use a condom during intercourse. She takes an oral contraceptive and her period is regular. She has no allergies. Her painful urination started 3 days ago.

ASSESSMENT

Primary survey
B: RR 15
C: HR 65 bpm, BP 100/70 mmHg
E: 37.3 °C
She noticed increased vaginal discharge 5 days ago, and painful urination started 3 days ago.

Cue

① What is the relationship between increased vaginal discharge and painful urination?

CONCEPT MAP 16.11 Nursing assessment for Vera

SAFETY IN NURSING ⚠

A urine sample for chlamydia is less invasive than a vaginal swab or a blood test for the patient.

16.13 PLANNING CARE FOR CHLAMYDIA

The planning of woman-centred care for a person with chlamydia will have the goals of:

- taking tests
- treating the infection
- health education.

Vera is a partner in the planning of her care. Box 16.5 lists the areas that are targeted in the planning stage of chlamydia care.

BOX 16.5   PLANNING CARE FOR CHLAMYDIA

- ➤ Urine test
- ➤ Health education and home care
- ➤ Referral to general practitioner for examination, antibiotic for both chlamydia and gonorrhoea

Concept map 16.12 outlines a plan for Vera's care.

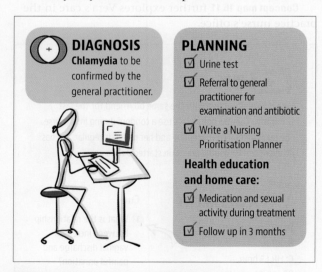

DIAGNOSIS
Chlamydia to be confirmed by the general practitioner.

PLANNING
- ☑ Urine test
- ☑ Referral to general practitioner for examination and antibiotic
- ☑ Write a Nursing Prioritisation Planner

Health education and home care:
- ☑ Medication and sexual activity during treatment
- ☑ Follow up in 3 months

CONCEPT MAP 16.12 Diagnosis and planning for Vera

16.14 NURSING INTERVENTIONS TO SUPPORT HEALTH CARE FOR CHLAMYDIA

Nursing interventions are implemented as part of woman-centred care to reverse the pathophysiology of chlamydia.

Concept map 16.13 explores Vera's healthcare journey.

INTERVENTIONS
1 Urine test
2 Referral to general practitioner for examination; Doxycycline for Vera and her partner, antibiotic for both chlamydia and gonorrhoea

Health education and home care:
- Abstain from sex while on antibiotic
- Always use a condom
- Follow up in 3 months

What further assessments should be initiated ?

CONCEPT MAP 16.13 Nursing interventions for Vera

EVIDENCE-BASED PRACTICE 🔍

To prevent antibiotic resistance, the entire course of the prescribed antibiotic must be taken. As part of patient education, the nurse will discuss with the patient that even though the person may feel better before the entire course of the antibiotic is completed, they must take all of the prescribed antibiotic.

16.15 EVALUATION OF CARE FOR CHLAMYDIA

Concept map 16.14 asks further questions in relation to Vera's management.

EVALUATION
Vera was able to explain what was required to ensure treatment was followed while her chlamydia infection was being resolved.

Plan:
Vera was able to see the general practitioner immediately after the consultation with the practice nurse.

Cue
1 What additional information would the general practitioner require to be able to differentiate chlamydia and gonorrhoea infections?

CONCEPT MAP 16.14 Evaluation and planning for Vera

16.16 DISCHARGE PLANNING AND COORDINATION OF CARE FOR CHLAMYDIA

Vera's infection requires ongoing management, and discharge planning is still an important component of Vera's care. **Concept map 16.15** explores discharge planning and coordination of care for Vera.

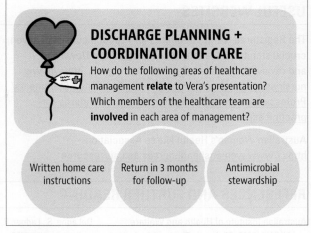

DISCHARGE PLANNING + COORDINATION OF CARE

How do the following areas of healthcare management **relate** to Vera's presentation? Which members of the healthcare team are **involved** in each area of management?

Written home care instructions

Return in 3 months for follow-up

Antimicrobial stewardship

CONCEPT MAP 16.15 Discharge planning and coordination of care for Vera

SUMMARY

When providing care to a woman with a disorder of female reproductive function, the nurse has the additional challenge of providing care to someone who may feel embarrassed about their reproductive health and concerned that private details of their life are known by the nurse.

CLINICAL SKILLS IN FEMALE REPRODUCTIVE HEALTH

The following clinical skills are required when managing a person with female reproductive conditions; consult your Clinical Skills resources, such as Tollefson and Hillman (2022), *Clinical Psychomotor Skills* (8th ed.).

- Temperature, pulse and respiration measurement
- Blood pressure measurement
- Monitoring pulse oximetry
- Pain assessment
- Focused female reproductive health history and physical assessment
- Oral medication
- Topical medication

PROBLEM-SOLVING SCENARIO

Using a concept map approach, how would you assist Wendy Cooper?

Wendy Cooper is a 39-year-old woman with two children. Wendy has had menorrhagia for the last six months and is feeling fatigued with abdominal fullness. Two large fibroids have been identified as the cause of the menorrhagia. A **hysterectomy** is performed.

1   What are the causes of menorrhagia?
2   What are the associated signs and symptoms of menorrhagia?
3   What is the nursing management for hysterectomy?
4   What is the self-care management for a hysterectomy in the home environment?

PORTFOLIO DEVELOPMENT

Wherever you practise nursing, you will need ongoing continuing professional development (CPD) to ensure that you are delivering current evidence-based nursing care that provides the best possible outcomes for the woman. As female reproductive care is based on evidence-based practice and ongoing clinical-based research, engaging in continuing professional development activities will enable the nurse to provide contemporary healthcare practice for women with reproductive conditions.

The useful websites below will assist in meeting CPD activities to meet the NMBA yearly registration requirements for a Registered Nurse.

USEFUL WEBSITES

The Registered Nurse Standards for Practice consist of seven crucial standards that all nurses must follow. Download and review the standards at the following link. https://www.nursingmidwiferyboard.gov.au/Codes-Guidelines-Statements/Professional-standards/registered-nurse-standards-for-practice.aspx

Australian Women's Health Nurse Association https://www.womenshealthnurses.asn.au/resource

The Royal Australian and New Zealand College of Obstetricians and Gynaecologists https://ranzcog.edu.au

Nursing and Midwifery Board of Australia, Decision-making framework for nursing and midwifery (2020) https://www.nursingmidwiferyboard.gov.au/codes-guidelines-statements/frameworks.aspx

REFERENCES AND FURTHER READING

Australian Institute of Health and Welfare [AIHW]. (2023, 27 June). *The health of Australia's females.* https://www.aihw.gov.au/reports/men-women/female-health/contents/how-healthy

Broyles, B., Reiss, B., Evans, M., Pleunik, S., Page, R., & Badoer, E. (2023). *Pharmacology in nursing* (4th ANZ ed.). Cengage Learning Australia.

Cunningham, P. (2016). Pathophysiology, diagnosis and treatment of polycystic ovary syndrome. *Nursing Standard, 31*(39), 44–51. DOI: 10.7748/ns.2017.e10595

DeLaune, S., Ladner, P., McTier, L., Tollefson, J., & Lawrence, J. (2024). *Fundamentals of nursing* (3rd ed.). Cengage Learning Australia.

Keeler, E., Collins Fantasia, H., & Morse, B. (2020). Interventions and practice implications for the management of endometriosis. *Nursing for Women's Health, 24*(6), 460–467. DOI: 10.1016/j.nwh.2020.09.011

Nadeau, C., McGhee, S., & Gonzalez, J. (2021). Endometriosis: a guide to investigations and treatment in the emergency department. *Emergency Nurse.* doi: 10.7748/en.2021.e2110

Neighbors, M., & Tannehill-Jones, R. (2023). *Human diseases* (6th ed.). Cengage.

Pereira, K., & Kreider, K. (2017). Caring for women with polycystic ovary syndrome. *The Nurse Practitioner, 42*(2), 39–47. DOI: 10.1097/01.NPR.0000480586.24537.64

Tollefson, J., & Hillman, E. (2022). *Clinical psychomotor skills: Assessment tools for nurses* (8th ed.). Cengage Learning Australia.

CHAPTER 17

MALE REPRODUCTIVE SYSTEM

Generally, reproductive health conditions in males do not occur by themselves; they are often associated with or are a result of a chronic condition. For example, urinary tract infections (UTIs) are far more frequent in males with benign prostate hypertrophy. Reproductive health conditions in males are common and represent a high social and economic cost (Andrology Australia, 2018).

Sexual health is, according to the World Health Organization, a state of physical, mental and social wellbeing in relation to sexuality. Included in the measurement of sexual health is the prevalence of sexually transmissible infections (STIs) and sexual difficulties (Australian Institute of Health and Welfare [AIHW], 2023).

In 2021, about 73 100 new cases of selected nationally notifiable STIs were reported for Australian males, with males accounting for more than half of all new STI cases at 56 per cent (AIHW, 2023).

In relation to sexual difficulties, this information is self-reported, and current data suggests more than half of men aged 18–55 have experienced some sexual difficulty that has lasted for at least three months in the last 12 months. Both of these aspects of sexual health for men have a significant impact on sexual wellbeing (AIHW, 2023).

LEARNING OBJECTIVES

After reading this chapter, you should have an understanding of the:
1 assessment required for a man with a male reproductive condition/disorder
2 prioritisation of key components in the development of a plan of care for a man with a urinary tract infection
3 prioritised and targeted nursing interventions required to promote recovery or prevent further deterioration of a man with a urinary tract infection
4 evaluation phase and how the prioritised and targeted nursing interventions inform further assessment, planning and collaboration with the healthcare team
5 discharge planning and coordination of care required in preparing the person for discharge and subsequent continuity of care between the person and their healthcare providers.

INTRODUCTION

The male reproductive system consists of primary and secondary organs. The primary organs are the testes, which are responsible for the secretion of hormones and the production of sperm. The secondary reproductive organs include the epididymis, the prostate gland, the scrotum and the penis. There are three primary roles for the male reproductive system:
1 transportation and production of sperm
2 secretion of hormones
3 depositing sperm into the female reproductive tract (Brown et al., 2019; Marieb & Hoehn, 2021).
  There are many common male reproductive conditions, including:

- urinary tract infections (UTIs), generally lower tract
- erectile dysfunction (ED)
- male infertility
- androgen or testosterone deficiency
- bloodborne viruses
- sexually transmitted infections (STIs)
- prostate cancer

- benign prostatic hyperplasia (BPH)
- testicular cancer
- testicular torsion
- epididymitis
- phimosis
- balanitis
- priapism.

EVIDENCE-BASED PRACTICE

Methamphetamine and priapism

Methamphetamine is a powerful stimulant drug that is known to have a number of negative side effects on the body. One of the most concerning side effects of methamphetamine use is the development of priapism, a condition characterised by a prolonged and painful erection that is not related to sexual arousal.

Priapism is a serious medical condition that can occur as a result of the use of certain drugs, including methamphetamine. This is because methamphetamine can cause abnormal blood flow to the penis, leading to an erection that lasts for an extended period of time. In some cases, the erection can last for several hours and can be extremely painful.

In addition to priapism, other potential side effects of methamphetamine use include increased heart rate,

high blood pressure and increased risk of heart attack or stroke. These side effects can be particularly dangerous for individuals with pre-existing heart conditions or hypertension.

According to a study conducted by the *Journal of Sexual Medicine*, priapism is a rare complication of methamphetamine use but has been reported in the literature. The study also reported the cases of priapism caused by methamphetamines have been associated with a high morbidity and the need for invasive treatments.

Another study conducted by the *Journal of Urology* found that the use of methamphetamine may be associated with an increased risk of priapism. The study also reported that individuals who use methamphetamine are more likely to develop priapism than those who do not use the drug (Kshatriya & Bello, 2020; Wayne et al., 2020).

It should be noted that reproductive or sexual health conditions in males do not generally occur in isolation from other chronic conditions – they are often associated with or serve as a predisposition to them. Some examples are

hypertension and erectile dysfunction, depression and other mental health conditions and the impact on sexual identity, infertility and hormonal imbalances (Andrology Australia, 2018).

17.1 ASSESSMENT OF A MALE REPRODUCTIVE CONDITION/DISORDER

The nursing assessment of the male reproductive system is a crucial component of providing comprehensive care to patients. The conditions vary greatly, so the foundation for all nursing assessment, intervention and evaluation will be on a physical assessment.

A patient history should be undertaken and should include information about the patient's sexual and reproductive history, including any previous surgeries or illnesses that may affect the reproductive system. This includes asking about the patient's sexual practices, including any history of STIs, and any history of infertility or impotence. It is also important to ask about any family history of reproductive or genetic disorders, as these can provide important information about the patient's risk for certain conditions, particularly cancers. See **Box 17.1** for the health assessment data collection areas.

The physical examination includes inspection and palpation of the testes, penis and scrotum, as well as assessment of the patient's secondary sexual characteristics. In many situations, this assessment may be undertaken by the medical officer, but in outpatient departments, or some acute care facilities, the nurse will need to undertake this physical assessment. When performing the physical examination, the testes should be inspected for size,

BOX 17.1 SUBJECTIVE ASSESSMENT

- ➤ History – medical and surgical, including psychosocial
- ➤ Past health history
- ➤ Family history
- ➤ Medications

Functional health patterns
- – Health perception and management
- – Nutritional and metabolic
- – Elimination
- – Activity and exercise
- – Sleep and rest
- – Cognitive and perceptual
- – Self-perception and concept
- – Sexuality and reproductive
- – Coping and stress
- – Values and beliefs
- ➤ Risk calculation

consistency and any masses or swelling. The penis should be inspected for any abnormalities, such as discharge or ulcers. The scrotum should be inspected for any masses or swelling, as well as any evidence of hernias. It is important to note that the examination should be conducted in a respectful and non-judgemental manner, with the patient's privacy and comfort in mind.

It is important for nurses to be familiar with the normal anatomy and physiology of the male reproductive system. This includes knowledge of the different types of testicular cancer, epididymitis, orchitis, varicocele and other conditions that may affect the reproductive system. This knowledge is essential for early detection and management of these conditions, and for evaluation and reporting findings to ensure patient safety and holistic care.

In addition to the physical assessment, nurses will likely need to provide psychological and emotional support to patients. Many men may feel embarrassment, shame or anxiety about discussing their reproductive health with a healthcare provider, and nurses should be able to provide a supportive and non-judgemental environment for these conversations (Andrology Australia, 2018; Brown et al., 2019; DeLaune et al., 2024).

Box 17.2 assists the nurse in the physical assessment of the male reproductive system.

BOX 17.2   PHYSICAL ASSESSMENT

➤ Vital signs
➤ Genitourinary assessment
➤ Diagnostic testing such as urinalysis
➤ Diagnostic investigations such as x-ray or CT
➤ Blood tests such as full blood count, hormones
➤ Blood glucose level (BGL)
➤ Swab if STI evident

17.2 ASSESSMENT FOR A URINARY TRACT INFECTION (UTI)

Presentation

Peter Carrington is a 58-year-old male who presented two days prior with an upper respiratory tract infection. He has developed urinary symptoms during his hospitalisation.

Concept map 17.1 further explores Peter's signs and symptoms while in hospital.

 PHx

Peter, a **58-year-old male**, day 2 on medical ward. Presented initially with upper respiratory tract infection, now complaining of difficulty in urinating, and an increase in urgency and frequency in urination.
PMHx – NKDA, Hypertension, COVID-19 May 2022, Asthma.
Meds – Telmisartan 20 mg, Atorvastatin 40 mg, Esomeprazole 20 mg, Salbutamol 2 puffs daily.

 ASSESSMENT

Primary survey
A: Patent
B: RR 16 bpm
C: Warm and well perfused
D: Alert
E: Nil concerns
F: Difficulty urinating
G: BGL 6.2 mmol/L

Secondary survey
CNS: E 4 V 5 M 6 = 15 PEARLA 3 mm
PAIN: C/o pain on urination 4/10
CVS: HR 90 bpm, BP 160/90 mmHg, T: 37.7 °C

RESP: RR 16 bpm, patent airway – spontaneous breathing, SpO$_2$ 98% RA, AE = on auscultation
GIT (Input): IVC to be placed, currently nothing running
RENAL (Output): C/o frequency, pain on urination, Pt reports blood passed on urination
SKIN/INTEG: Centrally warm and peripherally cooler. Cap refill time < 3 sec.
MUSCULOSKELETAL (Mobility): Steady gait, SOBOE prior to admission – RIB
BMI: 28.5

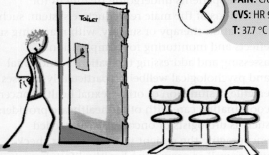

Cues

1 What are your priorities with this patient?

2 What other vital signs or bedside investigations would you perform?

3 What is the relationship between dysuria, frequency and urgency?

4 What is the pathophysiological relationship of UTI and frequency, dysuria and urgency?

5 What investigative or diagnostic procedures do you think would be relevant for this patient?

CONCEPT MAP 17.1 Nursing assessment for Peter

17.3 PLANNING CARE FOR A UTI

Planning for management of male reproductive conditions is broad as the causative factor/s needs to be identified. In any planning, the person is a partner in their care plan and needs to be able to contribute to their health care by following their plan of care and managing their condition in the home environment. **Box 17.3** indicates the areas that are targeted in the planning stage of male reproductive conditions.

BOX 17.3 PLANNING CARE FOR A UTI

- ❯ Lifestyle modifications – safe sex practices
- ❯ Diet – hydration/fluids
- ❯ Pain management
- ❯ Medication/s interactions
- ❯ Monitor blood pressure
- ❯ Impact of chronic conditions
- ❯ Previous history and impact from this
- ❯ Partner involvement

Any reproductive condition will affect every patient differently, and you will need to apply your observational skills, including collection of subjective and objective data to the patient. Patients will also respond differently to treatment and interventions in terms of symptom management, and this will also be reliant upon previous occurrences (such as UTIs or BPH) and medications used.

See **Concept map 17.2** for an outline of Peter's care plan.

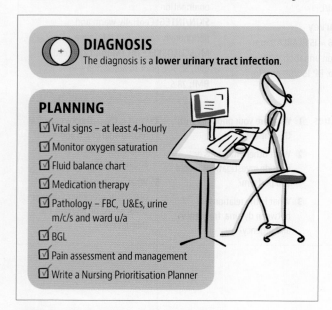

DIAGNOSIS
The diagnosis is a **lower urinary tract infection**.

PLANNING
- ☑ Vital signs – at least 4-hourly
- ☑ Monitor oxygen saturation
- ☑ Fluid balance chart
- ☑ Medication therapy
- ☑ Pathology – FBC, U&Es, urine m/c/s and ward u/a
- ☑ BGL
- ☑ Pain assessment and management
- ☑ Write a Nursing Prioritisation Planner

CONCEPT MAP 17.2 Diagnosis and planning for Peter

17.4 NURSING INTERVENTIONS TO SUPPORT HEALTH CARE FOR A UTI

Nursing care for the male reproductive system includes assessment and monitoring of the patient's testicles, penis and prostate gland. This may involve performing physical exams, taking vital signs and collecting laboratory samples.

Patients may also be taught about self-examination techniques for the testicles and how to identify signs of testicular cancer or other conditions. Patients with conditions such as prostate cancer or BPH may need education on the proper technique for performing prostate self-examination and the importance of regular check-ups. Nurses may also provide education on sexual health and the importance of safe sex practices, as well as the use of condoms to prevent STIs. Patients undergoing treatment for conditions of the male reproductive system, such as radiation therapy or surgery, may need assistance with managing side effects and monitoring for complications. Patients with conditions such as erectile dysfunction may need education on the use of erectile dysfunction medications, as well as counselling on the emotional and psychological effects of the condition.

Some nursing interventions for the male reproductive system include:

- ▪ assessing the patient's testicles, penis and prostate gland during physical exams and monitoring for any changes or abnormalities
- ▪ educating patients on self-examination techniques for the testicles and signs of testicular cancer
- ▪ providing education on sexual health and safe sex practices, including the use of condoms to prevent STIs
- ▪ assisting patients undergoing treatment for conditions of the male reproductive system, such as radiation therapy or surgery, with managing side effects and monitoring for complications
- ▪ assessing and addressing the patient's emotional and psychological wellbeing, particularly in cases of erectile dysfunction or other sexual health concerns
- ▪ coordinating care with other healthcare providers, such as urologists or oncologists, as needed
- ▪ encouraging the patient to have regular check-ups, as well as promoting healthy lifestyle such as regular exercise, healthy diet, and avoiding smoking and excessive alcohol consumption
- ▪ providing appropriate care for patients with conditions such as prostate cancer or benign prostatic hyperplasia, including medication management and monitoring for complications
- ▪ providing patient and family education about the disease process and the treatment options available, as well as the potential risks and benefits associated with each option

- encouraging patients to communicate openly and honestly with their healthcare providers and to be active participants in their care.

Additional diagnostic tests may include blood tests, imaging studies or a biopsy if needed. Blood tests can be used to assess the patient's testosterone levels, as well as to screen for any underlying medical conditions that may affect the reproductive system. Imaging studies, such as ultrasound or MRI, can be used to assess the size and structure of the testes and other reproductive organs. A biopsy may be performed if a mass or abnormal growth is detected during the physical examination.

Concept map 17.3 explores Peter's journey in the hospital.

INTERVENTIONS

1	Assess urinary symptoms with each void.	**5** Pain assessment and management
2	Fluid intake and output – fluid balance chart	**6** ISBAR handover preparation for end-of-shift handover – what would you be handing over regarding your patient's condition?
3	Nutrition status	
4	Vital signs	

What further assessments should be initiated

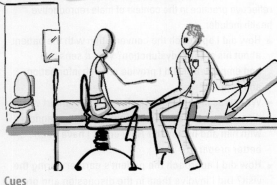

Cues

1. What are the symptoms relevant to a UTI here?
2. What patient education could you provide to Peter?
3. If the patient develops tachycardia and becomes more febrile what could this be evidence of?

CONCEPT MAP 17.3 Nursing interventions for Peter

17.5 EVALUATION OF CARE FOR A UTI

As part of the further assessment of Peter's condition, **Concept map 17.4** asks further questions in relation to his management.

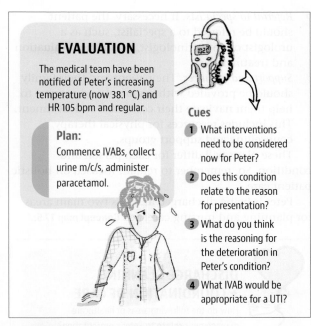

EVALUATION

The medical team have been notified of Peter's increasing temperature (now 38.1 °C) and HR 105 bpm and regular.

Plan:
Commence IVABs, collect urine m/c/s, administer paracetamol.

Cues

1. What interventions need to be considered now for Peter?
2. Does this condition relate to the reason for presentation?
3. What do you think is the reasoning for the deterioration in Peter's condition?
4. What IVAB would be appropriate for a UTI?

CONCEPT MAP 17.4 Evaluation and planning for Peter

17.6 DISCHARGE PLANNING AND COORDINATION OF CARE FOR A UTI

When discharging a male patient who has a disorder or injury related to the reproductive system, there are six nursing considerations that should be taken into account:

1. *Patient education.* It is important to provide the patient with detailed information about their condition and the treatment plan. This includes information about medications, follow-up appointments, and any lifestyle changes that may be necessary. The patient should also be educated about any potential complications that may arise and the signs and symptoms to look out for.

2. *Medication management.* The patient should be provided with the appropriate medications and instructions on how to take them. This includes information about dosages, side effects and potential interactions with other medications.

3. *Follow-up care.* The patient should be provided with information about follow-up appointments and any necessary tests or procedures. It is important to coordinate with the patient's GP or primary healthcare team to ensure continuity of care.

4. *Lifestyle changes.* Depending on the condition, the patient may need to make lifestyle changes to promote healing and prevent complications. For example, if the patient has a condition that affects their sexual function, they may need to avoid sexual activity until they are cleared by their healthcare provider.

5   *Referral to specialists.* If necessary, the patient should be referred to a specialist, such as a urologist or endocrinologist, for further evaluation and treatment.

6   *Support and resources.* The patient and their family should be provided with resources and support to help them navigate their condition and treatment. This includes resources for physical therapy, counselling and support groups.

These plans will differ for each person and condition. So, remember to remain focused on holistic patient care.

Peter is being discharged and has two main areas for planning and nursing care. See **Concept map 17.5.**

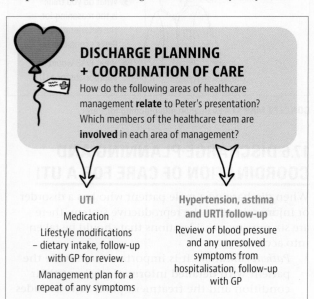

DISCHARGE PLANNING + COORDINATION OF CARE

How do the following areas of healthcare management **relate** to Peter's presentation? Which members of the healthcare team are **involved** in each area of management?

UTI

Medication

Lifestyle modifications – dietary intake, follow-up with GP for review.

Management plan for a repeat of any symptoms

Hypertension, asthma and URTI follow-up

Review of blood pressure and any unresolved symptoms from hospitalisation, follow-up with GP

CONCEPT MAP 17.5 Discharge planning and coordination of care for Peter

⚠ SAFETY IN NURSING

CHEMOTHERAPY – EXPOSURE TO CYTOTOXIC MEDICATIONS

Chemotherapy is used to destroy cancerous cells. It can be in a number of different formats, including oral medications. If you are treating a patient with any form of cancer, you need to be aware of the medications they are prescribed and what they are prescribed for. Chemotherapy can cause side-effects or symptoms to healthcare professionals who come in contact with bodily fluids from the person who is taking the chemotherapy.

For example, a patient with prostate cancer may be taking:

• oral chemotherapy
• oral hormone therapy (female hormones).

Each healthcare facility must have a process in place for the management, storage and disposal of cytotoxic agents. It is not always within the role of the ward RN or student RN to administer chemotherapy unless they have been provided with additional training to ensure safety.

More information regarding how to manage medication in cancer care can be found here: https://www.safetyandquality.gov.au/sites/default/files/2020-04/nsqhs_standards_user_guide_for_medication_management_in_cancer_care_april_2020.pdf

REFLECTIVE PRACTICE

Reproductive health – Male

Reflective practice is an important aspect of nursing education and professional development, as it allows nurses to critically examine their own actions and thought processes in order to improve their knowledge, skills and performance. In the context of male reproductive health, reflective practice can be used to explore various aspects of care such as patient education, communication with patients and other healthcare providers, and the management of specific conditions such as erectile dysfunction, infertility and testicular cancer. Reflective practice can also help nurses to identify and address any biases or misconceptions they may have about male reproductive health, and to develop a more inclusive and patient-centred approach to care.

Questions

Some examples of questions that a nurse might use for reflective practice in the context of male reproductive health include:

■ How did I approach the conversation with the patient about his erectile dysfunction? Was it sensitive and empathetic? Did I provide enough information and support?

■ What was my level of knowledge and comfort when discussing the patient's testicular cancer diagnosis with him and his family? How could I have been better prepared?

■ How did I approach the patient's partner during the visit? Did I involve them in the discussion and provide them with information and support? How could I have done better?

■ Did I feel comfortable discussing contraception options with the patient? Did I provide enough information and support? What could I have done better?

■ What was my attitude or preconceptions about the patient's infertility? Did it affect my interactions with him or his partner?

■ How well did I communicate with the other healthcare providers involved in the patient's care? Did I provide enough information and support? How could I have done better?

Answering these questions can help nurses to identify areas of strength and weakness in their practice, and to develop strategies for improvement.

SUMMARY

Nursing care for male reproductive health involves a wide range of responsibilities and interventions, including:

- Patient education: providing patients with accurate and up-to-date information about various conditions and treatments related to male reproductive health, such as erectile dysfunction, infertility, testicular cancer and STIs.
- Communication: building a rapport with patients and their partners and fostering an open and respectful dialogue about sensitive topics related to male reproductive health.
- Physical assessment: performing physical examinations, including testicular exams, and providing care for conditions such as testicular torsion, varicocele and epididymitis.
- Medication administration: administering medications and treatments, such as hormone replacement therapy.
- Coordination of care: collaborating with other healthcare providers, such as allied healthcare professionals and medical specialists, to coordinate and manage the patient's care.
- Support: providing emotional and psychological support for patients and their families and connecting them with relevant resources and support groups.
- Patient follow-up: monitoring patient's progress and providing ongoing follow-up care as needed.

Overall, the goal of nursing care for male reproductive health is to provide comprehensive, person-centred care that addresses the physical, emotional and psychological needs of the patient.

CLINICAL SKILLS IN MALE REPRODUCTIVE HEALTH

The following clinical skills are required when managing a person with male reproductive conditions; consult your Clinical Skills resources, such as Tollefson and Hillman (2022), *Clinical Psychomotor Skills* (8th ed.).

- Temperature, pulse and respiration
- Blood pressure measurement
- Monitoring pulse oximetry
- Pain assessment
- Focused male reproductive health history and physical assessment
- Neurovascular observations
- Oral medication
- Intravenous medication administration
- Venipuncture
- Urinalysis and collection of a sterile sample

PROBLEM-SOLVING SCENARIO

Using a concept map approach, how would you assist Jarrod Bennett?

Jarrod Bennett, 31 years old, has presented to the medical centre where you are on placement with increasing discharge from his penis, associated with pain on urination. Jarrod discloses that he has recently used methamphetamines and has had unprotected sex with multiple partners over the past few weeks. He states he takes no 'drugs or other stuff' and smokes 10 cigarettes a day.

1 With this information, what are some pathophysiological processes in place that could be occurring here?
2 What nursing considerations would you have for Jarrod?

PORTFOLIO DEVELOPMENT

Wherever you practise nursing, you will need ongoing continuing professional development (CPD) to ensure that you are delivering current evidence-based nursing care that provides the best possible outcomes for the man. As male reproductive care is based on evidence-based practice and ongoing clinical-based research, engaging in continuing professional development activities will enable the nurse to provide contemporary healthcare practice for men with reproductive conditions.

Healthy Male is a national organisation and it provides information for both healthcare professionals and healthcare consumers. It has a great array of CPD and other information for your ongoing portfolio development. It can be found here: https://www.healthymale.org.au.

The other useful websites below will assist in meeting CPD activities to meet the NMBA yearly registration requirements for a Registered Nurse.

USEFUL WEBSITES

Registered Nurse Standards for Practice
The Registered Nurse Standards for Practice consist of seven crucial standards that all nurses must follow. Download and review the standards at the following link. https://www.nursingmidwiferyboard.gov.au/Codes-Guidelines-Statements/Professional-standards/registered-nurse-standards-for-practice.aspx

Australasian Sexual Health & HIV Nurses Association Inc. (ASHHNA)
The ASHHNA is the peak reproductive, sexual and HIV nurses' professional organisation. Their aim is to share and develop knowledge and skills to improve the sexual and reproductive health of individuals and communities and support people living with HIV. https://ashhna.org.au

Prostate Cancer Foundation (Australia)
Prostate Cancer Foundation of Australia is a broad-based community organisation and the peak national body for prostate cancer in Australia. It has resources for professionals and patients and has specialised prostate cancer nurses available for patients to access. https://www.pcfa.org.au

Men's Health Collective
This website has information regarding men's sexual health including premature ejaculation, erectile dysfunction, testicular and prostate cancers and other male-specific conditions. https://menshealthcollective.au

REFERENCES AND FURTHER READING

Andrology Australia. (2018). *The current state of male health in Australia. Informing the development of the National Male Health Strategy 2020–2030.* https://consultations.health.gov.au/population-health-and-sport-division-1/online-consultation-for-the-national-mens-health-s/supporting_documents/Evidence%20Review%20%20Current%20state%20of%20male%20health%20in%20Australia.PDF

Australian Institute of Health and Welfare [AIHW]. (2023, 27 June). *The health of Australia's males.* https://www.aihw.gov.au/reports/men-women/male-health/contents/how-healthy

Brown, D., Edwards, H., Buckley, T., Aitken, R. L., Lewis, S. L., Bucher, L., McLean Heitkemper, M., Harding, M. M., Kwong, J., & Roberts, D. (2019). *Lewis's medical-surgical nursing ANZ* (5th ed.). Elsevier.

DeLaune, S., Ladner, P., McTier, L., Tollefson, J., & Lawrence, J. (2024). *Fundamentals of nursing* (3rd ed.). Cengage Learning Australia.

Kshatriya, D., & Bello, N. T. (2020). Central nervous system stimulants and drugs that suppress appetite. *Side Effects of Drugs Annual, 42,* 1–12.

Marieb, E. N., & Hoehn, K. N. (2021). *Human anatomy & physiology* (9th ed.). Pearson.

Tollefson, J., & Hillman, E. (2022). *Clinical psychomotor skills: Assessment tools for nurses* (8th ed.). Cengage Learning Australia.

Wayne, G., Weisberg, M., Monreal, A., Atri, E., Wong, V., Nieder, A. M., Caso, J., & Polackwich, A. S. (2020). Etiology of priapism in the community: local factors can help guide prevention and savings. *AME Medical Journal, 5.* https://amj.amegroups.com/article/view/5520

PART 03

INTERPROFESSIONAL APPROACHES TO CARE

INTERPROFESSIONAL
APPROACHES TO CARE

CHAPTER 18

CULTURALLY SAFE CARE

NMBA AND CATSINaM JOINT STATEMENT ON CULTURALLY SAFE CARE

Racial discrimination is well documented as a contributing factor to poor health outcomes for Aboriginal and Torres Strait Islander Australians (Australian Human Rights Commission, 2005, p. 10; Paradies et al., 2008). The Congress of Aboriginal and Torres Strait Islander Nurses and Midwives (CATSINaM) and the Nursing and Midwifery Board of Australia (NMBA) are committed to addressing racism and demonstrating leadership to nurses and midwives to ensure they value the needs of Aboriginal and/or Torres Strait Islander peoples, and promote and provide culturally safe care.

In order to effect change, CATSINaM and the NMBA know that regulations and codes establishing health professional standards must clearly communicate the requirement for cultural safety. The NMBA Code of conduct for nurses and Code of conduct for midwives (the codes), which are supported by CATSINaM:

* acknowledge that Australia has always been a culturally and linguistically diverse nation. Aboriginal and/or Torres Strait Islander peoples have inhabited and cared for the land as the First Peoples of Australia for millennia, and their histories and cultures have uniquely shaped our nation
* require nurses and midwives to understand and acknowledge the historic factors, such as colonisation and its impact on Aboriginal and/or Torres Strait Islander peoples' health, which help to inform care. In particular, Aboriginal and/or Torres Strait Islander peoples bear the burden of gross social, cultural and health inequality, and
* provide clear guidance and set expectations for nurses and midwives in supporting the health of Aboriginal and/or Torres Strait Islander peoples.

The codes also specifically require that nurses and midwives must:

* provide care that is holistic, free of bias and racism, challenges belief based upon assumption and is culturally safe and respectful for Aboriginal and/or Torres Strait Islander peoples
* advocate for, and act to facilitate, access to quality and culturally safe health services for Aboriginal and/or Torres Strait Islander peoples, and
* recognise the importance of family, community, partnership and collaboration in the healthcare decision-making of Aboriginal and/or Torres Strait Islander peoples, for both prevention strategies and care delivery.

The codes also advocate for culturally safe and respectful practice and require nurses and midwives to have knowledge of how their own culture, values, attitudes, assumptions and beliefs influence their interactions with people and families, the community and colleagues. CATSINaM and the NMBA believe that cultural safety and respectfulness is the responsibility of all nurses and midwives. By embracing this principle nurses and midwives provide leadership in building a health system free of racism and inequality, that is accessible for all.

Source: *NMBA and CATSINaM joint statement of culturally safe care* (2018). With permission of The Congress of Aboriginal and Torres Strait Islander Nurses and Midwives (CATSINaM) and the Nursing and Midwifery Board of Australia (NMBA).

LEARNING OBJECTIVES

After reading this chapter, you should have an understanding of:
1 cultural safety in Australia and New Zealand
2 the inequality in health outcomes for Aboriginal and Torres Strait Islander peoples
3 the importance of providing culturally safe and respectful care through all steps of the nursing process.

INTRODUCTION

Culture strongly influences our thoughts, beliefs, attitudes and behaviours. It impacts on the way we relate to others, the way we care for ourselves and our loved ones, the way we dress, eat, speak, write and live our lives. For this reason, a little cultural understanding or awareness can go a long way when caring for our patients from a different background to our own. Thus being mindful of race, culture and personal beliefs is crucial to any holistic nursing care. Cultural care involves the nurse ensuring that the person is the centre of their care, and that all care is holistic. Cultural care includes terms such as:

- cultural safety
- cultural competence
- cultural awareness.

Cultural care is inclusive of all these terms and applies to all patients in the healthcare domain. The term *cultural safety* is used more commonly in nursing and midwifery and is seen in Department of Health documents as well as Standards for Practice to further highlight the necessity of delivery of culturally safe care.

The importance of the nurse understanding their own personal beliefs and lived experience is highlighted in the Joint Statement between CATSINaM and NMBA and provides a basis for ongoing reflective practice in the delivery of culturally safe healthcare (NMBA & CATSINaM, 2018).

Cultures are constantly changing and developing over time. They are strongly influenced by:

- local environment; for example, weather: hot or cold, dry or wet
- geography: mountainous, near the sea, in the desert
- location: urban or rural
- local history and politics
- major events, both natural and made by humans
- interactions with other cultures.

Culture is a blueprint for living; that is, it determines ideas about appropriate values and behaviours. Our culture may determine when we sleep, how we bathe, what we wear and what we eat. It may tell us what is right and what is wrong, how to bring up our children, how to greet friends and address a stranger, what is polite and what is impolite. It may prescribe ways of grieving, ways to show affection and ways to cure illness (Best, 2021; Langton, 2018).

Human rights are shared by all people, whereas human needs are specific to our diverse cultural blueprints. Cultural aspects shared by one group of people, such as the way of performing activities of daily living, systems of belief and social code of conduct, may differ greatly from the cultural aspects of another group. No one way of getting ready in the morning, eating dinner at night, or bathing oneself is better or worse than any other way of doing the same task.

It is vital that we remember that cultural groups are made up of individuals, with each person being unique in his or her own way.

18.1 CULTURAL SAFETY IN AUSTRALIA AND NEW ZEALAND

Cultural safety is an evolving concept and began in the late 1980s in New Zealand (Ghys, 2008). At the forefront of this integration into health care was *Irihapeti Merenia Ramsden*, a registered general and obstetric nurse at Wellington Hospital. Her research outlined the concept of cultural safety, and this term has since been adopted worldwide. Her seminal work is still used as the basis for Nursing Standards within Australia and other countries (Ramsden, 2002). The term 'cultural safety' has been attributed in research to Hingerangi Mhi, who was a Māori nursing student (Heckenberg, 2020).

Cultural Safety for Indigenous Peoples began as a response to the colonial context in New Zealand where the Māori population were facing difficulties when accessing the western healthcare services (Papps & Ramsden, 1996). Due to this difficulty, New Zealand Māori nurse, Irahapeti Ramsden, went on to develop the concept of cultural safety. Ramsden's seminal work on cultural safety is based on five principles for health professionals to apply in their delivery of care:

1 incorporate reflection of one's own practice
2 minimise power differences
3 engage in communication with peoples
4 undertake a process of decolonisation through learning about the impact of colonisation
5 treat all peoples regardless of differences the same (Ramsden, 2002).

These five principles of cultural safety were further reiterated within the Australian healthcare context by Best and Fredericks (2021). In addition, cultural safety fosters the sharing of power between Indigenous peoples and healthcare professionals where the recipient of health care can determine how safe they feel during care delivery (Kurtz et al., 2018). In practice, cultural safety is applied to the Indigenous patient, not to a culture and its effectiveness is determined by the Indigenous patient, not the healthcare professional (Sherwood et al., 2021).

The wide dissemination of Ramsden's work has informed nursing and midwifery policy in providing culturally safe care for Indigenous peoples. For example, the Nursing Council of New Zealand outlines that cultural safety is 'a component of effective nursing practice, of a person, or family member from another culture, and is determined by that person or family' (Nursing Council of New Zealand, 2012, p. 13). Like the Māori experience in healthcare, cultural safety was instigated within the Australian health context due to the colonisation of health services and the delivery of health care using a western biomedical model (Best, 2021; Cox et al., 2021).

The implementation of cultural safety practices has the potential to improve health outcomes for Indigenous peoples, thus increasing their health span and life expectancy (Brooks-Cleator et al., 2018). To achieve this high standard of care, healthcare professionals at the bedside must identify cultural safety as an integral component of person-centred care when providing care for Indigenous peoples (Best, 2021; Moloney et al., 2023; Power et al., 2021; Sherwood et al., 2021).

Cultural safety requires the nurse to recognise that there is more than one way to achieve healthcare delivery, and during this process dignity, respect and basic human rights must be maintained (Williams, 1999). To further highlight the need for integration in healthcare practice, the Australian Health Practitioner Regulation Authority (Ahpra) has developed a cultural safety strategy that identifies four key points for health practitioners:

1 colonisation and systemic racism need to be acknowledged
2 acknowledgement of own biases, experiences, stereotypes and assumptions must be undertaken to ensure care is free of bias and racism
3 identify and recognise the importance of self-determination in decision making, while ensuring partnership with the person and their family
4 support the dignity and rights of Aboriginal and Torres Strait Islander peoples through a safe environment (Ahpra, 2020).

Cultural safety also aims to address the inherent power imbalance that exists within health care. While cultural safety is a component of care that the nurse/midwife needs to incorporate into their care, it is up to the patient to determine cultural safety. Any care or practice that disempowers, or diminishes the person including their wellbeing, is deemed as unsafe cultural practice (Nursing Council of New Zealand, 2011; Moloney et al., 2023).

Culture, as it applies to cultural competence and cultural safety includes, but is not restricted to:

■ age or generation
■ gender
■ sexual orientation
■ occupation and socioeconomic status
■ ethnic origin or migrant experience
■ religious and spiritual beliefs
■ disabilities (Phillips, 2015).

See how it encompasses so many facets of what makes us 'us'?

Cultural competence is the *mastery* of measurable skills, attitudes, knowledge and behaviours – which is inherent in our education and experience as a student in health care, and an active participant in society. You will notice that as you progress through your studies, more information surrounding cultural care will become available as it is a crucial part of holistic and person-centred care (Geia et al., 2020; Kurtz et al., 2018). Cultural safety is the practice of care that prioritises marginalised groups, and provides empowerment through challenging power imbalances that exist in health care (Moloney et al., 2023).

Cultural diversity differs from cultural safety but also needs to be valued and respected. Responding to cultural diversity is, therefore, fundamental to provision of culturally safe care. Valuing diversity means that we acknowledge and respect the cultural or religious background and previous experiences of all Australians, with respect to their gender, ethnicity and beliefs (Edwards et al., 2019; Geia et al., 2020; Kurtz et al., 2018; Phillips, 2015; Ramsden, 2002).

18.2 ABORIGINAL AND TORRES STRAIT ISLANDER HEALTH

Health has different meanings to people. For Aboriginal and Torres Strait Islander peoples it is holistic; meaning all physical and psychological aspects, including social, emotional, mental, cultural, spiritual and the inclusion of justice and equality (Best & Fredericks, 2021; Cox et al., 2021; Laverty et al., 2017). If any of these aspects go unaddressed, the person is seen as unwell (Lamp, 2018). Health and wellbeing are interrelated and often influenced by community, home and institutions such as hospitals or healthcare settings. They are also referred to as the *social determinants of health* (Phillips, 2015). Further, literature asserts that for holistic health to be achieved in Aboriginal and Torres Strait Islander peoples, aspects such as community capacity, governance and social wellbeing must be included in all healthcare delivery (Lutschini, 2005). This is inclusive of cultural determinants of health, which are crucial to wellbeing and holistic delivery of health to Aboriginal and Torres Strait Islander peoples (Garvey et al., 2021).

As asserted by Best and Fredericks (2021, p. 4), passing on knowledge relating to Aboriginal and Torres Strait Islander peoples' health and history can be difficult to understand and confronting in nature. The title of their book is a gifted word that means 'talking in a good way'. This wonderful notion of passing on knowledge regarding Country and experiences is incredibly apt for not only student nurses and midwives, but nurses and midwives who also need to practise talking in a good way for all patients, particularly Aboriginal and Torres Strait Islander peoples (Best & Fredericks, 2017). For this to occur, acknowledging the history of Aboriginal and Torres Strait Islander peoples of Australia is essential and, importantly, is in adherence to the Aboriginal and Torres Strait Islander Health and Cultural Safety Strategy 2020–2025 (Ahpra, 2020).

Racism is a determinant of health, and for Aboriginal and Torres Strait Islander peoples, this has significant impact upon their ability to live *well*; hence cultural safety is a philosophy of practice that is mindful of race as an important indicator of cultural diversity (Australian Institute of Health and Welfare [AIHW], 2017; Best, 2021; Power et al., 2021). Regarding life expectancy, this term is redundant as Aboriginal and Torres Strait Islander peoples have significantly shorter health-spans. The term 'health-span' relates to the quality of life rather than the length of it. For Aboriginal and Torres Strait Islander peoples, not living *well* aligns with racism, chronic conditions and diseases, and the culturally unsafe environment accessing health care can bring (Geia et al., 2020; Lamp, 2018). The overwhelming concept of Aboriginal and Torres Strait Islander peoples' health is presented by media as 'more bad news' or as 'problems to be solved'; which is ineffective in addressing the distinct power imbalance that exists for Aboriginal and Torres Strait Islander peoples (Best & Fredericks, 2021).

Health care becomes complex when there are historical factors that influence the access and equity principles of health care. Aboriginal and Torres Strait Islander peoples live with poorer overall health when compared to non-Aboriginal and Torres Strait Islanders, and this is evident in the morbidity and mortality data. There is data to suggest that Australian healthcare services are culturally unsafe for Aboriginal and Torres Strait Islander peoples to access and utilise, compared to higher rates of access by non- Aboriginal and Torres Strait Islanders, which further impacts upon their health-span (Artuso et al., 2013).

18.3 PROVIDING CULTURALLY SAFE CARE

Part of your role in health care will be to ensure that you maintain person-centred care, and more specifically, culturally safe care across all steps of the nursing process. Planning care around what your patient needs, rather than what you think or assume, sounds logical but there is inherent racism and stereotypes surrounding Indigenous peoples, and it requires healthcare professionals to constantly ensure that care is for the person, not the narrative.

Racism and prejudice comes in all colours, shapes and sizes. It can be as blatant as, for example, a society that passes laws that separate groups of people by their colour, or choosing which seat you take on a bus based on the person already sitting there. Most people experience prejudice at some time in their life, whether on the grounds of class, age, disability, sex, religion or race. Everyone makes choices based on personal prejudices; however, in healthcare, we are bound by our Standards for Practice, and this precludes us from aligning personal prejudice or stereotypes in our healthcare delivery. Therefore, cultural safety directs us to reflect on our biases and positions of power and address these in care. These concepts highlight the premise of cultural safety – in that it is subjective and derived by the person receiving the care (Gopal et al., 2022).

Racism can be expressed in many ways, such as being called derogatory names or even being served last in a shop despite being there first. Think about how this can relate to health care. In your role, you are not able to distinguish the priority of your cares based on someone's race, religion or appearance. This seems logical, doesn't it? Unfortunately, within Australia there are all too many examples of this not occurring. When planning your nursing care, remember it is *you* that is accountable for the provision of holistic care and patient outcomes; working collaboratively with the patient and their family and deriving care that is suitable and culturally safe for each patient.

REFLECTIVE PRACTICE

Coronial inquest

Aboriginal and Torres Strait Islander peoples are warned that this section contains the name of a deceased Aboriginal person.

Naomi Williams was a 27-year-old woman who died despite 18 presentations to a healthcare facility in the month prior to her death. Naomi was 22/40 pregnant at the time of her death, and her unborn son also died. This was Naomi's first pregnancy. Her presentations were for nausea, vomiting, dehydration and abdominal pain.

Naomi died from septicaemia.

1 Consider the above information. In terms of clinical safety, what do you think are some 'red flags' here?

Consider the addition of the following information from a coronial inquest:

Nurses assumed drug-seeking behaviour and lying about her level of pain despite no previous history of the same.

2 What is the subjective and objective data here?

Now consider the addition of this information:

Naomi was a Wiradjuri woman, and on her final visit (the 18th) with the same symptoms, with no referrals or follow-up from previous presentations, she was given 1 g of paracetamol, and no physical assessment or vital signs were recorded. She died 15 hours later.

3 Consider the joint statement from NMBA and CATSINaM for Cultural Safety – what should have occurred here?

4 How can you ensure you incorporate this into your ongoing practice?

The full coronial findings can be found here: https:// coroners.nsw.gov.au/coroners-court/download.html/ documents/findings/2019/Naomi%20Williams%20findings.pdf

In the delivery of cultural safety there will not be an easy-to-follow care plan – it will be individualised and unique for each person due to the very differences we are seeking to address. As with any assessment,

care or intervention, you will need to evaluate and re-assess throughout the provision of care. Establishing safe discharge planning is a component of any patient journey, but if your patient does not speak English, or speaks four other languages, you will need to ensure that information provided is appropriate and understood. The significance of English being a second, third or fourth language, coupled with past experiences of healthcare access and utilisation impacts greatly upon the ability for the nurse/midwife to deliver culturally safe care, and for the patient to receive adequate clinical care with cultural safety.

An example cited (Artuso et al., 2013, p. 5) outlines 'magic' occurring after an angioplasty procedure, with no follow-up treatment as the patient assumed that it was all 'fixed'. This led the patient to believe that there was no further treatment or intervention required. Safe clinical care requires the nurse or midwife to ensure that the patient and their family understand their health conditions and the subsequent treatment and follow-up required. Planning your nursing interventions will not ever be a 'one size fits all' approach in the delivery of culturally safe care. No two patients will have exactly the same requirements – even if you had a four-bed bay with all patients having the same surgical procedure. Holistic, and centred care is about the patient being a person, not the procedure that they have undergone or the illness they are currently recovering from.

Patients that are hospitalised are not able to follow their usual daily routines and this can be very disconcerting. They may miss the comforts of home and feel distressed at being in a strange place following orders instead of being independent. A person who is independent will find that being dependent on someone for assistance with activities of daily living increases their stress. Nurses should take into account the fact that anxiety may affect a person's ability to concentrate on what they are being told and thus they may not understand. When giving instructions to an anxious person, repetition or giving written instructions is one way of ensuring the patient actually receives the information.

Fear and stress in a patient can increase due to many factors, many of which the nurse can assist in mitigating. Uncertainty around diagnosis and treatment has a significant impact on fear and the physiological responses associated with it. Other factors to consider are privacy, dignity and the ability to meet cultural, family or spiritual requirements (Best & Fredericks, 2021; Edwards et al., 2019).

The combination of the above factors and illness can be very troubling for patients. The nursing role is to holistically review and assess our patients and ensure that we address each need. Ensuring patients know what to expect by providing adequate health promotion and education is an essential component of the nursing role. Consider the impact of not addressing cultural safety with the above factors. It is the responsibility of the healthcare professional to provide holistic and person-centred care.

Collaboration with the healthcare team is a vital component of holistic care. It is achieved through effective communication – written and verbal – and an insight into the patient's requirements gained from a thorough nursing assessment and focus on the patient's needs.

Holistic care entails looking at areas of the patient's requirements and addressing them. With a holistic approach, we can address areas of need or concern and ensure that our patient is getting the best person-focused care available. Holistic care involves ensuring cultural safety is maintained and always respected.

SUMMARY

It is essential for nurses and healthcare professionals to promote and provide culturally safe care in every variation of care delivery. We also provide care to the patient's family and significant others with the holistic framework. Holistic care involves utilising a multidisciplinary approach to health care, and ensuring that every need, no matter what discipline, is met.

USEFUL WEBSITES

Joint Statement on Culturally Safe Care – NMBA and CATSINaM
These codes advocate for culturally safe care and respectful practice and focus on how nurses and midwives must acknowledge their own culture, values, attitudes, assumptions and beliefs and their potential impact on healthcare delivery. https://www.nursingmidwiferyboard.gov.au/codes-guidelines-statements/position-statements/joint-statement-on-culturally-safe-care.aspx

Closing the Gap – 2022 Report
This report is an annual release from the Australian Prime Minister. It is also compiled by the Close the Gap Steering Committee and the Lowitja Institute. https://humanrights.gov.au/our-work/aboriginal-and-torres-strait-islander-social-justice/publications/close-gap-2022

CATSINaM
The Congress of Aboriginal and Torres Strait Islander Nurses and Midwives (CATSINaM) is the peak advocacy body for Aboriginal and Torres Strait Islander Nurses and Midwives in Australia. https://catsinam.org.au

Transforming EDs towards Cultural Safety (TECS) – Clinical excellence commission (Queensland Health)
https://clinicalexcellence.qld.gov.au/improvement-exchange/transforming-eds-towards-cultural-safety-tecs

Aboriginal and Torres Strait Islander Cultural Capability – Queensland Health
https://www.health.qld.gov.au/public-health/groups/atsihealth/cultural-capability

Registered Nurse Standards for Practice
The Registered Nurse Standards for Practice consist of seven crucial standards that all nurses must follow. Download and review the standards at the following link. https://www.nursingmidwiferyboard.gov.au/Codes-Guidelines-Statements/Professional-standards/registered-nurse-standards-for-practice.aspx

Australian Human Rights Commission
The Australian Human Rights Commission is an independent third party which investigates complaints about discrimination and human rights breaches. This website also houses resources and legislation relevant to Australia. https://humanrights.gov.au

Australian Commission on Safety and Quality in Health Care
They have provided a User Guide for Aboriginal and Torres Strait Islander Health which can be found at the following link. https://www.safetyandquality.gov.au/publications-and-resources/resource-library/nsqhs-standards-user-guide-aboriginal-and-torres-strait-islander-health

REFERENCES AND FURTHER READING

Artuso, S., Cargo, M., Brown, A., & Daniel, M. (2013). Factors influencing health care utilisation among Aboriginal cardiac patients in central Australia: a qualitative study. *Bmc Health Services Research, 13,* article 83. https://doi.org/10.1186/1472-6963-13-83

Australian Health Practitioner Regulation Agency (Ahpra). (2020). *Aboriginal and Torres Strait Islander cultural health and safety strategy 2020–2025.* AHPRA. https://www.ahpra.gov.au/About-Ahpra/Aboriginal-and-Torres-Strait-Islander-Health-Strategy/health-and-cultural-safety-strategy.aspx

Australian Human Rights Commission. (2005). *Social justice report 2005*. humanrights. gov.au/sites/default/files/content/ social_justice/sj_report/sjreport05/pdf/ SocialJustice2005.pdf

Australian Institute of Health and Welfare (AIHW). (2017). *Australia's welfare 2017*. https://www.aihw.gov.au/ getmedia/89b96698-1f50-449c-9260- 7c0243b109be/aihw-australias-welfare- 2017-chapter7-2.pdf.aspx

Best, O. (2021). The cultural safety journey: An Aboriginal Australian nursing and midwifery context. In O. Best & B. Fredericks (Eds.), *Yatdjuligin: Aboriginal and Torres Strait Islander nursing and midwifery care* (3rd ed., pp. 61–80). Cambridge University Press.

Best, O., & Fredericks, B. (2017). *Yatdjuligin: Aboriginal and Torres Strait Islander nursing and midwifery care* (2nd ed.). Cambridge University Press.

Best, O., & Fredericks, B. (2021). *Yatdjuligin. Aboriginal and Torres Strait Islander nursing and midwifery care* (3rd ed.). Cambridge Press.

Brooks-Cleator, L., Phillipps, B., & Giles, A. (2018). Culturally safe health initiatives for Indigenous peoples in Canada: A scoping review. *Canadian Journal of Nursing Research, 50*(4), 202–213. https://doi. org/10.1177/0844562118770334

Cox, L., Taua, C., Drummond, A., & Kidd, J. (2021). *Enabling cultural safety. In Potter & Perry's fundamentals of nursing* (6th ANZ ed.). Elsevier.

Edwards, H., Brown, D., Buckley, T., Aitken, R., & Plowman, E. (2019). *Lewis's medical- surgical nursing* (5th ANZ ed.). Elsevier.

Garvey, G., Anderson, K., Gall, A., Butler, T. L., Whop, L. J., Arley, B., Cunningham, J., Dickson, M., Cass, A., Ratcliffe, J., Tong, A., & Howard, K. (2021). The fabric of Aboriginal and Torres Strait Islander wellbeing: A conceptual model. *International Journal of Environmental Research and Public Health, 18*(15). https:// doi.org/10.3390/ijerph18157745

Geia, L., Baird, K., Bail, K., Barclay, L., Bennett, J., Best, O., Birks, M., Blackley, L., Blackman, R., Bonner, A., Bryant Ao, R., Buzzacott, C., Campbell, S., Catling, C., Chamberlain, C., Cox, L., Cross, W., Cruickshank, M., Cummins, A., … Wynne, R. (2020). A unified call to action from Australian nursing and midwifery leaders: ensuring that Black lives matter. *Contemporary Nurse, 56*(4), 297–308. https://doi.org/10.1080/10376178.2020. 1809107

Ghys, L. (2008). *Just journalism or just journalism: practising safe text* (Annual Conference of the Cultural Studies Association of Australia (CSAA), Issue. CSAA. http://www.kooriweb.org/foley/ resources/media/journalism%20or%20 just%20journalism.pdf

Gopal, D. P., Douglass, C., Wong, S., Khan, I., & Lokugamage, A. U. (2022). Reflexivity, cultural safety, and improving the health of racially minoritised communities. *The Lancet*. https://doi.org/10.1016/s0140- 6736(22)00459-7

Heckenberg, S. (2020). Cultural safety: A model and method that reflects us, respects us and represents us. *Journal of Australian Indigenous Issues, 23*(3–4), 48–66.

Kurtz, D. L. M., Janke, R., Vinek, J., Wells, T., Hutchinson, P., & Froste, A. (2018). Health sciences cultural safety education in Australia, Canada, New Zealand, and the United States: a literature review. *International Journal of Medical Education, 9*(9), 271–285. https://doi. org/10.5116/ijme.5bc7.21e2

Lamp, T. (2018). *The long history of indigenous nursing*. https://thelamp.com. au/specialities/general/the-long-history- %E2%80%A8of-indigenous-nursing/

Langton, M. (2018). *Welcome to Country: A travel guide to Indigenous Australia*. Hardie Grant Travel.

Laverty, M., McDermott, D., & Calma, T. (2017). Embedding cultural safety in Australia's main health care standards. *Medical Journal of Australia, 270*(1), 15–17. https://doi.org/doi:10.569/mja1700378

Lutschini, M. (2005). Engaging with holism in Australian Aboriginal health policy – a review. *Australian and New Zealand Health Policy, 2*(1), 15. https:// doi.org/0.1186/1743-8462-2-15

Moloney, A., Stuart, L., Chen, Y., & Lin, F. (2023). Healthcare professionals' cultural safety practices for indigenous peoples in the acute care setting – A scoping review. *Contemporary Nurse*, 1–22. https://doi.org/ 10.1080/10376178.2023.2271576

Nursing and Midwifery Board of Australia. (2016). *Registered Nurse Standards for Practice*. NMBA/AHPRA.

Nursing and Midwifery Board of Australia, & Congress of Aboriginal and Torres Strait Islander Nurses and Midwives. (2018). *NMBA and CATSINaM joint statement on culturally safe care*. https:// www.nursingmidwiferyboard.gov.au/ codes-guidelines-statements/position-

statements/joint-statement-on-culturally- safe-care.aspx

Nursing Council of New Zealand. (2011). *Guidelines for cultural safety, the Treaty of Waitangi, and Maori health in nursing education and practice*. https://www. nursingcouncil.org.nz/Public/Nursing/ Standards_and_guidelines/NCNZ/nursing- section/Standards_and_guidelines_for_ nurses.aspx

Nursing Council of New Zealand. (2012). *The code of conduct for nurses*. https://www. nursingcouncil.org.nz/Public/Nursing/ Standards_and_guidelines/NCNZ/nursing- section/Standards_and_guidelines_for_ nurses.aspx

Papps, E., & Ramsden, I. (1996). Cultural safety in nursing: the New Zealand experience. *International Journal for Quality in Health Care, 8*(5), 491–497. https://doi.org/intqhc/8.5.491

Paradies, Y., Harris, R., & Anderson, I. (2008). *The impact of racism on Indigenous health in Australia and Aotearoa: Towards a research agenda*. Cooperative Research Centre for Aboriginal Health Discussion Paper Series: No. 4.

Phillips, G. (2015). Dancing with power: Aboriginal health, cultural safety and medical education [PhD, Monash University]. Melbourne.

Power, T., Geia, L., Adams, K., Drummond, A., Saunders, V., Stuart, L., Deravin, L., Tuala, M., Roe, Y., Sherwood, J., Rowe Minniss, F., & West, R. (2021). Beyond 2020: Addressing racism through transformative Indigenous health and cultural safety education. *Journal of Clinical Nursing, 30*(7–8), E32–E35. https://doi.org/10.1111/jocn.15623

Ramsden, I. (2002). Cultural safety and nursing education in Aotearoa and Te Waipounamu. Unpublished doctoral dissertation, Victoria University of Wellington, Wellington, NZ. https://www. nccih.ca/634/Cultural_Safety_and_ Nursing_Education_in_Aotearoa_and_Te_ Waipounamu.nccih?id=1124

Sherwood, J., West, R., Geia, L., Drummond, A., Power, T., Stuart, L., & Deravin, L. (2021). 'Taking our blindfolds off' acknowledging the vision of First Nation peoples for nursing and midwifery. *Australian Journal of Advanced Nursing, 38*(1), 2–5. https://doi. org/https://doi.org/10.37464/2020.381.413

Williams, R. (1999). Cultural safety – what does it mean for our work practice? *Australian and New Zealand Journal of Public Health, 23*(2), 213–214. https://doi. org/10.1111/j.1467-842x.1999.tb01240.x

CHAPTER 19

RESPONDING TO THE DETERIORATING PATIENT

Early intervention and detection of the deteriorating patient are crucial in minimising further adverse events, and even death. Since the introduction of the early warning systems – with names such as 'between the flags', 'adult deterioration detection score', 'medical early warning score' – there have been thorough reviews and implementation of underpinning systems to ensure patient safety is maintained (Australian Commission on Safety and Quality in Health Care [ACSQHC], 2021b).

The Australian Commission on Safety and Quality in Health Care (ACSQHC) (2022) outlines within the Recognising and Responding to Acute Deterioration Standard that serious adverse events, such as unexpected death or cardiac arrest, are often preceded by observable clinical signs and symptoms such as physiological changes and clinical abnormalities. The warning signs, however, are not always identified or acted upon. Some of the biggest causes of clinical deterioration are:
- lack of physiological observations – in timing and consistency
- lack of knowledge that changes in observations could indicate a change in patient condition
- lack of skills to manage deteriorating patients
- failure to communicate clinical concerns
- lack of formal systems to respond and report/escalate deterioration (ACSQHC, 2022).

This national standard outlines the need to recognise acute deterioration, how to escalate care and how to respond to the deterioration. Visit the ACSQHC website for tools to use for observations, auditing and evaluation of systems in place at https://www.safetyandquality.gov.au/our-work/recognising-and-responding-deterioration/recognising-and-responding-acute-physiological-deterioration.

> **LEARNING OBJECTIVES**
> After reading this chapter, you should have an understanding of the:
> 1 assessment required for a person with physiological deterioration
> 2 prioritisation of key components in the development of a plan of care
> 3 prioritised and targeted nursing interventions required to promote recovery or prevent further deterioration
> 4 evaluation phase and how the prioritised and targeted nursing interventions inform further assessment, planning, and collaboration with the healthcare team.

INTRODUCTION

Recognition and response to the deteriorating patient has been a national priority since 2010. It remains, however, one of the areas in health care where there are still events of care not being escalated (Connell et al., 2021). Listening to our patients and escalating care regardless of the time of day or other 'things' occurring, are crucial aspects of nursing care and safe patient care. Every patient is a *person*, and they are *someone's favourite person* – we need to ensure they are cared for safely.

One patient, who nearly died in hospital after a series of failures to recognise or respond to her clinical deterioration, gives the following tips for nurses:
- listen to the patient, don't dismiss them
- introduce yourself properly, avoid saying 'I'm busy'
- be professional at all times
- take care to do vital signs observations properly
- don't label people – this can be hurtful and unhelpful
- don't make assumptions about your patient – act on evidence instead. If you want to know about your patient, ask your patient (ACSQHC, n.d.).

19.1 ASSESSMENT OF PHYSIOLOGICAL DETERIORATION

Recognition of the deterioration – physiological or psychological – in your patient is a component of your accountability and clinical judgement. The safety tools are created to ensure that patients do not enter the 'slippery slope' of deterioration to missed interventions and poor patient outcomes, including death. **Figure 19.1** illustrates the underlying safety factors of the Between the Flags program, the pilot project in NSW Health in 2010. Essentially, early recognition and intervention reduces the harm to patients and improves outcomes.

All healthcare facilities have guidelines based on the observation tools used that direct clinical staff to the frequency of vital signs. NSW Health has a recommendation for a minimum number and frequency for vital signs observations:

- for adult inpatients – the minimum requirement is four times per day at six-hourly intervals. The minimum set of vital signs include:
  - respiratory rate
  - oxygen saturation
  - heart rate
  - blood pressure
  - temperature
  - level of consciousness

- new onset of confusion or behaviour change
- and pain score (NSW Health, 2020).

All vital signs are important, but perhaps the most clinically relevant in adults is that of the respiratory rate. Many studies have highlighted that a respiratory rate greater than 27 breaths per minute is the most important predictor of cardiac arrest in hospital wards (Brown et al., 2019). Further studies (as cited in Brown et al., 2019) highlight that 25 per cent of patients with a respiratory rate of between 25–29 breaths per minute died in hospital, and patients with a respiratory rate of between 30–34 breaths per minute had a mortality rate of 35 per cent. The important factor here is the need for ongoing education around altered respiratory rate, and that it needs to be escalated for patient safety. When assessing the respiratory rate, the following components are also critical objective data:

- the work of breathing (effort it takes to breathe)
- the use of accessory muscles
- the position of the patient
- any nasal flaring
- the patient's colour/perfusion (including nail beds)
- oxygen saturation
- chest on auscultation – sounds heard, etc.

As you can see in **Figure 19.2**, respiratory rate is the first documented observation and is an immediate escalation if it is altered.

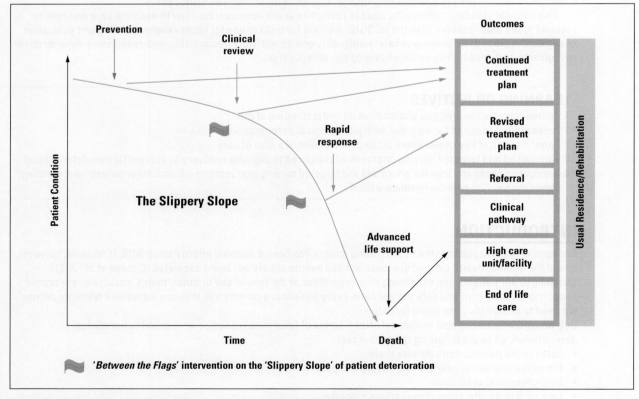

FIGURE 19.1 'Between the Flags' intervention on the 'slippery slope' of patient deterioration

SOURCE: © CLINICAL EXCELLENCE COMMISSION, 2014

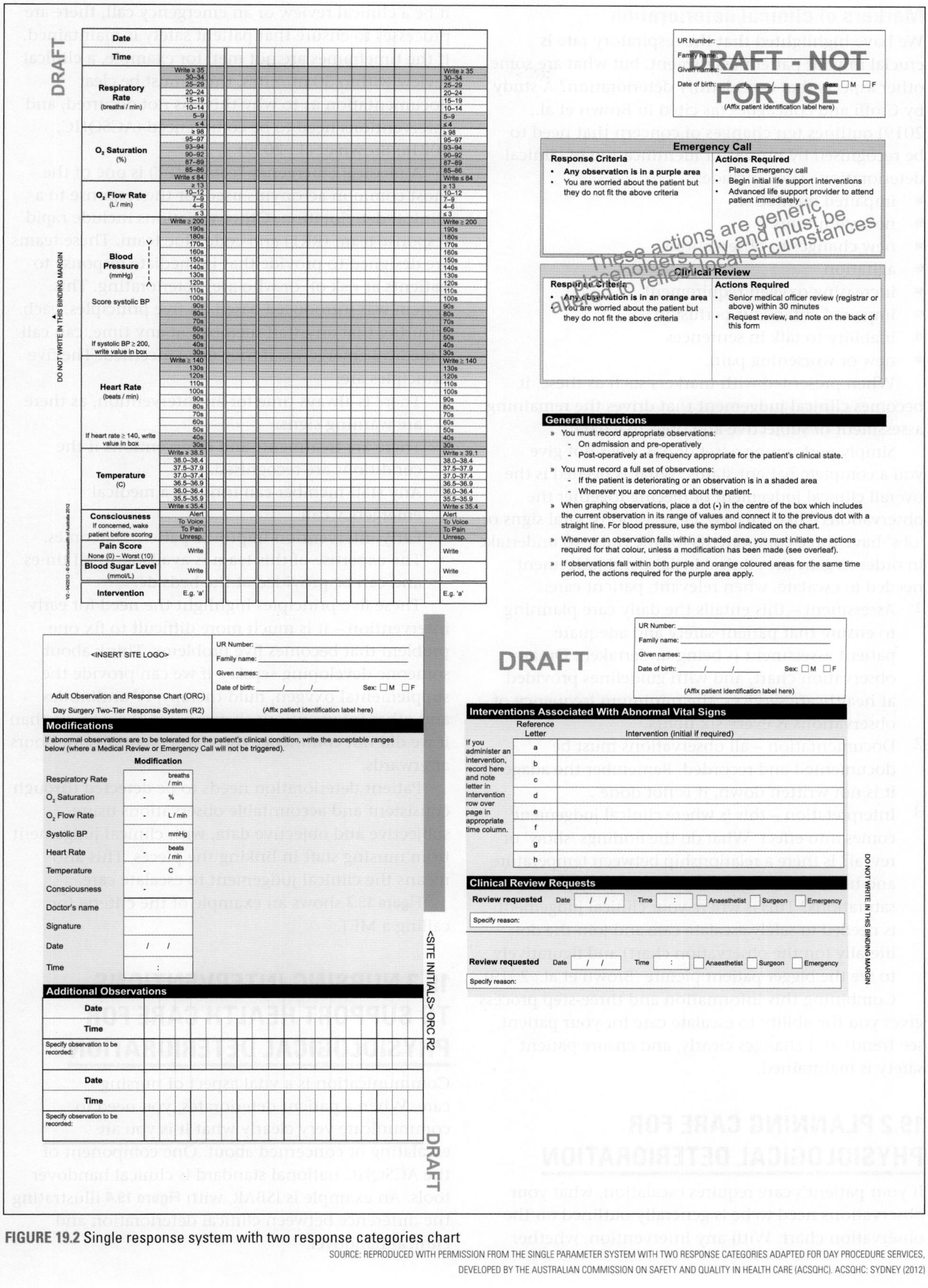

DRAFT

DRAFT - NOT FOR USE

These actions are generic placeholders only and must be adapted to reflect local circumstances

UR Number: _____
Family name: _____
Given names: _____
Date of birth: ___/___/___   Sex: ☐ M ☐ F
(Affix patient identification label here)

Date							
Time							

Respiratory Rate (breaths / min)	Write ≥ 35						Write ≥ 35
	30–34						30–34
	25–29						25–29
	20–24						20–24
	15–19						15–19
	10–14						10–14
	5–9						5–9
	≤ 4						≤ 4

O₂ Saturation (%)	≥ 98						≥ 98
	95–97						95–97
	93–94						93–94
	90–92						90–92
	87–89						87–89
	85–86						85–86
	Write ≤ 84						Write ≤ 84

O₂ Flow Rate (L / min)	≥ 13						≥ 13
	10–12						10–12
	7–9						7–9
	4–6						4–6
	≤ 3						≤ 3

Blood Pressure (mmHg)	Write ≥ 200						Write ≥ 200
	190s						190s
	180s						180s
	170s						170s
	160s						160s
	150s						150s
	140s						140s
	130s						130s
	120s						120s
Score systolic BP	110s						110s
	100s						100s
	90s						90s
	80s						80s
	70s						70s
	60s						60s
If systolic BP ≥ 200, write value in box	50s						50s
	40s						40s
	30s						30s

Heart Rate (beats / min)	Write ≥ 140						Write ≥ 140
	130s						130s
	120s						120s
	110s						110s
	100s						100s
	90s						90s
	80s						80s
	70s						70s
	60s						60s
If heart rate ≥ 140, write value in box	50s						50s
	40s						40s
	30s						30s

Temperature (C)	Write ≥ 38.5						Write ≥ 39.1
	38.0–38.4						38.0–38.4
	37.5–37.9						37.5–37.9
	37.0–37.4						37.0–37.4
	36.5–36.9						36.5–36.9
	36.0–36.4						36.0–36.4
	35.5–35.9						35.5–35.9
	Write ≤ 35.4						Write ≤ 35.4

Consciousness If concerned, wake patient before scoring	Alert						Alert
	To Voice						To Voice
	To Pain						To Pain
	Unresp.						Unresp.

Pain Score None (0) – Worst (10)	Write						Write
Blood Sugar Level (mmol/L)	Write						Write
Intervention	E.g. 'a'						E.g. 'a'

V2 - 04/2012 - © Commonwealth of Australia 2012

DO NOT WRITE IN THIS BINDING MARGIN

Emergency Call

Response Criteria	Actions Required
• Any observation is in a purple area • You are worried about the patient but they do not fit the above criteria	• Place Emergency call • Begin initial life support interventions • Advanced life support provider to attend patient immediately

Clinical Review

Response Criteria	Actions Required
• Any observation is in an orange area • You are worried about the patient but they do not fit the above criteria	• Senior medical officer review (registrar or above) within 30 minutes • Request review, and note on the back of this form

General Instructions

» You must record appropriate observations:
  - On admission and pre-operatively
  - Post-operatively at a frequency appropriate for the patient's clinical state.

» You must record a full set of observations:
  - If the patient is deteriorating or an observation is in a shaded area
  - Whenever you are concerned about the patient.

» When graphing observations, place a dot (•) in the centre of the box which includes the current observation in its range of values and connect it to the previous dot with a straight line. For blood pressure, use the symbol indicated on the chart.

» Whenever an observation falls within a shaded area, you must initiate the actions required for that colour, unless a modification has been made (see overleaf).

» If observations fall within both purple and orange coloured areas for the same time period, the actions required for the purple area apply.

<INSERT SITE LOGO>

Adult Observation and Response Chart (ORC)
Day Surgery Two-Tier Response System (R2)

UR Number: _____
Family name: _____
Given names: _____
Date of birth: ___/___/___   Sex: ☐ M ☐ F
(Affix patient identification label here)

Modifications

If abnormal observations are to be tolerated for the patient's clinical condition, write the acceptable ranges below (where a Medical Review or Emergency Call will not be triggered).

Modification

Respiratory Rate	-	breaths / min
O₂ Saturation	-	%
O₂ Flow Rate	-	L / min
Systolic BP	-	mmHg
Heart Rate	-	beats / min
Temperature	-	C
Consciousness	-	
Doctor's name		
Signature		
Date	/ /	
Time	:	

Additional Observations

Date							
Time							
Specify observation to be recorded:							

Date							
Time							
Specify observation to be recorded:							

<SITE INITIALS> ORC R2

DRAFT

DRAFT

UR Number: _____
Family name: _____
Given names: _____
Date of birth: ___/___/___   Sex: ☐ M ☐ F
(Affix patient identification label here)

Interventions Associated With Abnormal Vital Signs

	Reference Letter	Intervention (initial if required)
If you administer an intervention, record here and note letter in Intervention row over page in appropriate time column.	a	
	b	
	c	
	d	
	e	
	f	
	g	
	h	

Clinical Review Requests

Review requested   Date   / /   Time   :   ☐ Anaesthetist ☐ Surgeon ☐ Emergency
Specify reason: _____

Review requested   Date   / /   Time   :   ☐ Anaesthetist ☐ Surgeon ☐ Emergency
Specify reason: _____

DO NOT WRITE IN THIS BINDING MARGIN

FIGURE 19.2 Single response system with two response categories chart

SOURCE: REPRODUCED WITH PERMISSION FROM THE SINGLE PARAMETER SYSTEM WITH TWO RESPONSE CATEGORIES ADAPTED FOR DAY PROCEDURE SERVICES, DEVELOPED BY THE AUSTRALIAN COMMISSION ON SAFETY AND QUALITY IN HEALTH CARE (ACSQHC). ACSQHC: SYDNEY (2012)

Markers of clinical deterioration

We have highlighted that the respiratory rate is crucial in your patient assessment, but what are some other aspects that can identify deterioration? A study by Cioffi and colleagues (as cited in Brown et al., 2019) outlines ten changes of concern that need to be recognised by nurses for identification of clinical deterioration. They include:

- impaired mentation
- new symptoms
- new changes to observations
- agitation
- increasing oxygen requirement
- impaired cutaneous perfusion
- inability to talk in sentences
- new or worsening pain.

When presented with markers such as these, it becomes clinical judgement that drives the remaining assessment of subjective and objective data.

Simply performing a 'set of obs' does not give you a complete patient status. What is needed is the overall clinical judgement of piecing together the observations – like a jigsaw. Observations, vital signs or 'obs' have three components for the nurse to undertake in order to gain the clinical insight and judgement needed to escalate, when relevant, patient care:

1 Assessment – this entails the daily care planning to ensure that patient safety and adequate patient assessment is being undertaken. On any observation chart, and with guidelines provided at healthcare services, the minimum frequency of observations is every six hours.
2 Documentation – all observations must be documented and recorded. Remember the adage 'if it is not written down, it is not done'.
3 Interpretation – this is where clinical judgement comes into effect. What do the findings 'show' or reveal? Is there a relationship between temperature and heart rate? Respiratory rate and oxygen saturations? This is where your clinical judgement is needed to safely escalate care and join the dots literally (on the observation chart) and figuratively to see the bigger patient picture (Brown et al., 2019).

Combining this information and three-step process gives you the ability to escalate care for your patient, see trends and changes clearly, and ensure patient safety is maintained.

19.2 PLANNING CARE FOR PHYSIOLOGICAL DETERIORATION

If your patient's care requires escalation, what your observations need to be is generally outlined on the observation chart. With any intervention, whether it be a clinical review or an emergency call, there are processes to ensure that patient safety is maintained. If the timeframes are not met; for example, a clinical review within 30 minutes, there must be clear documentation as to why this has not occurred, and interventions need to be commenced (ACSQHC, 2021a; Brown et al., 2019).

A medical emergency team (MET) is one of the most common acronyms used for the response to a clinical deterioration. Other variations include rapid response team (RRT) and code blue team. These teams are designed to provide that immediate response to patients at risk of, or who are, deteriorating. This system was introduced based on five principles, each ensuring that any staff member, at any time, can call a medical emergency if they are concerned. The five principles are:

1 There is always time for an intervention, as there are warning signs.
2 There are treatments and interventions if the conditions are recognised.
3 Any staff member can intitiate a medical emergency call.
4 Early intervention improves patient outcomes.
5 The expertise of this team is available at all times and can be provided at the bedside.

These five principles highlight the need for early intervention – it is much more difficult to fix one problem that becomes five problems. Think about someone developing sepsis – if we can provide the supplemental oxygen, fluid therapy, IV antibiotics and other interventions they are less likely to die than if we did not commence those interventions for hours afterwards.

Patient deterioration needs to be detected through consistent and accountable observations using subjective and objective data, with clinical judgement from nursing staff in linking the pieces. This also means the clinical judgement to escalate care.

Figure 19.3 shows an example of the criteria for calling a MET.

19.3 NURSING INTERVENTIONS TO SUPPORT HEALTH CARE FOR PHYSIOLOGICAL DETERIORATION

Communication is a vital aspect of nursing care. When a patient deteriorates, you need to communicate very clearly what it is you are escalating or concerned about. One component of the ACSQHC national standard is clinical handover tools. An example is ISBAR, with **Figure 19.4** illustrating the difference between clinical deterioration and clinical handover.

CLINICAL	
MEDICAL EMERGENCY TEAM (MET) CALLING CRITERIA	
All Cardiac and Respiratory Arrests Any patient that breaches the 'RED ZONE' And all conditions listed below	
ACUTE CHANGES IN:	**PHYSIOLOGY**
AIRWAY	Threatened
BREATHING	**All Respiratory arrests** Respiratory rate < 5 or > 30 SpO_2 < 90% and/or increase in O_2 requirement
CIRCULATION	**All cardiac arrests** Pulse rate < 40 or > 140 SBP < 90 or > 200
NEUROLOGY	**Sudden fall in level of consciousness** (Fall in GCS of > 2 points) (P) or (U) on AVPU scale Repeated or prolonges seizures
WORRIED	Any patient who you are seriously worried about that does not fit the above criteria
CALL A MET – DIAL 2222 from any internal phone State clearly the patient or person's location – Building/floor/department	

FIGURE 19.3 Example medical emergency team calling criteria

SOURCE: © STATE OF NEW SOUTH WALES NSW MINISTRY OF HEALTH. FOR CURRENT INFORMATION GO TO WWW.HEALTH.NSW.GOV.AU.

COMMUNICATING WITHIN YOUR HEALTH CARE TEAM

CLINICAL DETERIORATION	CLINICAL HANDOVER
INTRODUCTION • Introduce yourself, your role and location • Identify the patient	**INTRODUCTION** • Introduce yourself, your role and location • Identify team leader • Clearly identify patient and family and carer if present
SITUATION • State the immediate clinical situation	**SITUATION** • State the immediate clinical situation • State particular issues, concerns or risks • Identify risks - Deteriorating patient, Falls risk, Allergies, limitation to resuscitation
BACKGROUND • Provide relevant clinical history and background • Presenting problems and clinical history	**BACKGROUND** • Provide relevant clinical history referring to medical record and/or eMR
ASSESSMENT • Work through A-G physical assessment • What clinical observations are of particular concern? • What do you think the problem is? • Remember to have current observations and information ready!	**ASSESSMENT** • Work through A-G physical assessment • Refer to observations, medication and other patient charts • Summarise current risk management strategies • Have observations breached CERS criteria?
RECOMMENDATION • What do you want the person you have called to do? • What have you done? • Be clear about what you are requesting and the timeframe • Repeat to confirm what you have heard	**RECOMMENDATION** • Recommendations for the shift • Refer to medical record or eMR • Provide expected date of discharge • What further assessments and actions are required by who and when • State expected frequency of observations • Request that receiver read back important actions required

FIGURE 19.4 Communicating with your healthcare team: Clinical deterioration and clinical handover

SOURCE: SYDNEY LOCAL HEALTH DISTRICT.

19.4 EVALUATION OF CARE FOR PHYSIOLOGICAL DETERIORATION

You will need to rely upon your foundation anatomy and physiology, and the application of this, to your patient's condition and to their current deterioration in physiological condition. There are known risk factors; for example, after a surgical procedure the most common ones are bleeding or infection. To monitor for these, we are looking at changes to homeostasis; for instance, if blood pressure drops and heart rate increases, we are likely looking at hypovolaemia. For infection we would expect to see an increase in temperature and heart rate. These are all parts of a 'jigsaw' that you will need to assemble for each and every patient. Just like the assessment of pain, there are no two patients who will respond to an operation in the same way, recover the same way, or have the same observations postoperatively.

Using your clinical insight, judgement and communication skills you will be able to maintain patient safety, escalate care and recognise and respond to the deteriorating patient.

SUMMARY

Failure to recognise and manage appropriate care and interventions to deterioration in a patient's physiological and psychological status is a significant contributing factor in the majority of adverse events in hospitals and healthcare organisations globally.

Recognition of the deteriorating patient is enabled using standardised observation tools and reporting structures to ensure patient safety is maintained.

USEFUL WEBSITES

Registered Nurse Standards for Practice
The Registered Nurse Standards for Practice consist of seven crucial standards that all nurses must follow. Download and review the standards at the following link. https://www.nursingmidwiferyboard.gov.au/Codes-Guidelines-Statements/Professional-standards/registered-nurse-standards-for-practice.aspx

Australian Commission on Safety and Quality in Health Care
National standards and clinical guidelines for safe and consistent care in all healthcare settings. https://www.safetyandquality.gov.au

Clinical Excellence Commission – NSW Health
Lead agency supporting safety and quality improvement in the NSW health system. https://www.cec.health.nsw.gov.au

The National Safety and Quality Health Service (NSQHS) standards
All eight are essential, but for this chapter, Communicating for Safety Standard and Recognising and Responding to Acute Deterioration Standard. https://www.safetyandquality.gov.au/standards/nsqhs-standards

REFERENCES AND FURTHER READING

Australian Commission on Safety and Quality in Health Care (ACSQHC). (2021a). *National safety and quality health service standards*. https://www.safetyandquality.gov.au/sites/default/files/2021-05/national_safety_and_quality_health_service_nsqhs_standards_second_edition_-_updated_may_2021.pdf

Australian Commission on Safety and Quality in Health Care (ACSQHC). (2021b). *National consensus statement – Essential elements for recognising and responding to acute physiological deterioration*. https://www.safetyandquality.gov.au/sites/default/files/2021-12/essential_elements_for_recognising_and_responding_to_acute_physiological_deterioration.pdf

Australian Commission on Safety and Quality in Health Care (ACSQHC). (2022). *Recognising and responding to acute deterioration standard*. https://www.safetyandquality.gov.au/standards/nsqhs-standards/recognising-and-responding-acute-deterioration-standard

Australian Commission on Safety and Quality in Health Care (ACSQHC). (n.d.). *Fact sheet – Tips from the real world: A patient's story*. https://www.safetyandquality.gov.au/sites/default/files/migrated/Learning-from-a-patients-experience.pdf

Brown, D., Edwards, H., Buckley, T., Aitken, R. L., Lewis, S. L., Bucher, L., McLean Heitkemper, M., Harding, M. M., Kwong, J., & Roberts, D. (2019). *Lewis's medical-surgical nursing ANZ* (5th ed.). Elsevier.

Connell, C. J., Endacott, R., & Cooper, S. (2021). The prevalence and management of deteriorating patients in an Australian emergency department. *Australasian Emergency Care, 24*(2), 112–120. https://doi.org/https://doi.org/10.1016/j.auec.2020.07.008

NSW Health. (2020). *Recognition and management of patients who are deteriorating*. https://www1.health.nsw.gov.au/pds/ActivePDSDocuments/PD2020_018.pdf

CHAPTER **20**

PERIOPERATIVE CARE

Surgery is a planned procedure encompassing three phases which are referred to as the perioperative period. This is the period that includes patient admission for surgery, performing the surgery and recovery from surgery. The nurse is responsible for providing comfort and safety throughout these periods, from admission to a patient's safe discharge to home.

LEARNING OBJECTIVES

After reading this chapter, you should have an understanding of:

1 the three phases of the perioperative period
2 preparing a person for surgery
3 immediate postanaesthetic care
4 postoperative care
5 discharge planning.

INTRODUCTION

Perioperative care is the care provided when a person is scheduled for a surgical procedure. Surgical procedures are also 'day procedures' where the patient is admitted and discharged on the same day as the surgery/procedure. There are three phases in the perioperative period: **preoperative**, **intraoperative** and **postoperative**. Patients requiring surgery could either be inpatients or outpatients. Outpatient procedures are day surgeries, which means patients do not require an overnight stay. Outpatients present themselves on the day of surgery and they are discharged on the same day after the surgery.

The patient flow in the perioperative period is shown in **Figure 20.1**.

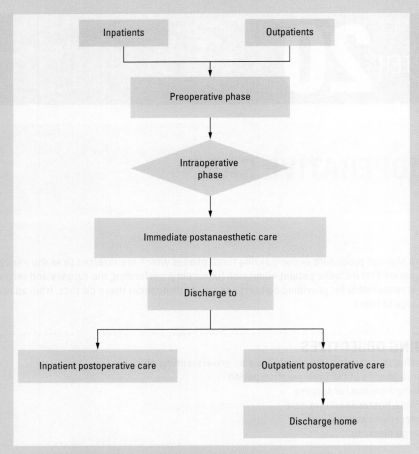

FIGURE 20.1 The patient flow in the perioperative period

20.1 PREOPERATIVE PHASE

In the preoperative phase, the patient is prepared for surgery. The preoperative phase starts when the patient is booked for surgery and ends when the patient is transferred to theatre. The goal of the preoperative period is to prepare the patient physically and mentally, and take care of other psychosocial needs, if needed. Preoperative care assessment can occur in the hospital for inpatients. For outpatients, preoperative care planning occurs in an outpatient clinic either face to face or through a telephone conversation. Some facilities have outpatient clinics that pre-screen patients prior to surgery for assessment and diagnostics prior to admission. For example, John is an inpatient and Peter is an outpatient, and both are scheduled for surgery. John will have his preoperative care assessment in the ward. On the other hand, Peter will have his preoperative care assessment in an outpatient clinic either face to face or via a telephone interview a few days before the surgery.

On the day of surgery and before the patient is brought to theatre, the nurse must complete a preoperative checklist as a safety guide. The checklist may vary from one organisation to another. A sample of a preoperative checklist is shown in **Figure 20.2**.

Preoperative assessment
Concept map 20.1 is an example of an inpatient preoperative assessment and **Concept map 20.2** is an example of an outpatient preoperative assessment.

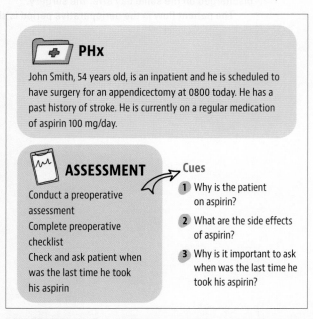

PHx

John Smith, 54 years old, is an inpatient and he is scheduled to have surgery for an appendicectomy at 0800 today. He has a past history of stroke. He is currently on a regular medication of aspirin 100 mg/day.

ASSESSMENT

Conduct a preoperative assessment
Complete preoperative checklist
Check and ask patient when was the last time he took his aspirin

Cues

1 Why is the patient on aspirin?

2 What are the side effects of aspirin?

3 Why is it important to ask when was the last time he took his aspirin?

CONCEPT MAP 20.1 Preoperative assessment for an appendicectomy

Sample preoperative checklist

Safety Check			
Patient Identification (ID) Correct name Correct hospital number Correct date of birth	☐ Yes		
Valid consent	☐ Yes		
Allergies If yes, is allergy band in situ	☐ Yes	☐ NKA	Details of allergies
Is fasting required	☐ Yes	☐ N/A	Date/time food Date/time fluids
Is bowel prep required	☐ Yes	☐ N/A	
Any infectious diseases	☐ Yes		Details
Teeth Dentures, caps, crowns, bridges, loose teeth	☐ Yes ☐ Nil		Details
Jewelleries Jewellery removed/taped	☐ Yes ☐ No		Details
Nail polish, make-up, tampon, contact lenses	☐ Yes ☐ Nil		Details
Any artificial things inside the body Prosthesis, pacemaker, cataract implants	☐ Yes ☐ No		Details
Does the patient smoke	☐ Yes ☐ No		Details
Does the patient drink alcohol	☐ Yes ☐ No		Details
List of current medications – prescribed and unprescribed drugs including herbal medicines.			
Document patient valuables and lock belongings	☐ Yes ☐ Nil		
Recent Observations and Baseline Vital Signs			
Neurological Observation: Time			
Neurovascular observation			
Weight			
Height			
Respiration rate			
Heart rate			
Temperature			
Sa0$_2$			
Blood pressure			
Blood glucose level (BGL)			

FIGURE 20.2 Sample preoperative checklist

PHx

Peter Jones, 35 years old, is an outpatient and has presented to Day Procedure Unit for colonoscopy at 0800 hours. Preoperative care planning was done one week before his interventional procedure via telephone interview. He was consented via phone.

ASSESSMENT

Conduct a preoperative assessment

Complete preoperative checklist

Check consent form

Cues

1 What is a valid consent?
2 What is phone consent?
3 What are the legal requirements for a valid consent?

CONCEPT MAP 20.2 Diagnostic procedure – assessment for a colonoscopy

SAFETY IN NURSING ⚠

CONSENT

A patient cannot be taken to theatre without a valid consent. Although it is a surgeon's responsibility to get the patient's consent, the nurse should check that the consent is valid. The nurse asks the patient what surgery the patient is having. This is to ascertain that the patient has full knowledge of the procedure to be performed and that it matches what is written in the consent. The nurse must ensure that the consent is signed and dated by both the patient and the surgeon. If the consent is not valid, then the nurse should inform the surgeon.

PATIENT IDENTIFICATION (ID)

A patient must not be brought to theatre without correct ID in place. The nurse must ensure that the patient's name, date of birth and hospital number are correct.

ALLERGIES

Allergies to prescription, non-prescription drugs, food, latex and any other allergies should be documented, including the patient's reactions and the severity. The appropriate allergy band (ID band) must be applied to the patient prior to the transfer to the operating theatre.

MEDICATIONS

Some medications, such as aspirin and anticoagulants, increase the risk of surgery, including bleeding, and need to be discontinued several days before the surgery.

Preoperative patient education

Preoperative patient education provides necessary information for both the patient and their carer. For outpatients, this can be done face to face in a pre-admission clinic or via a telephone conversation. Preoperative education can be broken down into different components:

1 Before coming for their surgery, the nurse ensures that the patient is informed of:
   - their arrival time for the surgery
   - when to stop eating and drinking
   - medications they need to stop taking or need to take as per doctor's instructions
   - instructions and toiletries required for preoperative shower and skin preparation
   - what to bring, such as x-rays or blood tests
   - what to leave at home, such as jewellery and other valuables
   - how they must arrange for somebody to pick them up when ready to go home and a responsible adult to stay with them overnight.

2 Upon arrival for the surgery, the patient will be admitted by a nurse who will complete the checklist for surgery and take vital signs and the patient will be asked to change into a hospital gown.

3 After surgery the nurse educates the patient about their recovery period. If the patient is going home on the same day, they will be given discharge information concerning what they can do and cannot do, pain medications, follow-up appointments and a telephone number for them to call if they have questions.

4 Postoperative and discharge cares will include planning for return to work or normal daily activities. Some patients will require a medical certificate and this needs to be included with discharge planning. If the patient is staying overnight, they will be transferred to a ward for ongoing care and their family will be informed upon arrival in the ward.

20.2 INTRAOPERATIVE PHASE

The intraoperative phase begins when the patient is transferred to the operating room and ends when the patient is transported to the recovery room for immediate postanaesthetic care.

Intraoperative nursing roles

Intraoperative nurses have specialised skills to perform throughout the surgery. These roles include anaesthetic nurse, scrub nurse and scout nurse.

Anaesthetic nurse

The anaesthetic nurse assists the anaesthetist. They:
- prepare and check the anaesthetic machines
- obtain anaesthetic drugs and document
- escort patient into the operating theatre
- reassure and maintain patient comfort and safety
- assist anaesthetist where appropriate
- help monitor patient's vital signs.

Scrub nurse

The scrub nurse is also referred to as an instrument nurse. They:
- assist the doctor throughout the surgical procedure
- prepare instruments, supplies and equipment for the procedure
- ensure aseptic technique is practised
- are responsible for handing the instruments to the surgeon while maintaining aseptic technique
- are responsible for ensuring the instrument and needle count (including gauze and packing materials) are correct prior to skin closure.

Scout nurse

The scout nurse is also referred to as the circulating nurse. They:
- maintain cleanliness of the operating room
- ensure sterile supplies and instruments are available
- ensure that instruments and other equipment are working and safe to use
- checks with scrub nurse that all materials and equipment are accounted for before the surgical site is closed.

20.3 IMMEDIATE POSTANAESTHETIC CARE

Once the surgery is finished, the patient is transferred for immediate postanaesthetic care. This is usually provided in the postanaesthetic care unit (PACU). The nursing role in PACU includes, but is not limited to, the following:
1 assessment of:
  - Airway: keep artificial airway in place until the patient is awake. Assess for any noises and suction any secretions

  - Breathing: respiratory rate, work of breathing, rhythm, oxygen therapy and delivery mode
  - Circulation: assess pulses for rate, rhythm and strength; temperature, skin colour, capillary refill, oxygen saturation, blood pressure
  - Disability: assess for consciousness (alert, responding to voice, responding to pain, unresponsive), gross motor function
  - Exposure/extra: assess for wounds, drains, dressings, etc.
  - Blood loss: assessment of surgical wounds, drains and bedding. Documenting blood loss and escalating care as required
2 Postoperative pain: pain management commenced as required
3 Postoperative nausea and vomiting (PONV): PONV management commenced as required.

Remember John Smith who had an appendicectomy? **Concept map 20.3** illustrates a PACU nursing assessment for John.

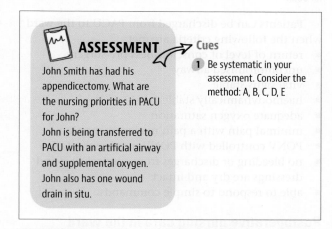

ASSESSMENT

John Smith has had his appendicectomy. What are the nursing priorities in PACU for John?

John is being transferred to PACU with an artificial airway and supplemental oxygen. John also has one wound drain in situ.

Cues

1 Be systematic in your assessment. Consider the method: A, B, C, D, E

CONCEPT MAP 20.3 PACU nursing assessment for John (appendicectomy)

20.4 POSTOPERATIVE PHASE

Patients can be discharged from PACU to the ward after meeting certain criteria. It is the responsibility of the nurse in charge of escorting the patient from PACU to ensure that the patient is safe to be transferred to the ward. The nurse can refuse to take the patient back to the ward if the criteria are not met or if there are concerns about the patient's condition. The patient will be reviewed by a doctor as to whether the patient can be safely discharged from PACU. Some criteria may be modified by the doctor who then documents the time when the modification was made, the modified parameters for the vital signs, and the duration of the modification.

Concept map 20.4 considers John's discharge to the ward.

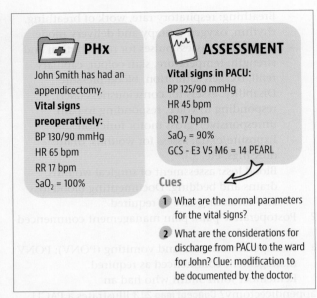

CONCEPT MAP 20.4 Considerations for discharge from PACU to ward for John

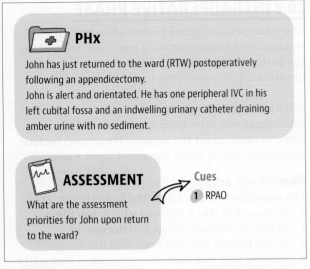

CONCEPT MAP 20.5 Postoperative assessment in the ward for John

Patients can be discharged from PACU to the ward when the following criteria are met:

- return of level of consciousness pre-surgery
- uncompromised airway
- vital signs stable
- haemodynamically stable
- adequate oxygen saturation
- minimal pain with a pain management plan
- PONV controlled with PONV management plan
- no bleeding or discharges from surgical sites and dressings are dry and intact
- able to respond to simple commands.

Postoperative nursing care in the ward

Upon a patient's return to the ward, the nurse conducts a routine postanaesthetic observation (RPAO) as per hospital's protocols. The frequency of observation must be adjusted depending on the patient's condition or medical advice.

Routine postanaesthetic observation (RPAO)

- 15 minutes for the first hour
- 30 minutes for the second hour
- 1 hourly for the next 2 hours
- Then 4 hourly for the next 48 hours
- Drain tubes must be monitored and documented for drainage as per hospital's protocol or as directed by the doctor/surgeon.

Concept map 20.5 considers John's postoperative assessment in the ward.

Postoperative patient assessment and interventions continue until the patient is discharged from the unit.

Nursing assessment and interventions include, but are not limited to:

- pain management:
  - analgesia as prescribed by the doctor
  - monitor patient-controlled analgesia (PCA) if applicable and epidural observations if the PCA is an epidural
- wound care:
  - assess for bleeding
  - dressings are dry and intact
  - monitor drains for volume loss, type, colour and consistency if applicable
- IV monitoring:
  - assessment and management of IV site
  - monitoring of fluids
- diet and fluid intake:
  - unless the doctor has specified that the patient is nil by mouth (NBM), the patient should be given food and fluids 4–6 hours postoperatively (highly dependent on type of surgery)
  - monitor for nausea and vomiting
- elimination:
  - monitor urine output
  - monitor bowel function
- ambulation:
  - early ambulation should be encouraged unless contraindicated
  - educate patient for deep breathing, coughing and leg exercises
  - observe and supervise patients the first time they get out of bed after surgery
- medications:
  - administer medications as prescribed
  - ensure venous thromboembolism (VTE) prophylaxis as per National Inpatient Medication Chart (NIMC) has been administered and adhered to.

Complications

It is important to recognise signs of complications and to intervene accordingly. **Table 20.1** lists the areas of assessment and expected normal findings in the postoperative phase. The potential postoperative problems that may occur are defined as abnormal findings.

TABLE 20.1

Initial postoperative assessment: normal and abnormal findings

AREA OF ASSESSMENT	NORMAL FINDINGS	ABNORMAL FINDINGS
Airway and respiratory status: • adequacy of airway and return of gag, cough and swallowing reflexes • type of artificial airway • rate, rhythm and depth of respirations • symmetry of chest wall movements and use of accessory muscles • breath sounds • colour of mucous membranes • pulse oximeter readings • amount and method of oxygen administration • if awake, ability to breathe deeply and cough.	The person is able to: • expel an oral airway; exhibit return of gag reflex • breathe deeply and cough freely with normal rate for age, without use of accessory muscles, and exhibit chest wall symmetry; show breath sounds present in all lobes; show pink mucous membranes • show pulse oximeter reading between 96% and 100% • demonstrate proper use of incentive spirometer, if awake.	• Upper airway obstruction: stridor, retractions, asymmetrical chest movement • Laryngospasm: high-pitched squeaky sounds • Dyspnoea: shortness of breath or difficulty in breathing • Diminished breath sounds, wheezing, rales or rhonchi • Residual neuromuscular blockage: weak inspiratory effort, inability to lift head or inadequate muscle strength
Circulatory status: • apical and peripheral pulses • blood pressure (BP) • nail bed and skin colour and temperature • capillary refill • Homans' sign (assess for DVT: dorsiflex each foot, assess for calf/popliteal pain). Monitoring devices: • cardiac monitor (ECG) • pressure readings (arterial BP or central venous pressure).	The person has: • normal apical rate and peripheral pulses • BP within 20 mmHg of baseline measurements • pink nail beds; warm and dry skin • capillary refill < 3 s • negative Homans' sign • normal ECG rhythm.	• Hypotension: BP < 20 mmHg of baseline; rapid, weak pulse; bluish nail beds; capillary refill < 3 s • Haemorrhage/hypovolaemic shock: rapid, weak pulse; increasing respirations; restlessness; hypotension; cold, clammy skin; pallor; urinary output < 30 mL/h • Positive Homans' sign (calf pain present on dorsiflexion of foot) • ECG pattern: dysrhythmias; signs of cardiac ischaemia
Neurologic status: • Level of consciousness (Glasgow Coma Scale) • eye opening • verbal response • motor response.	The person: • spontaneously opens eyes • is orientated • obeys commands (Glasgow Coma Scale of 15, highest rating).	• Glasgow Coma Scale score of under 15 indicates some alteration in consciousness; a score of 7 is considered coma
Fluid and metabolic status: • intake and output • palpate for bladder distension • patency of intravenous (IV) infusion (type, rate and amount) • signs of dehydration (skin integrity and turgor) or overload (oedema) • patency, amount and character of drainage (catheters, drains or tubes) • inspect operative dressing (type, colour and amount of drainage) • auscultate for bowel tones in all four quadrants and inspect for abdominal distension.	Fluid intake balanced with total output and electrolytes within normal limits, considering replacement of blood volume lost during surgery. The person has: • IV fluids infusing per doctor's order • absence of bladder distension • good skin turgor • absence of oedema • drains and other tubing patent and intact • dressing dry and intact • bowel tones faint or absent during the immediate recovery phase • absence of nausea and vomiting.	• Signs of deficient fluid volume (thirst, poor skin turgor, low-grade temperature, tachycardia, respirations ≥ 30, a 10–15 mmHg decrease in systolic BP, slow venous filling, urinary output, < 25 mL/h) • Bright red blood on operative dressing • Signs of excess fluid volume (increased central venous pressure and oedema, pulmonary or peripheral)
Level of discomfort or pain: • location, intensity and duration • type and amount of analgesia administered and person's response.	The person is free from pain.	• Pain not relieved by analgesia
Wound management: • inspect the dressing • if drainage is present, reassess in 15-minute intervals.	Dressing is dry and intact.	• Clot dislodged: bright red drainage on the dressing

SOURCE: DELAUNE, S., LADNER, P., MCTIER, L., TOLLEFSON, J., & LAWRENCE, J. (2024). *FUNDAMENTALS OF NURSING* (3RD ED.). CENGAGE LEARNING AUSTRALIA.

20.5 DISCHARGE PLANNING

A patient is ready for discharge when:
- vital signs are stable
- tolerating fluids or diet
- no nausea and vomiting
- wound dressings are dry and intact with no sign of bleeding or swelling
- adequate oral analgesia
- mobilising independently
- home support arranged.

Discharge planning commences during the preoperative phase. Discharge planning should include the patient and, where appropriate, their family or carer/s.

- Patients undergoing day surgery should be escorted home by a responsible adult and should have a responsible adult stay with them overnight unless the patient was only given local anaesthetics.
- For patients admitted to the ward, patients and their families should be advised of the expected date and time of discharge as soon as it is known.

- When possible, discharge prescriptions should be completed and sent to pharmacy a day prior to discharge.
- Equipment required for discharge should be arranged and be available prior to discharge.
- Medical certificate if required.
- A copy of relevant patient instructions to be given to help patients and their carers understand about the surgery.
- Follow-up appointments if required.
- Provide patients with emergency and postoperative contact numbers.

Each patient's postoperative discharge planning will vary depending upon their recovery and response to interventions. All patients will require education regarding their pain management (analgesia), limitations to movement, activities or abilities such as driving, continuing VTE prophylaxis and follow-up specialist and general practitioner appointments.

SUMMARY

Perioperative nursing care involves caring for the patient from the time they are admitted for surgery until the patient is discharged from surgery. During the three phases of perioperative care, the perioperative nurse reassures the patient and tries to maintain patient comfort and safety during the whole process.

CLINICAL SKILLS IN PERIOPERATIVE NURSING

The clinical skills in perioperative nursing are aligned with the Nursing and Midwifery Board of Australia (NMBA) (2021) Registered Nurse Standards for Practice 1.1, 1.4, 1.5, 1.6, 2.1, 2.2, 2.6, 2.7, 3.2, 3.4, 4.1, 4.2, 5.1, 5.5, 6.1, 6.2, 6.5, 7.1, 7.2 and 7.3.

For further information, consult your Clinical Skills resources, such as Tollefson and Hillman (2022), *Clinical Psychomotor Skills* (8th ed.).

- Preoperative care, including:
  - Performs hand hygiene
  - Introduces self to patient
  - Performs patient identification
  - Maintains patient privacy at all times
  - Checks consent
  - Explains procedure to the patient
  - Performs patient assessment
  - Completes preoperative checklist
  - Conducts preoperative education
  - Documents procedure
- Postanaesthesia care and handover, including:
  - Performs hand hygiene
  - Introduces self to patient
  - Performs patient identification
  - Assessment of patient airway

  - Accurately and appropriately records vital signs
  - Assesses patient consciousness
  - Assesses surgery sites
  - Assesses patient pain score
  - Assesses patient postoperative nausea and vomiting
  - Assesses patient's safe discharge from PACU
  - Documents procedure
- Postoperative care, including:
  - Performs hand hygiene
  - Introduces self to patient
  - Identifies patient
  - Obtains consent
  - Reviews postoperative orders
  - Maintains patient privacy at all times
  - Assesses conscious state
  - Accurately and appropriately records vital signs
  - Assesses surgery sites
  - Assesses patient pain score
  - Assesses patient postoperative nausea and vomiting
  - Assesses ability to ambulate
  - Assesses oral intake and hydration status
  - Documents procedure

PROBLEM-SOLVING SCENARIO

Using a concept map approach, how would you help Frank?
Frank has had his open cholecystectomy and returned to your ward from PACU. He has a PCA attached to his IVC.

1   What are the nursing care priorities for Frank in your ward?

2   Frank is complaining of severe pain. How would you manage his pain?

3   Frank is attempting to get out of bed. How would you assist him in getting up to ambulate?

PORTFOLIO DEVELOPMENT

Perioperative nursing care is based on best practice or evidence-based practice (EBP). Therefore, perioperative nursing care can change from time to time based on EBP. The Joanna Briggs Institute is one of the organisations that monitors EBP. Joanna Briggs Institute's COVID-19 special collection for the management of infected patients in perioperative settings can be viewed at https://jbi.global/covid-19.

The information gained from reading the given link can add to your continuing professional development (CPD) hours.

USEFUL WEBSITES

Australian College of Perioperative Nurses (ACORN): Information on perioperative nursing roles https://www.acorn.org.au/nursing-roles

NSW Health: the Perioperative Toolkit is a step-by-step guide to perioperative care https://www1.health.nsw.gov.au/pds/ActivePDSDocuments/GL2018_004.pdf

NSW Agency for Clinical Innovation: Perioperative Patient Information Booklet and Checklist https://aci.health.nsw.gov.au/__data/assets/pdf_file/0014/344201/Appendix_7_Perioperative_Patient_Information_Booklet_including_Outcome.pdf

The Perioperative Toolkit https://aci.health.nsw.gov.au/resources/anaesthesia-perioperative-care/the-perioperative-toolkit/the-perioperative-toolkit-webpage

The Perioperative Toolkit: Patient Information Checklist https://aci.health.nsw.gov.au/__data/assets/pdf_file/0008/342692/Appendix_8_for_Perioperative_Toolkit.pdf

Australian and New Zealand College of Anaesthetists (ANZCA): Guideline for the perioperative care of patients selected for day stay procedures https://www.anzca.edu.au/getattachment/021e4205-af5a-415d-815d-b16be1fe8b62/PS15-Guideline-for-the-perioperative-care-of-patients-selected-for-day-stay-procedures

Position statement on the post-anaesthesia care unit: Background Paper https://www.anzca.edu.au/getattachment/fc82bdc3-ea8b-43c9-b6c5-aa857fc81e23/PS04BP-Statement-on-the-post-anaesthesia-care-unit-Background-Paper

Victorian Department of Health: Mobility and self-care in discharge planning https://www.health.vic.gov.au/patient-care/mobility-and-self-care-in-discharge-planning

JBI – COVID-19 special collection: Evidence-based resources for health professionals and health organisations https://jbi.global/covid-19

REFERENCES AND FURTHER READING

Australian College of Operating Room Nurses. (2020). *Standards for perioperative nursing in Australia* (16th ed., vol. 2). https://www.acorn.org.au/standards

DeLaune, S., Ladner, P., McTier, L., Tollefson, J., & Lawrence, J. (2024). *Fundamentals of nursing* (3rd ed.). Cengage Learning Australia.

Johnstone, J. (2020). How to provide preoperative care to patients. *Nursing Standard. 35*(12), 72–76. DOI: http://dx.doi.org/10.7748/ns.2020.e11657

Liddle, C. (2018). An overview of the principles of preoperative care. *Nursing Standard, 33*(6). DOI: 10.7748/ns.2018.e11170

Nursing and Midwifery Board of Australia. (2016). *Registered nurse standards for practice.* https://www.nursingmidwiferyboard.gov.au/codes-guidelines-statements/professional-standards/registered-nurse-standards-for-practice.aspx

CHAPTER 21

COMPLEX CARE

I remember nursing two patients who came in on the same day with a stroke. Both were male. There was not a great deal of difference in their ages and they both had a right-sided CVA. The first patient, Joe, had aphasia and left-sided weakness, but could still move his arm. The second patient, Tom, had no aphasia and very minimal weakness to his left side. He could still dress himself and mobilise – with an obvious deficit – but he could still do so. The big differences between the two were Joe had diabetes and hypertension, and Tom had previously had an MI but had no other medical conditions.

It was very interesting to see the different needs of both patients and their outcomes from a very similar occurrence. Joe required a great deal of rehabilitation, whereas Tom, from memory, went home with assistance from community nurses.

Bella, 30, CN

LEARNING OBJECTIVES
After reading this chapter, you should have an understanding of the:
1 assessment of a person with complex needs
2 prioritisation of key components in the development of plans of care for a person with the complex care problems of:
   – COVID-19
   – coronary artery graft surgery
   – shock and disseminated intravascular coagulation
   – acute respiratory distress syndrome
3 planning of nursing care for patients with common complex disorders and conditions
4 evaluation of interventions and the reassessment for the patient with complex care needs
5 discharge planning and coordination of care required in preparing the person for discharge and subsequent continuity of care between the person and their healthcare providers.

INTRODUCTION

Complex nursing is more than just chronic disease. It is nursing patients with a significant illness or injury and the potential presence of co-morbidities such as ischaemic heart disease, diabetes or respiratory conditions. Each person responds differently to disease, illness, surgery, or condition such as a stroke, and complex nursing care looks at all the intricacies that make up our patients. Complex nursing involves the nursing process, holistic care and critical thinking.

21.1 ASSESSMENT OF COMPLEX CARE

Patient assessment is an ongoing process that becomes, very quickly, part of your routine in patient care. The introduction 'Hi Mr Grohl, my name is Andrew, and I am your nurse today' gives you a great deal of information. If Mr Grohl responds verbally, and can breathe, talk and acknowledge your statement, you can cross off ABC in your primary survey. Even when performing vital signs (temperature, pulse, blood pressure, respiratory rate and oxygen saturations) you can assess a great deal about a patient. Are they breathing rapidly because of an underlying respiratory condition? Do they have abdominal pain from longstanding reflux or constipation? Do they have chest pain from angina or reflux? All these aspects are little signs that we are well able to objectively observe, and then ask questions to get further subjective data from the patient. For each body system there are specific assessments we can undertake, as shown in **Table 21.1**. What you will soon notice is that the body's homeostatic mechanism is the driving force that causes many compensatory mechanisms when there are chronic conditions in place. For example, an 80-year-old patient with COPD has baseline oxygen saturations of 88%. This reading is the person's baseline or normal. (Gray et al., 2019; Joustra & Moloney, 2019; Rizzo, 2015).

TABLE 21.1
Body systems and their type of assessment

BODY SYSTEM	ASSESSMENT	INFORMATION OBTAINED	DISEASE THAT MAY BE INDICATED	SKILLS FOR ASSESSMENT
Nervous system	Glasgow Coma Scale	Assesses the person's conscious state	Brain injury	2.7 Neurological observation
	Reflexes for infants (adults if required)	Assesses neurological function	Brain or spinal cord injury	As described in assessment procedures of the facility for individuals
Cardiovascular system	Pulse	Assesses the rate, volume and pattern the heart is working at	Heart failure Atrial fibrillation Cardiac arrhythmias	2.3 Temperature, pulse and respiration (TPR) measurement
	Blood pressure	Assesses the amount of pressure exerted by the blood on the arterial wall	Hypertension	2.4 Blood pressure measurement
	Electrocardiogram	Assesses the electrical conduction of the heart	Heart failure Atrial fibrillation Cardiac arrhythmias Conduction problems	2.10 12-lead ECG recording
Respiratory system	Respirations	Assesses how often the client breathes in and out. One inspiration and one expiration = one respiration	Neurological function Respiratory disease-COPD, asthma	2.3 Temperature, pulse and respiration (TPR) measurement
	O_2 saturation level	Assesses how much oxygen a single RBC is carrying on each haemoglobin molecule	Respiratory disease-COPD, asthma Anaemia	2.5 Pulse oximetry
	Peak flow measures	Assesses the amount of air the client can move into and out of their airways in one expiration	Asthma	As described in assessment procedures of the facility for individuals
Urinary system	Urinalysis	Tests for abnormal constituents of urine	For all clients	3.8 Urinalysis and urine specimen collection
	Mid-stream specimen of urine	Urine will be collected from the midstream for micro and culture to identify bacteria (a doctor needs to authorise this test)	Suspected urinary tract infection	3.8 Urinalysis and urine specimen collection

BODY SYSTEM	ASSESSMENT	INFORMATION OBTAINED	DISEASE THAT MAY BE INDICATED	SKILLS FOR ASSESSMENT
Digestive system	Weight	Assesses the person is at a healthy weight	Obesity and nutritional state	As described in assessment procedures of the facility for individuals
	BMI	Assesses if body mass index is within normal levels	Obesity and nutritional state	As described in assessment procedures of the facility for individuals
	Waist circumference	Assesses if the waist measurement falls within normal levels	Obesity and nutritional state	As described in assessment procedures of the facility for individuals
	Stool chart	Assesses if normal bowel motion – usually against the Bristol Stool Chart	Absorption disorders of the gut Constipation/diarrhoea Crohn's disease/IBS GIT bleeding	3.9 Faeces assessment and specimen collection
Endocrine system	BGL measurement	Assesses if blood glucose levels are within normal levels	Diabetes	2.6 Blood glucose measurement
Musculoskeletal system	Gait	Assesses if the person is able to move in normal pattern	Strength and coordination – related to intact joints, muscles and bones	2.8 Neurovascular observation 3.14 Active and passive exercises
	Falls risk assessment	Assesses if the person is at risk of falling	Strength and coordination – related to intact joints, muscles and bones	As described in assessment procedures of the facility for individuals 3.14 Active and passive exercises
Integumentary system	Skin assessment: – Norton – Waterloo – Braden	Assesses whether the person has an intact skins-barrier to infection, maintenance of internal systems	Pressure areas Skin infections Chronic wounds Traumatic wounds	As described in assessment procedures of the facility for individuals
Immune system	Temperature	Assesses if within normal parameters	If the person is at risk of infection or other disease processes	2.3 Temperature, pulse and respiration (TPR) measurement
Lymphatic system	Check for peripheral oedema	Assesses if circulatory system is functioning well. Assesses electrolyte balance	Cardiac failure Hormonal diseases such as Addison's disease	As described in assessment procedures of the facility for individuals

As discussed in Chapter 19, the National Safety and Quality Health Service (NSQHS) Standards has Recognising and Responding to Acute Deterioration as the eighth standard to ensure that the acute deterioration of an individual requiring health care is recognised promptly and is treated appropriately to provide optimal health outcomes (Australian Commission on Safety and Quality in Health Care [ACSQHC], 2022).

SAFETY IN NURSING

NORMAL RANGES

Throughout your educational program you will work within normal ranges for vital signs. This becomes a grey area when you have patients who have multiple co-morbidities and, as such, their 'normal' ranges are affected. As we age, our blood pressure does drop, partly due to decreased contractility from the left ventricle. So, someone who is 90 years old may have a blood pressure of 90/60 mmHg and not be symptomatic with this. The other aspect to consider is children – they also have varying ranges for age groups. The important thing to always consider in your assessment is that you are looking *at the patient* with these findings. For example, if you are performing vital signs and you observe:

- Caitlyn-Rose, 28-year-old female
  - T 38.2 HR 90 & reg BP 100/65 mmHg RR 24 SpO$_2$ 95% RA

• Emma, 72-year-old female
  – T 38.2 HR 120 & reg BP 80/40 mmHG RR 30 SpO$_2$ 90% RA
  Both patients have a temperature, but look at the differences in compensation here. Would you expect Caitlyn-Rose to have any cyanosis? Emma? Underlying conditions also impact the vital signs. When you are taking vital signs, it is not a task – it is an assessment – your assessment – and needs to be taken in line with the patient, not the normal parameters.

Presentation

Caitlyn-Rose is a 28-year-old female who has presented to the emergency department via ambulance for increased shortness of breath, fever and coughing. **Concept map 21.1** further explores Caitlyn-Rose's initial care in the emergency department.

 PHx

Caitlyn-Rose, a 28-year-old female with a 2/7 history of shortness of breath, non-productive cough, subjective fevers, fatigue, and headache. Works in retail.
No medical or surgical history.
Presents via ambulance, who were called to her workplace due to increased SOB and coughing.

 ASSESSMENT

Primary survey
A: Patent
B: RR 24
C: Warm
D: ALOC GCS 14
E: T 38.2°C
F: IVF @ 166 ml/hr voided
G: BGL 6.5 mmol/L

Secondary survey
CNS (Cognition): E 4 V4 (disorientated to time/person/place) M 6 = 14 PEARL 4 mm
PAIN: c/o headache, not rating pain
CVS: HR 90 bpm and reg, BP 100/65 mmHg, pedal pulses bounding. A 12-lead electrocardiogram showed sinus rhythm

with no abnormalities. T 38.2 °C (has had paracetamol 1 g 60 mins ago)
RESP: RR 24, SpO$_2$ 94%, patent airway – spontaneous breathing, increased work of breathing, spontaneous cough, non-productive. AE decreased BB
GIT (input): IVF 166 mL/hr. Abdo soft, non-tender, BS audible in all quadrants
RENAL (output): voided via pan, 240 mL – some sediment, amber coloured
SKIN/INTEG: Centrally warm and peripherally cooler
MUSCULOSKELETAL (mobility): RIB currently due to confusion
BMI: 23.0

Cues ① What are your priorities with this patient?
② What is the significance of her temperature?
③ What is the relationship between work of breathing and respiratory rate?
④ What is the pathophysiological relationship between a viral infection, such as COVID-19, and multi-organ dysfunction?
⑤ What are some concerns in relationship to the GCS assessment in this patient?
⑥ What physiological impact can a prolonged fever cause?
⑦ What investigative or diagnostic procedures would you think would be relevant for this patient?

CONCEPT MAP 21.1 Nursing assessment for Caitlyn-Rose

21.2 PLANNING FOR COMPLEX CARE

Nursing interventions have been a constant element of your learning so far. Nursing interventions are actioned after a health assessment and are often predetermined care plans or **clinical pathways**. These clinical pathways are an essential component of the nursing process and contain a summary of care requirements, goals and specific interventions for each individual patient. Some clinical pathways are generic; for example, postoperative hip replacement.

This is because, generally, most patients follow the same recovery path. Nursing care plans are usually formulated between many members of the healthcare team. They are often evidence-based and are reviewed at specified dates to ensure clinical currency.

An example of nursing interventions based on a clinical pathway would be guidelines for measurement of vital signs postoperatively. Routine management will be subject to an accurate nursing assessment of each individual patient and may vary accordingly. Nursing assessment is outlined in **Figure 21.1**.

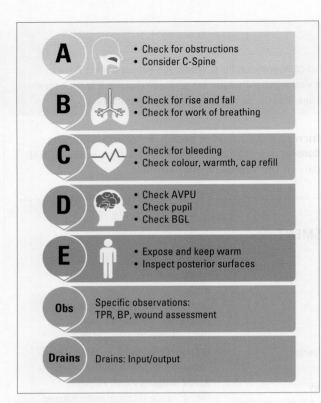

FIGURE 21.1 Nursing assessment

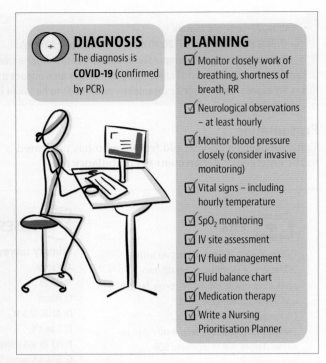

CONCEPT MAP 21.2 Diagnosis and planning for Caitlyn-Rose

Some operations; for example, a femoral popliteal bypass graft, require pedal pulses checked with each set of observations to assess the patency of the graft. A carotid endarterectomy would require neurological observations performed with each set of vital signs to assess pupillary response to light and to observe any complications from reperfusion of the carotid artery. Post-caesarean section, you would need to check the fundus and any PV loss. Despite the nature of the operation, the basics of vital signs are required in all cases, with additional specified observations as required by the surgery undertaken.

Generally, vital signs (and specific observations) are performed half hourly for 2 hours, hourly for 2 hours and then fourth hourly until the condition of the patient is stable. The timing of this is from when the patient returns to the ward.

Concept map 21.2 outlines a plan for Caitlyn-Rose's care.

There are many nursing interventions that are required for each patient, regardless of their presentation or clinical condition. It becomes even more involved when planning for safe and effective nursing care when there are co-morbidities (such as preexisting heart conditions, diabetes, asthma). This is where working as part of a multidisciplinary team is essential.

Perform nursing interventions based on predetermined care plans

Each patient is unique and that makes each nursing care plan or clinical pathway individualised and holistic. Holistic caring is looking at the patient and providing the needs that they cannot meet or need assistance with – no matter how small it may seem to you – it may be a very serious or very important concern for the patient.

The argument does exist that clinical pathways do not allow for this – as they are all the same. The refuting comments would be that the clinical pathways are designed as a guideline and there are many spots to enter a variance or alteration in the care plan.

Nursing care plans or clinical pathways should always be adapted to the patient as an individual. They should always address the needs outlined in **Figure 21.2**.

Concept map 21.3 shows interventions appropriate for Caitlyn-Rose.

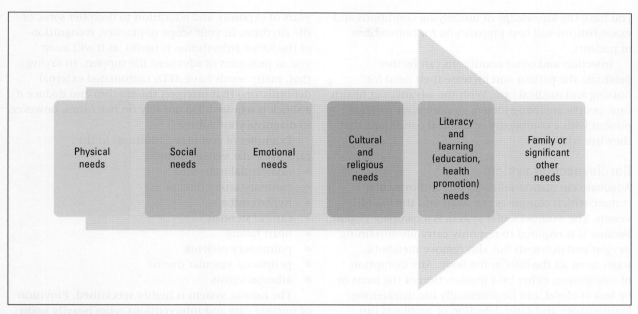

FIGURE 21.2 Holistic care planning

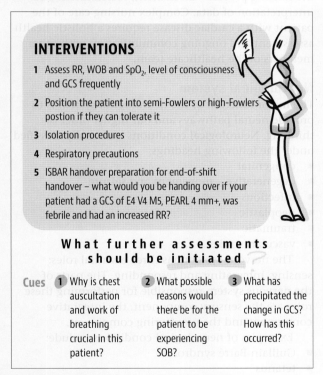

INTERVENTIONS

1 Assess RR, WOB and SpO$_2$, level of consciousness and GCS frequently

2 Position the patient into semi-Fowlers or high-Fowlers postion if they can tolerate it

3 Isolation procedures

4 Respiratory precautions

5 ISBAR handover preparation for end-of-shift handover – what would you be handing over if your patient had a GCS of E4 V4 M5, PEARL 4 mm+, was febrile and had an increased RR?

What further assessments should be initiated

Cues

1 Why is chest auscultation and work of breathing crucial in this patient?

2 What possible reasons would there be for the patient to be experiencing SOB?

3 What has precipitated the change in GCS? How has this occurred?

CONCEPT MAP 21.3 Nursing interventions for Caitlyn-Rose

21.3 COMMON DISORDERS AND CONDITIONS

As your experience grows, you will notice that there are several chronic conditions that are common reasons for admission to hospital. For example, an exacerbation of chronic obstructive pulmonary disease (COPD), infective bronchitis, acute or chronic renal failure, or worsening of congestive cardiac failure. What will also be evident is how disease affects each person

differently. You could have four patients with the same illness – let's say pneumonia. If we observed the process of pneumonia in the patients, we would see different recovery periods, as it would affect all four differently. Some would take days to recover, others weeks. It would depend on other variables such as age, other illnesses/conditions, medications and general state of wellbeing.

There are many complex conditions that require nursing interventions and care. The list is exhaustive, and some examples only are given here. The focus of nursing care should always be to provide holistic and individualised care, via thorough patient assessment and data collection, then evaluation and reassessment.

Respiratory system

There are many health problems that affect the lower respiratory tract, including COPD and asthma. Respiratory tract infections are also common, and respiratory tract disease and pneumonia account for a significant number of deaths annually.

Disorders and diseases include:

- pneumonia
- pleurisy
- viral and bacterial infections
- Legionnaire's tuberculosis
- pulmonary embolism
- airway obstruction due to structural abnormality or neoplasm growth
- haemothorax
- pneumothorax
- traumatic problems.

Current emphasis is placed also on influenza and COVID-19, both of which have a significant impact upon the respiratory system.

Respiratory conditions are often chronic with acute exacerbations or infective processes. Ensuring that you have the knowledge of underlying conditions and exacerbations will best prepare you for holistic care of patients.

Infection and other conditions can further debilitate the patient and increase their need for nursing and medical care. With the advances in health care, people are living longer, so numerous patients present with a complexity of medical conditions that they live with daily.

Cardiovascular system

Adequate circulation relies on the cardiovascular system, which comprises the heart and the blood vessels. The cardiovascular system is a complex system because it is required to not only carry life-sustaining oxygen and nutrients but also remove metabolic waste from all the cells in the body. Any disruption of this system, either by a malfunction of the heart or by loss of blood, can be potentially life threatening. Maintenance and early detection of problems can improve patient outcomes.

Cardiovascular assessment is imperative and is assessed as shown in **Figure 21.3**.

The 12-lead ECG recording is performed on all patients who present with suspected cardiac conditions to provide a comprehensive view of the electrical activity occurring in the heart. It will be a very common intervention – performing an ECG – so knowing how to do it is crucial. It is essential that you know how to place the leads correctly. A misplaced lead can distort the reading and lead to inappropriate actions or mismanagement. ECG interpretation involves an understanding of electrical conduction and myocardial contractility.

Interpretation of the ECG is ultimately up to the medical officer. It is a highly specialised skill that takes

years of exposure and education to decipher some of the rhythms. In your scope of practice, recognition of the lethal arrhythmias is useful, as it will assist you in provision of advanced life support. In saying that, many wards have AEDs (automated external defibrillators) that interpret the rhythm and deduce if a shock is required. Do not rely on machines, however, to diagnose your patient.

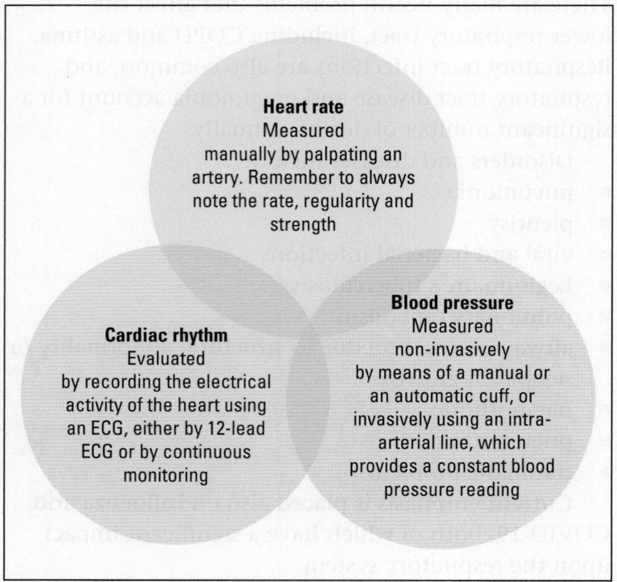

Examples of complex conditions in the cardiovascular system include:

- myocardial ischaemia
- coronary artery disease
- hypertension
- carotid stenosis
- heart failure
- pulmonary oedema
- peripheral vascular disease
- atherosclerosis.

The cardiac system is highly specialised. Provision of nursing care and interventions relies heavily upon the nursing process – assessment, reassessment and interpretation of data. Complex nursing care of the patient with a cardiac disease requires a holistic health assessment and ongoing communication with other members of the healthcare team.

Neurological system

The major function of the neurological system is to provide neural pathways and our higher order of thinking. Neurological conditions are usually classified under the following headings:

- congenital
- degenerative – movement and seizure
- infectious
- neoplastic
- traumatic
- vascular (stroke).

The nervous system has three essential roles: sensing, integrating and responding. The parts of the nervous system responsible for performing these roles are the sensory component, the integrative component and the monitoring component.

Examples of neurological conditions include:

- Guillain-Barré syndrome
- tetanus
- brain tumours
- head injury
- spinal cord injury
- epilepsy
- meningitis
- stroke.

One key factor in assessing any patient with a neurological condition is the Glasgow Coma Scale (GCS). The GCS was designed originally to assess the level of consciousness in people who had sustained head injuries, but it is now used in several different

Heart rate
Measured manually by palpating an artery. Remember to always note the rate, regularity and strength

Cardiac rhythm
Evaluated by recording the electrical activity of the heart using an ECG, either by 12-lead ECG or by continuous monitoring

Blood pressure
Measured non-invasively by means of a manual or an automatic cuff, or invasively using an intra-arterial line, which provides a constant blood pressure reading

FIGURE 21.3 Cardiovascular assessment

settings. The lowest score is 3, while a score of 15 is the highest and indicates a fully alert, orientated patient.

As you can see, the care plans our patients require are intricate and dependent upon the disease or injury process and their response to interventions. Each body system affected also adds to the very complex nature of nursing.

Gastrointestinal (GI) system

The major function of the GI system is to supply nutrients to the body's cells. The principles of nursing assessment and data collection continue in this body system, and along with objective and subjective data, will provide you with information to plan nursing care.

GI system disorders include problems related to:
- nutrition
- malnutrition
- obesity
- upper and lower GI system disorders
- the liver, biliary tract and pancreas.

Diet and nutrition play a critical role in the cause of illness, disability and death – either premature or related to ageing. Conditions such as stroke, hypertension, coronary heart disease and hyperlipidaemia are all directly related to modifiable risk factors such as diet and nutrition. Diabetes is another example of the need for a balanced diet – when patients do not comply with a lower glycaemic index diet, their blood sugar levels are erratic, which has further impact upon the body. While diet and nutrition are not the sole factor at play here, it certainly accounts for a great deal in terms of risk factors for disease.

This complex interrelationship between diet and other risk factors and disease needs to be recognised in your role of providing care and resources on nutritional practices for patients. It also highlights the intricacies that are involved in patient care.

Some GI diseases/conditions are also a direct effect of medication/s; for example, reflux.

Endocrine system

The endocrine system is one of the major components in homeostasis and the maintenance of it. The endocrine system is responsible for hormone secretion, which is something that can affect all body cells. Think of the flight or fight response – where adrenaline is released to increase our focus on self-preservation. The adrenaline causes an increase in heart rate and blood pressure, and its effects carry on to other systems.

Diabetes is the most common disorder of the endocrine system. Diabetes affects every person differently and it has potential long-term complications that can affect the kidneys, eyes, heart, blood vessels and nerves. It is absolutely a disease that is not 'one size fits all' and it has many contributing factors. You also need to consider if the person is compliant with their medication or treatment. Their family history and age also play a factor.

Other types of endocrine disorders include:
- hyperthyroidism
- cancers
- Cushing's syndrome
- Addison's disease.

Care of endocrine disorders is comprehensive and ever changing. Much of endocrine pathophysiology relies on assessment skills and interpretation of subjective and objective data. Experience and teamwork will enable this information to be discovered, coupled with diagnostic tests.

Integumentary system

Our skin is our largest organ. Skin can be compromised in many ways – from allergic reactions to skin cancers, to ulcers and pressure area sores to burns. The nursing care of skin is always focused upon restoring its integrity. Due to the nature of skin conditions, you will need to focus on the cause – is it infective, related to pressure or heat? Then you can assess and determine the most appropriate plan of care for your patient; bearing in mind all the other conditions that can affect recovery, healing and treatment.

Musculoskeletal system

Musculoskeletal disorders are a group of conditions that affect the musculoskeletal system. These conditions result in a dysfunction of the body's bones, joints or muscles. The effect of these can impact upon your patient's performance of activities of daily living (ADLs) due to reduced mobility or pain. Some examples of conditions you could expect to provide nursing care for are:
- arthritis
- fracture or bony injury
- bursitis
- gout
- infection.

Most of the nursing care and interventions required for musculoskeletal illness or injury is, again, patient specific. You will need to assess the person based upon co-morbidities, contributing factors or injuries, and level of pain. Pain relief (analgesia) is extremely important in the rehabilitation and care of the person with a musculoskeletal injury/ disorder/illness.

REFLECTIVE PRACTICE

The one-armed man

On my first placement in acute care, I was working in an orthopaedic ward. I was allocated four patients with my buddy nurse. One patient was in a car accident and he had his left arm fractured in about three places. It meant that he had only one arm to use to attend to his ADLs. He was 18 and was incredibly embarrassed. I remember asking him when I was assisting him with his ADLs how we could work it so he could get as much done as possible without needing someone to help or see him exposed. The solution was to put on a singlet that was slightly too big (easy to get on) and for him to wear boxer shorts as they were (coupled with his other injuries) easiest to get on. So, always ask what you can do to help the patient perform the task rather than assuming they have an injury and cannot do any of it.

Josh, 42, RN

Haematological system

Haematology is the branch of biology that is concerned with the study of blood, the blood-forming organs and blood diseases. Haematology also includes the study of the aetiology, diagnosis, treatment, prognosis and prevention of blood disease. Blood diseases affect the production of blood and its components – blood cells, haemoglobin, blood proteins and the mechanism of coagulation.

Nursing interventions and care will need a complete health history and assessment. This involves subjective and objective data. Haematological disorders are complex and are individualised. Treatment modalities are ever changing, and this requires clinical currency and best practice to ensure the patient is receiving the most appropriate care. Haematological disorders are intricate – as they are the very basis of our being, and the disturbances are far reaching.

A component of assessing not only the haematological system, but also all systems, is blood tests. This is undertaken through venipuncture.

Urinary/reproductive system

As with all assessment processes, the collection of important health information begins with an interview. This is where subjective data is obtained about past health history, medications, surgery or other treatments, health perception and management, nutritional-metabolic, elimination, activity-exercise, sleep-rest, cognitive-perceptual, self-concept, role-relationship and sexual-reproductive patterns are ascertained. Objective data is also collected through physical examination and diagnostic studies that contribute to the information gathered.

The most common urinary and reproductive disorders are related to infectious processes; as well, there are cancers, urinary calculi, renal failure and hormonal imbalances.

Nursing intervention and care can require the management of urinary drainage bags and the insertion of indwelling catheters. The need for an indwelling catheter can be as simple as a decreased level of consciousness, or as complex as a debilitating illness or long-standing condition.

21.4 EVALUATION OF CARE FOR COMPLEX CARE

The nursing process provides nurses with a systematic, interrelated five-step method of problem solving, as discussed in Chapters 1 and 2 and shown in **Figure 21.4**. Nurses utilising the nursing process must use critical thinking and clinical reasoning skills to collect, review and validate patient data to plan, implement and then evaluate patient care based on evidence-based nursing practice.

Nursing practice is always changing, and as new knowledge becomes available nurses need to challenge traditional ways of doing things and discover new interventions that are the most effective and have high scientific relevance, ultimately resulting in better patient outcomes. The nursing process is a traditional critical thinking competency that allows nurses to make clinical judgements and take actions based on reason. A process is a series of steps or components taken to achievement of a goal.

While performing nursing cares, you will soon discover your ability to assess both forms of data – objective and subjective. With this data, you will relate it to the patient and make planned interventions and unplanned ones. For example, if a patient has low blood pressure – let's say 90/60 – you will first review the baseline observations or previous observations to see what they have 'been'. From here, you would question the patient – 'Are you dizzy?', 'How do you feel?' and with this information, you would formulate your next intervention/s.

Conversely, if a patient has planned interventions that are not appropriate, you will need to communicate this clearly and effectively to both the patient and your team leader. This could include simple things such as ADL cares – the patient may wish to have the cares completed at another time. Another example could be refusal to comply with the intervention, all of which requires documentation and explanation to the multidisciplinary team.

There will always be changes in healthcare delivery. Equipment, processes, and procedures will

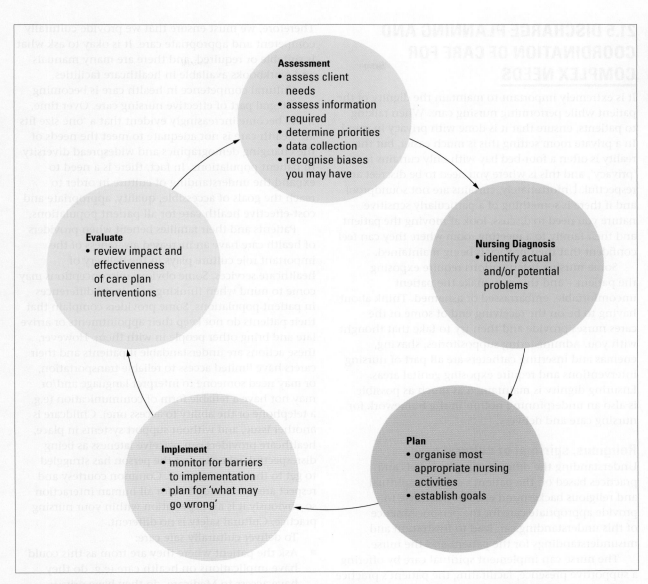

FIGURE 21.4 The nursing process and critical thinking. At any time in the care of a patient, a nurse may move back and forth from one step of the process to another should new information emerge.

change based on evidence-based practice. An element of your role will be to remain up to date with clinical practice relevant to your area of nursing. It is quite clear that observation ranges do not alter – what alters are the methods of nursing care and interventions. Complex nursing requires the nurse to be aware of many conditions, and, more importantly, their potential impact on the patient and their wellbeing and recovery. Utilising a holistic approach, and through obtaining data from the patient, you will be well able to assess and manage all patients with complex nursing requirements.

As part of the further assessment of Caitlyn-Rose's ongoing condition, **Concept map 21.4** asks further questions in relation to her management.

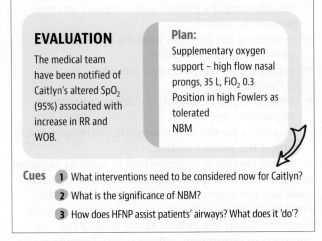

EVALUATION

The medical team have been notified of Caitlyn's altered SpO$_2$ (95%) associated with increase in RR and WOB.

Plan:
Supplementary oxygen support – high flow nasal prongs, 35 L, FiO$_2$ 0.3
Position in high Fowlers as tolerated
NBM

Cues
1. What interventions need to be considered now for Caitlyn?
2. What is the significance of NBM?
3. How does HFNP assist patients' airways? What does it 'do'?

CONCEPT MAP 21.4 Evaluation and planning for Caitlyn-Rose

21.5 DISCHARGE PLANNING AND COORDINATION OF CARE FOR COMPLEX NEEDS

It is extremely important to maintain the dignity of the patient while performing nursing care. When talking to patients, ensure that it is done with privacy in mind. In a private room setting this is much easier, but the reality is often a four-bed bay with only curtains for 'privacy', and this is where you need to be discreet and respectful. Unfortunately, curtains are not soundproof and if there is something of a particularly sensitive nature you need to discuss, look at moving the patient and their family to a meeting room where they can feel confident that their privacy is being maintained.

Some nursing interventions require exposing the patient – and this may make the patient uncomfortable, embarrassed or ashamed. Think about having to be on the receiving end of some of the cares nurses provide and then try to take that thought with you. Administering suppositories, shaving, enemas and inserting catheters are all part of nursing interventions and require exposing genital areas. Ensuring dignity is maintained as much as possible is also an underpinning notion in the framework for nursing care and delivery.

Religious, spiritual or cultural care

Understanding the difference in the beliefs and practices based on the patient's cultural, spiritual and religious background enables the nurse to provide appropriate care for the person. Absence of this understanding can lead to frustration and misunderstandings for the patient and the nurse.

The nurse can implement spiritual care by offering a supportive presence, facilitating the patient's practice of religion, and resolving conflicts between treatments (e.g. timing) and spiritual activities.

You can do this by:

- familiarising the patient with religious services within the facility
- respecting the patient's need for privacy during prayer or spiritual activity
- arranging for the patient to receive sacraments if desired
- attempting to best meet any dietary restrictions or preferences
- arranging for the priest, minister, pastor or rabbi to visit if the patient wishes.

When looking at issues related to cultural, religious and spiritual beliefs, it is important to identify what these are. For example, not all Muslims follow the same practices regarding health care. This is, in part, because religion and culture factor heavily into our approach to health care and *our beliefs*. Religion is practised by so many people – but never is it identical.

Therefore, we must ensure that we provide culturally competent and appropriate care. It is okay to ask what is suitable or required, and there are many manuals and workbooks available in healthcare facilities.

Cultural competence in health care is becoming an integral part of effective nursing care. Over time, it has become increasingly evident that a 'one size fits all' health care is not adequate to meet the needs of the changing demographics and widespread diversity in patient populations. In fact, there is a need to expand the understanding of culture in order to reach the goals of accessible, quality, appropriate and cost-effective health care for all patient populations.

Patients and their families benefit when providers of health care have an increased awareness of the important role culture plays in the delivery of healthcare services. Some obvious misconceptions may come to mind when thinking of cultural differences in patient populations. Some providers complain that their patients do not keep their appointments or arrive late and bring other people in with them. However, these actions are understandable if patients and their carers have limited access to reliable transportation, or may need someone to interpret language and/or may not have a reliable form of communication (e.g. a telephone or the ability to access one). Childcare is another issue, and without support systems in place, healthcare providers can perceive lateness as being disrespectful, when in fact the person has struggled to get to their appointment. Common courtesy and respect are the foundation for all human interaction so obviously it is an expectation within your nursing practice. Cultural safety is no different.

To deliver culturally safe care:

- Ask the patient where they are from as this could have implications on health care (e.g. do they have access to Medicare, do they have private health insurance)
- Ask the patient what language is spoken at home. Is English a second language? If so, ascertain the level of actual language comprehension early in your encounter. Allowing a family member or friend to accompany the patient to translate for them during the examination should be a last resort. Instead, arrange a hospital-provided interpreter to ensure that the correct and full information is given to the patient and reported back to you. The family member or friend can stay as a support person.
- Ask the patient if they have a specific dietary pattern.
- Ask the patient if their religion prohibits or restricts any medical treatments or interventions; for example, use of blood products, fasting or timing of interventions.

Being able to determine what support mechanisms are in place in the patient's family and/or significant others is important to the nursing process. The patient may be a first generation Australian and have no family support and feel quite isolated. Chronic and complex medical conditions require support of family/carers or health professionals to maintain the patient's health status.

Encourage patient involvement in their own care during care interventions

There are many nursing interventions that a patient can be encouraged to be involved with. For example, a patient who is being discharged with a wound. You can start preparing the patient for caring for the wound themselves through education, demonstration and health promotion. If the patient is assessed in hospital on the management of their wound, education or learning gaps can be addressed immediately to avoid any possible complications.

While it is always a positive to have the patient complete their own cares, you are still accountable for the patient while they are in hospital. So, you still need to assess and implement nursing care as required. For example, if a patient is emptying their catheter bag and not following safe and effective infection control measures, you need to address this with the patient and their carers.

The nursing process involves education, assessment, constant review and addressing the holistic needs of the patient. Practising holistic care ensures that these needs are incorporated into the nursing care as they all interrelate and impact on health outcomes. A patient who is not having their emotional or psychosocial needs met is at risk of not being able to meet the physical demands of the nursing interventions. For example, a patient may have no social support networks or be unable to afford the required home care after discharge. Also consider the emotional needs of the patient, as some people may not communicate these needs. How do you know if these needs are being met? How would you ensure that these needs are met? By taking a holistic approach and referring the patient to appropriate healthcare professionals is how.

In planning for Caitlyn-Rose's discharge, Concept map 21.5 explores the considerations for her care.

Rehabilitation

Rehabilitation is a dynamic process in which an individual is helped to achieve optimal function and independence within their limitations (if any). Rehabilitation is what is involved in hospital care – after surgery, or during periods of illness, the aim of acute care provision is to rehabilitate the patient to their previous level of functioning if possible, or to assist the patient and their family to adjust to new care requirements. For example, a patient is in hospital for a hernia repair. Rehabilitation will include deep breathing exercises, education regarding lifting and wound care, and nursing assessment to determine the physical status of the patient. The patient will be discharged with physical limitations in the short term. An example that is far more complex is a patient who has experienced a cerebrovascular accident (CVA) or stroke. The patient may have residual deficits, such as hemiparesis, aphasia or dysphagia. These conditions will require ongoing and long-term health care intervention, assessment and management. The patient and their family will need to be supported throughout the entire process.

Rehabilitation:

- recognises the worth of the individual
- must be an integral component of care offered by the healthcare facility
- means a comprehensive rehabilitation plan is arranged through active participation and coordination of all healthcare team members
- requires active participation by the individual with a disability to achieve their optimal rehabilitation potential
- should always actively involve the individual and their significant others involved with rehabilitating the individual through all five parameters of health
- aims to achieve the highest level of independence possible for the individual.

DISCHARGE PLANNING + COORDINATION OF CARE

How do the following areas of healthcare management **relate** to Caitlyn-Rose's presentation? Which members of the healthcare team are **involved** in each area of management?

Respiratory – increased work of breathing, shortness of breath, hypoxia
Medication
Spirometry
Follow-up review with physiotherapist

Deep breathing and cough exercises
Worksheet for patient
Physiotherapy

Infection control measures
Contact tracing
Advice on presentation for testing if symptomatic
Vaccination information for when well again
Follow-up with GP

CONCEPT MAP 21.5 Discharge planning and coordination of care for Caitlyn-Rose

Nursing interventions and the patient's rights

It is important to remember that when performing nursing interventions, or any nursing cares, all of the patient's healthcare rights need to be protected.

- Be aware of the patient's healthcare rights.
- Respect the dignity of each patient and their family/significant others.
- Respect the patient's right to refuse treatment.
- Listen attentively to patients and their family. Convey any of their concerns to the registered nurse.
- Unless otherwise instructed, answer the patient's questions completely and provide information as would normally be provided by the health care professional responsible.
- Respect the right of confidentiality of information.
- On admission, inform the patient of the facility's policies, rules and regulations.
- Assist patients to maintain their rights to freedom and to make decisions.

Every day nurses observe behaviour. Behaviour of colleagues, patients and their relatives. A component of nursing assessment is assessing the patient's behaviour. If the patient is aggressive or abusive it is clearly not appropriate, but it may be that they are acting in this manner due to a need not being met. Never doubt the power of a simple observation in an interaction with your patient. Asking the patient how they are is often overlooked. As nurses, it can be easy to fall into a 'task orientated' approach and work towards crossing tasks off your worksheet rather than listening to a patient's concerns and assessing *them*.

From assessment of behaviours, you can incorporate any need deficits into the care plan and then identify if your nursing interventions are satisfying an expressed need of the patient. The difficult task is determining from the expressed behaviour what the patient's actual deficits of needs are. Again, this is where a multifaceted and holistic approach to patient care is essential in ensuring all needs are met.

Underlying all nursing interventions are the professional, legal and ethical standards that are our scope of practice. It is essential that all nursing staff are aware of their professional requirements as well as their specific organisational requirements. In any situation, no matter how urgent, all nurses must act within their scope of practice.

It is essential that nurses report and record all responses to nursing interventions, regardless of whether they have been effective. It is important that these responses are noted in the daily care notes, so a timeline of responses can be viewed. It is not always appropriate to document these at the end of the shift.

For example, vital signs are documented at the time they are performed and a response to an intervention that is identified by a nurse should also,

in most cases, be recorded at the time. There are many situations where responses/reactions should be reported to the team leader or another appropriate person prior to commencing written records; for example, if the patient's pain management is not effective or the patient is showing adverse medical reactions.

Effective responses are just as important to report and document as non-effective ones. For example, a patient that was going to be discharged is still nauseous. An antiemetic is then administered, and the patient feels better and decides they would like to leave. In this case, ensure that you document the effect of the antiemetic and any education or information regarding follow-up treatment for nausea you have provided.

Additional nursing interventions may be planned for a patient but may not be needed if a positive/effective response from other treatments occurs prior to these planned interventions. Reporting and recording patient responses assists in ensuring that unnecessary interventions are not undertaken.

Nursing care is provided by a team so all members of the team contribute to the sharing of information where appropriate. In the handover, the nurse should report all care given and the patient's responses.

REFLECTIVE PRACTICE

Nursing interventions

So much can be gained by recognising that all patients are unique and are individuals. We all have a certain way we brush our teeth or hair, or the time of day we choose to shower. Imagine being told when to shower, or when to perform oral hygiene? As a nurse, you should always remember this. Even if someone has suffered a stroke, it does not mean they have to shower when they are 'told' to. Always factor in the individual aspects of nursing care. This is definitely one of the rewarding aspects of nursing – working with a person to return them to health. Assisting them through times of illness, injury or prolonged rehabilitation. Empowering them to take part in their health care. So, my only advice is always remember that that patient is a person.
Hope, RN, 35

We will now consider three further concept map sequences for patients with complex care needs: a 78-year-old man requiring coronary artery bypass graft surgery; a 55-year-old man suffering from shock and disseminated intravascular coagulation; and a 36-year-old man with acute respiratory distress syndrome.

21.6 ASSESSMENT FOR CORONARY ARTERY BYPASS GRAFT SURGERY

In the collection of subjective data, previous and current person-reported information is important in the determination of complex care problems symptoms. See **Box 21.1** for the health assessment data collection areas.

The collection of objective data is informed by the health history and is highlighted in the physical assessment and diagnostic studies for the respiratory and cardiac systems (see **Box 21.2**). This chapter acknowledges that patients are presenting with complex health needs, and the physical assessment will be guided by the person's health history.

Presentation

John Kennedy is a 78-year-old man that has been admitted to the emergency department (ED) with chest pain and breathlessness for the last two hours. He is pale and sweaty and is admitted to the monitored area of the ED.

As part of John's health assessment, **Box 21.1** and **Box 21.2** components are employed for a person-centred health assessment, and since John has type 2 diabetes an endocrine system assessment will also be prominent in the physical assessment. See **Concept map 21.6** to further explore John's initial care in the ED.

BOX 21.1   SUBJECTIVE ASSESSMENT

➤ History of illness
➤ Past health history
➤ Family history
➤ Medications
➤ Surgery

Functional health patterns:
– Health perception and management
– Nutritional and metabolic
– Elimination
– Activity and exercise
– Sleep and rest
– Cognitive and perceptual
– Self-perception and concept
– Role relationship
– Sexuality and reproductive
– Coping and stress
– Values and beliefs
➤ Risk calculation

BOX 21.2   OBJECTIVE ASSESSMENT

➤ Inspect nose and nasal cavity
➤ Palpate frontal and maxillary sinuses
➤ Complex care problems rate
➤ Inspection of the thorax
➤ Palpation of the thorax
➤ Percussion of the thorax
➤ Auscultation of the lungs
➤ Diagnostic tests – pulse oximetry, sputum, arterial blood gases, chest x-ray, computed tomography, magnetic resonance imaging, pulmonary ventilation-perfusion scan, bronchoscopy, thoracentesis
➤ Peripheral vascular system
➤ Vital signs
➤ Inspect skin, hair, venous pattern and oedema
➤ Palpate upper and lower extremities for temperature, moisture, pulses and capillary refill
➤ Auscultation of the arteries
➤ Thorax
➤ Inspection of bony structures, heart valves, epigastric area and PMI
➤ Palpation of bony structures, heart valves, epigastric area and PMI
➤ Auscultate heart sounds
➤ Diagnostic tests – cardiac biomarkers, biochemistry, blood glucose measurement, C-reactive protein, full blood count, clotting profile, cardiac natriuretic peptide markers, serum lipids, homocysteine, chest x-ray, electrocardiogram, exercise testing, echocardiogram, nuclear cardiology, cardiovascular magnetic resonance imaging, cardiac computed tomography, cardiac catheterisation
➤ Other body systems as appropriate

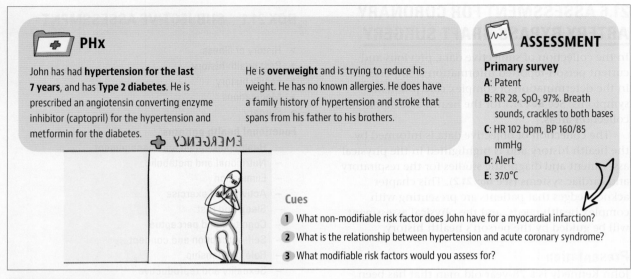

PHx

John has had **hypertension for the last 7 years**, and has **Type 2 diabetes**. He is prescribed an angiotensin converting enzyme inhibitor (captopril) for the hypertension and metformin for the diabetes.

He is **overweight** and is trying to reduce his weight. He has no known allergies. He does have a family history of hypertension and stroke that spans from his father to his brothers.

ASSESSMENT

Primary survey

A: Patent
B: RR 28, SpO$_2$ 97%. Breath sounds, crackles to both bases
C: HR 102 bpm, BP 160/85 mmHg
D: Alert
E: 37.0°C

Cues

1 What non-modifiable risk factor does John have for a myocardial infarction?

2 What is the relationship between hypertension and acute coronary syndrome?

3 What modifiable risk factors would you assess for?

CONCEPT MAP 21.6 Nursing assessment for John

21.7 PLANNING CARE FOR CORONARY ARTERY BYPASS GRAFT SURGERY

Planning for the nursing care for acute coronary artery bypass graft surgery has the goals of:

- increasing coronary artery patency
- pain relief
- collecting physical assessment data, including pathology and radiographic investigations
- patient education and consent to surgery
- self-care in relation to physical activity for the first week after surgery
- cardiac rehabilitation and ensuring a safe home environment with no adverse effects from therapy.

John is a partner in his care plan and contributes to his health care by following his plan of care and managing his condition in the home environment. **Box 21.3** lists the areas that are targeted in the

planning stage of acute coronary artery bypass graft surgery management.

> **BOX 21.3   PLANNING FOR ACUTE CORONARY ARTERY BYPASS GRAFT SURGERY**
>
> - Cardiovascular function
> - Pain relief
> - Oxygenation
> - Tests
> - Reperfusion therapy
> - Medication
> - Respiratory function
> - Psychosocial care
> - Self-care

Concept map 21.7 outlines a plan for John's care.

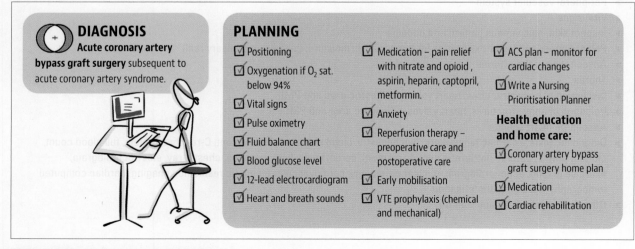

DIAGNOSIS
Acute coronary artery bypass graft surgery subsequent to acute coronary artery syndrome.

PLANNING

- ☑ Positioning
- ☑ Oxygenation if O$_2$ sat. below 94%
- ☑ Vital signs
- ☑ Pulse oximetry
- ☑ Fluid balance chart
- ☑ Blood glucose level
- ☑ 12-lead electrocardiogram
- ☑ Heart and breath sounds

- ☑ Medication – pain relief with nitrate and opioid , aspirin, heparin, captopril, metformin.
- ☑ Anxiety
- ☑ Reperfusion therapy – preoperative care and postoperative care
- ☑ Early mobilisation
- ☑ VTE prophylaxis (chemical and mechanical)

- ☑ ACS plan – monitor for cardiac changes
- ☑ Write a Nursing Prioritisation Planner

Health education and home care:

- ☑ Coronary artery bypass graft surgery home plan
- ☑ Medication
- ☑ Cardiac rehabilitation

CONCEPT MAP 21.7 Diagnosis and planning for John

21.8 NURSING INTERVENTIONS TO SUPPORT HEALTH CARE FOR CORONARY ARTERY BYPASS GRAFT SURGERY

Nursing interventions are implemented as part of person-centred care, which includes John's coronary artery blood flow to be augmented by a coronary artery bypass graft.

Concept map 21.8 explores John's journey in the ED, coronary care unit, operating room and intensive care unit (ICU) therapy before discharge to home.

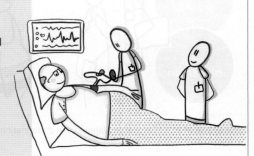

INTERVENTIONS

1 Position upright
2 Oxygen if O_2 sat. below 94%
3 Vital signs and pulse oximetry
4 Continuous cardiac monitoring
5 Fluid balance chart
6 Blood glucose level
7 Sublingual glyceryl trinitrate
8 Morphine
9 Heart and breath sounds
10 Blood tests
11 12-lead ECG
12 Monitor for stress and anxiety
13 Psychosocial support
14 Medication – aspirin, heparin, captopril and metformin
15 VTE prophylaxis
16 Prepare for coronary artery bypass graft surgery
17 Post surgical management in ICU

Health education and home care:
• Cardiac rehabilitation plan

What further assessments should be initiated

CONCEPT MAP 21.8 Nursing interventions for John

SAFETY IN NURSING ⚠

Consider the risk of cardiac tamponade. Monitor for increased heart rate, decreased blood pressure, increased central venous pressure, decreased intercostal catheter output, decreased urine output, muffled heart sounds and decreased peripheral pulses.

21.9 EVALUATION OF CARE FOR CORONARY ARTERY BYPASS GRAFT SURGERY

As part of the further assessment of John's presentation, **Concept map 21.9** asks further questions in relation to John's management.

EVALUATION

John has responded well to coronary artery bypass graft surgery.

Plan:
John has joined the hospital's cardiac rehabilitation program, and will be reviewed by the cardiac surgeon in 3 weeks.

Cues

 Why is it important that John attend the cardiac rehabilitation program?

 John has non-modifiable and modifiable risk factors for cardiac disease. What can he do to address the modifiable risk factor for cardiac disease?

CONCEPT MAP 21.9 Evaluation and planning for John

EVIDENCE-BASED PRACTICE 🔍

If you are unable to palpate pulses or auscultate blood pressure, use a Doppler ultrasound to evaluate blood flow.

21.10 DISCHARGE PLANNING AND COORDINATION OF CARE FOR CORONARY ARTERY BYPASS GRAFT SURGERY

John's coronary artery graft surgery requires discharge planning and further management at home – see **Concept map 21.10**.

21.11 ASSESSMENT FOR SHOCK AND DISSEMINATED INTRAVASCULAR COAGULATION

Presentation

Subra Manorama is a 55-year-old man who was brought into the ED by ambulance. Subra fell off a ladder while pruning an apple tree. He landed on his left side and the blade of the open secateurs pierced his upper left thigh. His daughter, who has a first aid certificate, applied a compression bandage to the bleeding wound. When paramedics arrived to assess Subra, considerable blood seepage was occurring around the bandage and there was a pool of blood on the ground. Paramedics applied a further compression pad before transporting Subra to the ED.

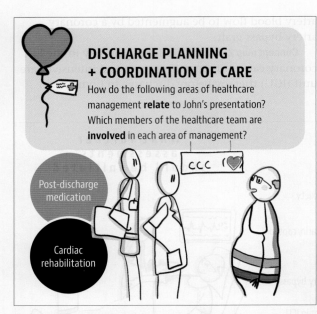

DISCHARGE PLANNING + COORDINATION OF CARE

How do the following areas of healthcare management **relate** to John's presentation? Which members of the healthcare team are **involved** in each area of management?

Post-discharge medication

Cardiac rehabilitation

CONCEPT MAP 21.10 Discharge planning and coordination of care for John

Initial and ongoing assessment is important, especially for people with complex care needs. Please refer to **Box 21.1** and **Box 21.2** as a guide to Subra's health assessment.

See **Concept map 21.11** to further explore Subra's initial care in the ED, before transfer to the operating theatre and the surgical ward for further care.

REFLECTIVE PRACTICE

Always consider potential drug interactions between herbal medicines and over-the-counter (OTC) drugs, as quite often patients do not consider herbal medicines and OTC drugs important to mention.

21.12 PLANNING CARE FOR SHOCK AND DISSEMINATED INTRAVASCULAR COAGULATION

Planning person-centred care for a patient with shock and disseminated intravascular coagulation has the goals of:
- oxygenation
- controlling bleeding
- wound repair.

Box 21.4 lists the areas that are targeted in the planning stage for caring for the person with shock and disseminated intravascular coagulation.

BOX 21.4 PLANNING FOR SHOCK AND DISSEMINATED INTRAVASCULAR COAGULATION

- ➤ Respond to severity of symptoms
- ➤ Bleeding
- ➤ Oxygenation
- ➤ Pain management
- ➤ Diagnostic tests – full blood profile, electrolytes, renal function, liver function
- ➤ To the operating theatre for exploration of wound
- ➤ Admit to surgical ward
- ➤ Health education and home care:
  - wound care
  - physical activity
  - medication

Concept map 21.12 outlines a plan for Subra's care.

 PHx

Subra has enjoyed good health which he attributes to being a gardener and walker. He takes ginger for a healthy immune system and cardiac strength aspirin for his heart. He has no allergies. He takes aspirin as his family has a history of heart disease.

 ASSESSMENT

Primary Survey
A: Patent
B: RR 22, pulse oximetry 97% on room air, breath sounds normal
C: HR 118 bpm, BP 130/80 mmHg, skin pale. Wound on left thigh oozing blood through compression bandage
D: Alert and orientated
E: 36.7°C

F: IV to be commenced, wound ooze
G: BGL 5.7 mmol/L

Secondary Survey
CNS: Alert and orientated. GCS E 4 V 5 M 6 = 15.
CVS: BP 130/80 mmHg, HR 118 bpm, T 36.8°C, centrally and peripherally cool
Resp: RR 20, SpO₂ 96%

GIT: Bowel sounds present with a non-tender abdomen.
Renal: Urine concentrated but no abnormalities detected
Metabolic: BGL 5.7 mmol/L
Integumentary: Cool dry skin
Musculoskeletal: equal limb strength with pain at the wound site.
Left thigh x-ray and chest x-ray to be reviewed.

CONCEPT MAP 21.11 Nursing assessment for Subra

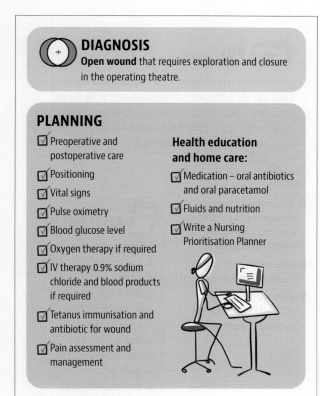

DIAGNOSIS

Open wound that requires exploration and closure in the operating theatre.

PLANNING

☑ Preoperative and postoperative care

☑ Positioning

☑ Vital signs

☑ Pulse oximetry

☑ Blood glucose level

☑ Oxygen therapy if required

☑ IV therapy 0.9% sodium chloride and blood products if required

☑ Tetanus immunisation and antibiotic for wound

☑ Pain assessment and management

Health education and home care:

☑ Medication – oral antibiotics and oral paracetamol

☑ Fluids and nutrition

☑ Write a Nursing Prioritisation Planner

CONCEPT MAP 21.12 Diagnosis and planning for Subra

INTERVENTIONS

1 Positioning – Fowlers

2 Vital signs 4 hourly

3. Pulse oximetry 4 hourly

4 Blood glucose level

5 Oxygen therapy if required

6 IV therapy 0.9% sodium chloride 8/24

7 Cross-match and group and hold - confirm these have been taken

8 Benzylpenicillin 1.2 g QID IV

9 Paracetamol 1 g QID oral for pain

10 Wound care

11 Prepared for the operating theatre and consent for procedure given

Health education and home care:

• Postoperative exercises

• Medication – oral antibiotics and paracetamol 1 g prn

• Fluids and nutrition

What further assessments should be initiated?

CONCEPT MAP 21.13 Nursing interventions for Subra

21.13 NURSING INTERVENTIONS TO SUPPORT HEALTH CARE FOR SHOCK AND DISSEMINATED INTRAVASCULAR COAGULATION

Nursing interventions are implemented as part of person-centred care and include responding to unanticipated patient responses.

Concept map 21.13 explores Subra's journey from the ED to the operating room to the surgical ward.

21.14 EVALUATION OF CARE FOR SHOCK AND DISSEMINATED INTRAVASCULAR COAGULATION

As part of the further assessment of Subra's response to therapy, **Concept map 21.14** asks further questions in relation to Subra's management.

EVALUATION

During the cleansing and closing of the wound in theatre, the wound would not stop oozing. Subra was transferred to the ICU for monitoring, fluid maintenance and wound management. Subra's wound is still oozing and his vital signs show tachypnoea, tachycardia and borderline hypotension. Subra states he is feeling anxious, and wonders if he will ever see his garden again.

Plan:
To take blood sample for full blood count and clotting profile.

Cues

1 Why is Subra deteriorating?

2 What is the medical management for disseminated coagulopathy?

3 What nursing interventions would you instigate for Subra?

CONCEPT MAP 21.14 Evaluation and planning for Subra

21.15 DISCHARGE PLANNING AND COORDINATION OF CARE FOR SHOCK AND DISSEMINATED INTRAVASCULAR COAGULATION

The discharge planning for Subra's shock and disseminated intravascular coagulation has the foci of further management in the ICU ward then discharge to the home, with a follow-up appointment in the hospital's outpatient clinic – see **Concept map 21.15**.

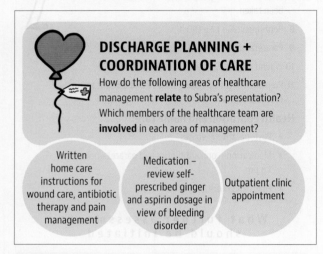

DISCHARGE PLANNING + COORDINATION OF CARE

How do the following areas of healthcare management **relate** to Subra's presentation? Which members of the healthcare team are **involved** in each area of management?

- Written home care instructions for wound care, antibiotic therapy and pain management
- Medication – review self-prescribed ginger and aspirin dosage in view of bleeding disorder
- Outpatient clinic appointment

CONCEPT MAP 21.15 Discharge planning and coordination of care for Subra

21.16 ASSESSMENT FOR ACUTE RESPIRATORY DISTRESS SYNDROME

The assessment for acute respiratory distress syndrome is ongoing; please refer to **Box 21.1** and **Box 21.2** to select and conduct appropriate assessments.

Presentation

Juan Montoya is a 36-year-old plumber who went to the general practitioner with an infected cut on his right calf. Juan was prescribed antibiotics for the infected wound and has been taking them for the last two days. This morning he woke up flushed and sweaty, and feels very nauseated. His mother brought him to the ED. Juan has noticed that his breathing has quickened.

Concept map 21.16 further explores Juan's initial care in the ED.

21.17 PLANNING CARE FOR ACUTE RESPIRATORY DISTRESS SYNDROME

The planning of person-centred care for a patient with septic shock and acute respiratory distress syndrome will have the goals of:

 PHx

Juan sustained a cut on his calf while digging up drainage pipes 7 days ago. The cut became inflamed so he went to the general practitioner 2 days ago, and was prescribed antibiotics. Apart from the antibiotics he is not taking medications and has no allergies. He is an occasional drinker. He plays soccer on the weekends.

Cues

1. What is the relationship between the high respiratory and heart rates and the normal blood pressure?
2. What do the diminished breath sounds indicate?
3. What tests should be obtained to confirm a diagnosis of septic shock?

 ASSESSMENT

Primary survey

A: Patent
B: RR 30
C: HR 120 bpm, BP 135/75 mmHg warm dry flushed skin, scattered fine crackles in lower lobes R-L. Pulse oximetry 95% on room air.
D: Alert and orientated
E: 38.1 °C
ABG – mild respiratory alkalosis

CONCEPT MAP 21.16 Nursing assessment for Juan

- increasing oxygenation
- relieving pain
- providing rest.

Juan is a partner in the planning of his care.

Box 21.5 lists the areas that are targeted in the planning stage of septic care.

Concept map 21.17 outlines a plan for Juan's care.

BOX 21.5   PLANNING FOR SEPTIC SHOCK AND ACUTE RESPIRATORY DISTRESS SYNDROME

➤ Wound management
➤ Medication
➤ Respond to severity of symptoms, and airway maintenance
➤ Diagnostic tests – wound culture and sensitivity, blood cultures, arterial blood gases (ABGs), chest x-ray

DIAGNOSIS
Sepsis from calf wound, progressing to **early septic shock**. Respiratory function deteriorating towards **acute respiratory distress syndrome** (ARDS).

PLANNING

☑ Positioning

☑ Vital signs

☑ Pulse oximetry

☑ Blood glucose level

☑ Lung sounds, cough, sputum

☑ Oxygen therapy, consider non-invasive ventilation or high flow oxygen therapy for deterioration of respiratory function. Admission to ICU.

☑ IV therapy 0.9% sodium chloride

☑ Initial antibiotic therapy regimen for unidentified microorganism – benzylpenicillin and azithromycin

☑ Medication – intravenous antibiotics and paracetamol

☑ Fluids and nutrition

☑ Write a Nursing Prioritisation Planner

CONCEPT MAP 21.17 Diagnosis and planning for Juan

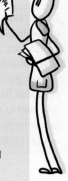

INTERVENTIONS

1 Positioning – high Fowlers

2 Oxygen via mask to keep oxygen saturation above 94%

3 Vital signs hourly

4 Pulse oximetry hourly

5 Blood glucose level

6 Arterial blood gases as indicated

7 Lung sounds 4 hourly. Chest x-ray shows scattered interstitial filtrates.

8 Respiratory care, including physiotherapy

9 IV therapy 0.9% sodium chloride 8/24

10 Urinary catheter

11 Fluid balance

12 Benzylpenicillin 1.2 g QID IV; azithromycin 500 mg daily IV over 1 hour

13 Paracetamol 500 mg QID IV

14 Psychosocial support for a very unwell patient

What further assessments should be initiated❓

CONCEPT MAP 21.18 Nursing interventions for Juan

21.18 NURSING INTERVENTIONS TO SUPPORT HEALTH CARE FOR ACUTE RESPIRATORY DISTRESS SYNDROME

Nursing interventions are implemented as part of person-centred care and to reduce or reverse signs and symptoms and the associated pathophysiology of a septic shock and acute respiratory distress syndrome.

Concept map 21.18 explores Juan's journey from the ED to the ICU.

21.19 EVALUATION OF CARE FOR ACUTE RESPIRATORY DISTRESS SYNDROME

As part of the further assessment of Juan's presentation, Concept map 21.19 asks further questions in relation to his respiratory function.

EVALUATION

Juan is developing a cough, his work of breathing is increasing and oxygenation has deteriorated to 90% and is not physiologically responding to the increased FiO$_2$.

Plan:
For endotracheal intubation and mechanical ventilation to address deteriorating oxygen levels.

Cues

1 What additional information should we obtain about Juan's respiratory status?

CONCEPT MAP 21.19 Evaluation and planning for Juan

REFLECTIVE PRACTICE

Acute respiratory distress syndrome normally occurs within 48 hours of a predisposing illness (signs and symptoms). In this case, septic shock is the predisposing illness due to a wound infection. The pathogen that has caused the wound infection activates an immunological response that includes severe inflammatory responses that lead to altered vascular permeability that lead to pulmonary oedema and culminates in the complication of acute respiratory distress syndrome.

21.20 DISCHARGE PLANNING AND COORDINATION OF CARE FOR ACUTE RESPIRATORY DISTRESS SYNDROME

Juan's septic shock and acute respiratory distress syndrome will be cared for in the ICU. Once Juan begins to recover and does not require mechanical ventilation he will be transferred to the ward – see Concept map 21.20.

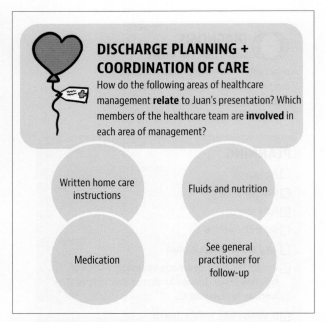

DISCHARGE PLANNING + COORDINATION OF CARE
How do the following areas of healthcare management **relate** to Juan's presentation? Which members of the healthcare team are **involved** in each area of management?

- Written home care instructions
- Fluids and nutrition
- Medication
- See general practitioner for follow-up

CONCEPT MAP 21.20 Discharge planning and coordination of care for Juan

SUMMARY

Many patients require complex care due to their existing health concerns or conditions. Pneumonia, for instance, will affect every person differently due to factors such as age, gender, previous medical history and existing chronic conditions. What do you think the impact of pneumonia would be on a 4-week-old baby? A 90-year-old male with COPD? A 32-year-old female with a PE and pneumonia who is 28/40 pregnant? Patients' responses to disease, injury or illness are as unique as they are.

CLINICAL SKILLS IN COMPLEX CARE PROBLEMS

The following clinical skills are required when managing a person with complex care conditions; consult your Clinical Skills resources, such as Tollefson and Hillman (2022), *Clinical Psychomotor Skills* (8th ed.).
- Temperature, pulse and respiration measurement
- Blood pressure measurement
- Monitoring pulse oximetry
- Pain assessment
- Focused cardiovascular health history and physical assessment
- 12-lead electrocardiogram
- Focused respiratory health history and physical assessment

- Blood glucose measurement
- Nasogastric tube insertion
- Oral medication
- Topical medication
- Intravenous medication
- Preoperative care
- Postoperative care
- Oxygen therapy via nasal cannula or various masks
- Oropharyngeal and nasopharyngeal suctioning
- Artificial airway suctioning
- Tracheostomy care

PROBLEM-SOLVING SCENARIO 1

- Emma James, 72-year-old female
- T 38.2 °C HR 120 bpm & reg BP 80/40 mmHG RR 30 SpO2 90% RA
- PMHx – T2DM, Asthma, COPD, HTN, TIAs, Angina
Consider Emma's PMHx. What, if any, impact do you see here on her observations?

1   If Emma is normally hypertensive, is her current blood pressure significant?
2   What information would auscultation of Emma's chest provide? Would this be useful for your assessment?
3   Are these observations within normal limits?

4   Is there a relationship between the T and HR?

5   What PPE would you be required to use if Emma had a diagnosis of tuberculosis? COVID-19? Influenza? Varicella?

6   Emma has a +ve PCR for COVID-19, unknown variant, awaiting further testing. How would you explain this to Emma?

PROBLEM-SOLVING SCENARIO 2

Using a concept map approach, how would you assist Jeanne Aldridge?

Jeanne Aldridge is a 29-year-old woman who has had a history of sudden chest pain and dyspnoea for the last 2 hours. A chest x-ray and spiral CT scan revealed a pulmonary embolism.

1   What are the causes of pulmonary embolism?

2   What are the associated signs and symptoms of pulmonary embolism?

3   What is the medical management for pulmonary embolism?

4   What is the nursing management for pulmonary embolism?

PROBLEM-SOLVING SCENARIO 3

Using a concept map approach, how would you assist Jasmine Harrison?

Jasmine Harrison is a 31-year-old female who has been hospitalised for the past 4 weeks post a motor vehicle accident. She sustained significant head injuries and has been in the rehabilitation unit for 1 week. Jasmine has developed a pressure injury on her left heel. The wound has a cavity, the size of a 10-cent piece, and involves subcutaneous tissue. The wound has previously not been documented so the length of time it has existed is unknown.

1   What stage pressure area injury does this wound sound like?

2   What factors could be contributing to the wound developing?

3   What would you document regarding finding this wound?

PORTFOLIO DEVELOPMENT

Complex conditions and their management are based on best practice or evidence-based practice (EBP). Therefore, complex care management can change from time to time based on EBP. The Joanna Briggs Institute is one of the organisations that monitors EBP. Within their resources are current peer-reviewed journals and guidelines that are applicable to nursing care. The COVID-19 section has free resources regarding hand hygiene, transmission and reuse of disposable masks (or extended use) and can be viewed at https://jbi.global/covid-19#professionals.

This information can contribute to your annual continuing professional development (CPD). Simply note a reflection from your learning/reading and you will have some CPD accrued.

USEFUL WEBSITES

Australian Commission on Safety and Quality in Health Care, the National Safety and Quality Health Service (NSQHS) Standards https://www.safetyandquality.gov.au/standards/nsqhs-standards

Australian Commission on Safety and Quality in Health Care, the Australian Charter of Healthcare Rights https://www.safetyandquality.gov.au/our-work/partnering-consumers/australian-charter-healthcare-rights

Agency for Clinical Innovation: Resources https://aci.health.nsw.gov.au/resources

Department of Health and Aged Care, Chronic conditions https://www.health.gov.au/health-topics/chronic-conditions

Department of Health and Aged Care, Chronic conditions in Australia https://www.health.gov.au/health-topics/chronic-conditions/chronic-conditions-in-australia

Cardiac Society of Australia and New Zealand https://www.csanz.edu.au/for-professionals/position-statements-and-practice-guidelines

Heart Foundation https://www.heartfoundation.org.au

Nursing and Midwifery Board of Australia, Decision-making framework for nursing and midwifery (2020) https://www.nursingmidwiferyboard.gov.au/codes-guidelines-statements/frameworks.aspx

REFERENCES AND FURTHER READING

Australian Commission on Safety and Quality in Health Care (ACSQHC). (2022). *Recognising and responding to acute deterioration standard*. https://www.safetyandquality.gov.au/standards/nsqhs-standards/recognising-and-responding-acute-deterioration-standard

Broyles, B., Reiss, B., Evans, M., Pleunik, S., Page, R., & Badoer, E. (2023). *Pharmacology in nursing* (4th ANZ ed.). Cengage Learning Australia.

DeLaune, S., Ladner, P., McTier, L., Tollefson, J., & Lawrence, J. (2024). *Fundamentals of nursing* (3rd ed.). Cengage Learning Australia.

DiSilvio, B., Young, M., Gordon, A., Malik, K., Singh, A., & Cheema, T. (2019). Complications and outcomes of acute respiratory distress syndrome. *Critical Care Nursing Quarterly, 42*(4), 349–361. DOI: 10.1097/CNQ.0000000000000275

Epley, D. (2000). Pulmonary emboli risk reduction. *Journal of Vascular Nursing, 18*(2), 61–68. https://doi.org/10.1016/S1062-0303(00)90029-3

Gray, S., Ferris, L., White, L. E., Baumle, W., & Duncan, G. (2019). *Foundations of nursing: enrolled nurses* (2nd ANZ ed.). Cengage Learning Australia.

Joustra, C., & Moloney, A. (2019). *Clinical placement manual*. Cengage Learning Australia.

Khajian Gelogahi, Z., Aghebati, N., Mazloum, S., & Mohajer, S. (2018). Effectiveness of nurse's intentional presence as a holistic modality on depression, anxiety, and stress of cardiac surgery patients. *Holistic Nursing Practice, 32*(6), 296–306. DOI: 10.1097/HNP.0000000000000294

Lucchini, A., Bambi, S., Mattiussi, E., Elli, S., Villa, L., Bondi, H., Rona, R., Fumagalli, R., & Foti, G. (2020). Prone position in acute respiratory distress syndrome patients: A retrospective analysis of complications. *Dimensions of Critical Care Nursing, 39*(1), 39–46. DOI: 10.1097/DCC.0000000000000393

Mousavi Malek, N., Zakerimoghadam, M., Esmaeili, M., & Kazemnejad, A. (2018). Effects of nurse-led intervention on patients' anxiety and sleep before coronary artery bypass grafting. *Critical Care Nursing Quarterly, 41*(2), 161–169. DOI: 10.1097/CNQ.0000000000000195

Neighbors, M., & Tannehill-Jones, R. (2023). *Human diseases* (6th ed.). Cengage.

Pinto, L., de Oliveira, K., Lucena, A., Moretti, M., Haas, J., Moraes, R., & Friedman, G. (2020). Septic shock: Clinical indicators and implications to critical patient care. *Journal of Clinical Nursing, 30*, 1607–1614. https://doi.org/10.1111/jocn.15713

Rizzo, D. C. (2015). *Fundamentals of anatomy and physiology* (4th ed.). Cengage Learning.

Rolving, N., Bloch-Neilsen, J., Brocki, B., & Andreasen, J. (2020). Perspectives of patients and health professionals on important factors influencing rehabilitation following acute pulmonary embolism: A multi-method study. *Thrombosis Research, 196*, 283–290. https://doi.org/10.1016/j.thromres.2020.09.016

Singh, P., & Schwartz, A. (2020). Disseminated intravascular coagulation: A devastating systemic disorder of special concern with COVID-19. *Dermatological Therapy, 33*(6), e14053. https://doi.org/10.1111/dth.14053

Tollefson, J., & Hillman, E. (2022). *Clinical psychomotor skills: Assessment tools for nurses* (8th ed.). Cengage Learning Australia.

CHAPTER 22

CANCER CARE

Cancer remains a major or significant cause of death and illness within Australia and has considerable social and economic impact on not only the person with cancer, but their families and the surrounding community. Males were estimated to represent more than 50 per cent of the new cancer diagnoses in 2022, with a total figure estimated to be more than 160000 cases. It is estimated that some 50000 people died from cancer in 2022 (Australian Institute of Health and Welfare (AIHW), 2022).

Cancer, while a specialty in nursing, is something that almost every ward or department will come across, with past medical histories, acute or chronic conditions or exacerbations, or hospitalisations required for problems other than cancer care.

LEARNING OBJECTIVES

After reading this chapter, you should have an understanding of the:
1. assessment required for a person with cancer conditions
2. prioritisation of key components in the development of a plan of care for people who have:
   - colorectal cancer
   - lung cancer
3. prioritised and targeted nursing interventions required to promote recovery, rehabilitation or palliation or prevent further deterioration
4. evaluation phase and how the prioritised and targeted nursing interventions inform further assessment, planning and collaboration with the healthcare team
5. discharge planning and coordination of care required in preparing the person for discharge and subsequent continuity of care between the person and their healthcare providers.

INTRODUCTION

Cancer can be described as a group of diverse diseases which are characterised by abnormal cells. Cells are the building blocks of the body and cancer cells tend to grow rapidly and invade and destroy body tissues and organs. They can metastasise (spread) to a distant site via the blood vessels, lymph vessels or by invading other organs. The most frequent sites of metastasis are the lungs, brain, bone, liver and adrenal glands (Brown et al., 2019; DeLaune et al., 2024; Rizzo, 2015).

Most cancers do not occur or result from inherited genes but are acquired from damage to genes occurring over the person's lifetime. A mutation is passed on to all cells that develop from that single cell, so even if the damaged cell dies, the cell replicates into daughter cells, each carrying the same genetic alteration – the cancer (Craft & Gordon, 2019).

Nurses play a vital role in caring for cancer patients and by implementing health education can help to reduce not only the incidence of cancer in our society but also the fear and anxiety that comes with a diagnosis of cancer, thereby focusing on holistic health.

A **neoplasm** can be either benign or malignant. A benign tumour has certain characteristics which differ from a malignant tumour. For example, a benign tumour is normally localised, enclosed in a capsule and does not spread or metastasise. Examples of benign tumours include cysts, fibroids or a wart. On the other hand, malignant tumours are cancerous growths that do not remain localised to their site of origin. They invade neighbouring tissues and organs and can spread through the lymph system or bloodstream to other parts of the body and form new growths known as secondaries or metastases. Even if the primary tumour is removed by surgery, the disease sometimes recurs in the form of secondaries which have detached from the primary tumour before being arrested. Death results when this growth interferes with vital life processes (Rizzo, 2015).

Neoplasms are divided into three categories – carcinomas, sarcomas and blood and lymph neoplasms.

- Carcinomas or solid tumours: arise from epithelial tissue from the external and internal body surfaces. May be initially confined to a specific tissue or organ. As the tumour grows, cells are shed which travel through blood and lymph to produce metastasis in distant sites.
- Sarcomas: less common than carcinomas, they arise from supportive and connective structures such as bone, fat, muscle and cartilage.
- Haematological cancers: involve the blood and lymph systems and are scattered throughout the body. Leukaemias arise from the body's blood and form tissues within the bone marrow. The abnormal tissue proliferates, crowding out normal blood-forming cells and releases large quantities of abnormal white blood cells called leucocytes into the circulating blood (Craft & Gordon, 2019; DeLaune et al., 2024; Rizzo, 2015).

Neoplasms are a disease process where in many cases the actual cause is unknown. It is believed that mutations occur often within the body; however, the immune response destroys the abnormal cells as soon as they occur. Genetics are linked to some common cancers such as breast and bowel/colorectal. In other cancers, viruses may be the cause. For example, a virus appears to be more common in individuals with cervical cancer. Carcinogens such as tobacco smoke and exposure to ultraviolet rays of the sun have also been linked to cancers (AIHW, 2022).

Pathologists grade neoplasms using a microscope to determine the anatomical extent of the disease by stages. There are usually four stages.

- Stage/Grade 1. Tumour cells are localised and closely resemble normal tissue
- Stage/Grade II. Limited local spread
- Stage/Grade III. Extensive local and regional spread
- Stage/Grade IV. Metastasis/es.

Persons with grade 1 tumours typically have a high survival rate, whereas persons with grade IV have a much poorer likelihood of survival (Craft & Gordon, 2019).

Nurses play a fundamental role in providing education for cancer prevention and detection. Education in the following areas will assist patients to identify early signs and symptoms of cancer:

- techniques of breast self-examination
- techniques of testicular self-examination
- dietary modifications and weight control
- decreasing alcohol intake
- smoking cessation
- techniques of skin self-examination and protective measures against sun exposure
- the importance of screening tests
- the importance of early detection.

Cancer progression, diagnosis and presentation is unique for every patient. Specific cancers, however, do have hallmark warning signs. Now let's look at the assessment of a person with colorectal cancer.

22.1 ASSESSMENT FOR COLORECTAL CANCER (CRC)

The nursing assessment of the person with colorectal cancer (CRC) will rely upon subjective and objective data, and symptom severity and objective findings will differ.

Signs and symptoms of CRC will differ dependent upon the location of the tumour/primary cancer. For example, a patient with cancer in the transverse colon will exhibit pain, obstruction, change in bowel habits and anaemia, while the descending colon patients will display pain, change in bowel habits, bright red blood in their stool and likely obstruction (Craft & Gordon, 2019).

Other considerations that will be relevant in a patient presenting with CRC are:

- psychosocial issues
- medications
- past medical history
- self-care issues
- any other information relevant to the cancer, or other chronic conditions.

Presentation

The patient presenting with CRC is Darby Fuller, a 78-year-old male. Concept map 22.1 further explores Darby's presentation.

PHx

Darby is a 78-year-old male who is presenting post a rectal bleed this a.m. Darby describes the bleed as 'bright red and a lot'. He reports infrequent defecation, with associated lower abdominal pain. He has a history of COPD, HTN and obesity.

Cues

1. What are your priorities with this patient?.
2. What is the significance of tachycardia post rectal bleeding?
3. What is the relationship between bleeding and anaemia?
4. What is the pathophysiological relationship between CRC and anaemia?
5. What are some concerns in relationship to the GIT assessment in this patient?
6. What physiological impact does tachypnoea, tachycardia and temperature have on the patient?
7. What investigative or diagnostic procedures do you think would be relevant for this patient?

CONCEPT MAP 22.1 Nursing assessment for Darby

 ASSESSMENT

Primary survey
A: Patent
B: RR 24
C: Warm centrally
D: Alert
E: T 38 °C
F: IVT to commence, dark urine
G: BGL 6.2 mmol/L

Secondary survey
CNS: (E4 V5 M6 = 15, PEARLA 3 mm). Febrile @ 38 °C
PAIN: Abdo pain LLQ 6/10. Headaches infrequently.
CVS: HR 105 bpm, irregular and thready, NIBP 100/80 mmHg, ECG – sinus arrythmia

RESP: RR 24, patent airway – spontaneous breathing, SpO$_2$ 90%
GIT: Nausea and vomiting, abdo tender in LLQ, BS on auscultation hypoactive. Faecal odour on breath. Blood in faeces reported.
RENAL (output): Pt reports no changes to habits. Dark, urine, await ward UA
SKIN/INTEG: Centrally warm, peripherally cooler. Skin intact, however, fragile
MUSCULOSKELETAL (mobility): strict RIB, with VTE prophylaxis
BMI: 31.0

22.2 PLANNING CARE FOR CRC

Planning for rectal bleeding, secondary to CRC, will have the goals of:

- maintenance of cardiovascular function within normal parameters
- diagnostic investigations to determine the source and site of bleeding.

Darby is a partner in his care plan and can contribute to his health care by following his plan of care and managing his condition in the home environment. **Box 22.1** lists the risk factors for CRC.

Darby's assessment will be aligned to further diagnostic interventions including full blood count, abdominal x-ray, CT abdo, as well as a digital rectal examination.

See **Concept map 22.2** for an outline of Darby's care plan.

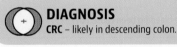 **DIAGNOSIS**
CRC – likely in descending colon.

PLANNING
☑ Diagnostic tests – x-ray abdo, CT scan
☑ For theatre – for bowel resection +/- -ostomy
☑ Conservative treatment if the cancer has spread and is inoperable
☑ Write a Nursing Prioritisation Planner

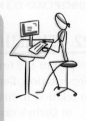

CONCEPT MAP 22.2 Diagnosis and planning for Darby

BOX 22.1 RISK FACTORS FOR CRC

- Lifestyle modifications
- Weight reduction
- A diet high in red or processed meat
- Obesity
- Physical inactivity
- Long-term smoking
- Low intake of fruits and vegetables
- Genetics – 5–10 per cent of all cancers or predispositions are inherited from parents (Brown et al., 2019)

22.3 NURSING INTERVENTIONS TO SUPPORT HEALTH CARE FOR CRC

Nursing interventions are implemented as part of person-centred care and to reduce or reverse signs and symptoms and the associated condition. In Darby's case, he has presented with new onset of rectal bleeding, associated with weight loss, change in bowel habits and abdominal pain. He has also presented with cardiovascular compromise, and is anaemic and hypoxic. Darby will require surgery to determine the level of his cancer, and the aim will be for a bowel resection, with the likelihood of an ostomy formation.

An ostomy is a surgical procedure which allows the contents of the bowel out through an opening in the skin – the opening is called a stoma. It will mean that Darby will not defecate using his rectum, all of his faeces will exit through the stoma (Brown et al., 2019; Craft & Gordon, 2019).

Concept map 22.3 explores Darby's journey prior to surgery.

INTERVENTIONS

1 Assess bowel function

2 Assess pain, fluid balance and cardiovascular function regularly

3 ISBAR handover preparation for end-of-shift handover – what would you be handing over if your patient was due for theatre in 30 mins?

What further assessments should be initiated

Cues 1 What specific preoperative requirements does Darby have?

2 What possible reasons would there be for the patient to report pain?

3 What has the bleeding been caused by?

CONCEPT MAP 22.3 Nursing interventions for Darby

22.4 EVALUATION OF CARE FOR CRC

As part of the further assessment of Darby's presentation, Concept map 22.4 asks further questions in relation to his management.

In Darby's case, he has had a stoma formed due to cancer in his colon. The operation involved a double-barreled stoma, with both proximal and distal ends to the stoma, reversible. His post-op care will depend greatly upon his response to the surgery and the psychological process of adjusting to a stoma. Nursing care will also be focused on assessment of the stoma – is it passing flatus, fluid? What is the colour? There is a significant component of grief and loss with stoma formation, and there will be a need for a stomal therapist who will ensure that Darby can apply bags, manage his ostomy and care for himself postoperatively.

Nursing management of the patient undergoing chemotherapy and radiation therapy includes

EVALUATION

The medical team have been notified of Darby's decreasing blood pressure (90 mmHg systolic) and increasing HR – 120 bpm, irregular and weak.

Plan:
While Darby is being prepared for OT for a bowel resection, his vital signs deteriorate. He is yet to have the nasogastric tube (NGT) that was ordered inserted.

Cues

1 What interventions need to be considered now for Darby?

2 Does this deterioration relate to his presentation?

3 Why do you think an NGT is required?

4 If there was a delay in inserting the NGT, what impact do you think this could have had on Darby's pain?

CONCEPT MAP 22.4 Evaluation and planning for Darby

knowledge of the side effects and problems caused by this form of treatment.

Nursing care can be a component of the new diagnosis of cancer, such as in Darby's case, or in an ongoing case of cancer care and treatment in someone who has had, for example, a haematological cancer with varying treatments.

22.5 DISCHARGE PLANNING AND COORDINATION OF CARE FOR CRC

Darby presented initially with rectal bleeding, which has led to a diagnosis of CRC, and the requirement of surgical intervention to resect his bowel. Postoperatively, Darby has continued to demonstrate cardiovascular compromise and has had postoperative anaemia. Darby has also shown very little interest in learning about how to manage his stoma and has requested his room be left 'dark' almost all the time. He has withdrawn from his family and is expressing considerable frustration with his inability to 'go to the toilet normally' or 'be a man' and care for himself.

Your aim in your nursing management will be to holistically support Darby and his family in his recovery. The addition of stoma and a cancer diagnosis is something that will require each person to adjust to and even process feelings of loss and grief. In previous

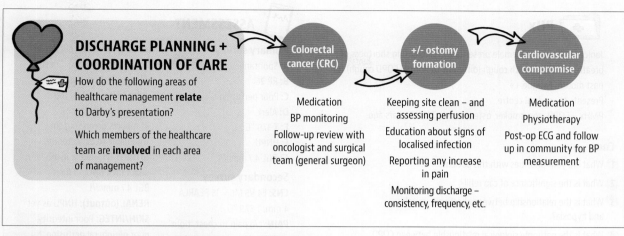

CONCEPT MAP 22.5 Discharge planning and coordination of care for Darby

---

NASOGASTRIC TUBES

Nasogastric tubes (NGTs) are a crucial intervention for the CRC patient if they are presenting with abdominal pain. This pain is likely due to the compression of the stomach from the bowel obstruction. If your patient is exhibiting nausea, or is vomiting, this is also an excellent interventional tool to alleviate symptoms and to also obtain objective information regarding their symptoms.

'Putting off' insertion of an NGT can compromise patient care. While an NGT cannot clear a bowel obstruction, it can provide comfort and further insight into the type of blockage. If the NGT aspirate or contents for example are faecal, then it can identify preoperatively other precautions that the patient will require (Brown et al., 2019; DeLaune et al., 2024).

Cancer care nursing

You have been allocated EOL (end of life) for two patients. One is an 18-year-old female, Georgia, who has breast cancer and is in the terminal phase. The second patient is Bille, a 78-year-old female, who has end stage lung cancer.

Consider the aetiology for each type of cancer:
» one patient has smoked heavily for ~5 years
» one patient has never smoked.

Questions

1 Which patient do you think is the non-smoker? Why?
2 Do you have any preconceived notions around lung cancer and the patient's past history? What about for breast cancer?
3 Do you think lung cancer patients experience stigma?

---

chapters, such as Chapter 11, we have outlined the process for feedback, health education and health promotion. This same process needs to be applied to Darby to ensure that he not only recovers from his surgery, but that he also recovers quality of life and has self-determination regarding his health care.

Concept map 22.5 explores discharge planning and coordination of care for Darby.

22.6 ASSESSMENT FOR LUNG CANCER

In Australia, more than 13 250 people will be diagnosed with lung cancer annually. The majority of these people (85%) will be diagnosed with lung cancer at a late stage and therefore lung cancer is the most common cause of cancer death in Australia (Lung Foundation Australia, 2022).

Assessment of the patient who has lung cancer will show many, if not all, the following symptoms:

- cough
- hoarseness of voice
- chest pain or shoulder pain
- weight loss or loss of appetite
- shortness of breath
- low albumin on full blood count
- crackles/creps on chest auscultation
- decreased peripheral perfusion – cool clammy peripheries
- hypoxia
- presence of fever
- barrel chest
- lymphadenopathy
- pleural effusion
- deep vein thrombosis (DeLaune et al., 2024; Derrickson et al., 2021; Edwards et al., 2019; Lung Foundation Australia, 2022).

PHx

Janice, a 55-year-old female presents with increasing shortness of breath, associated with cough (different to normal COPD cough) for past month. Fatigue ++
Presents to medical centre.
PMHx – COPD, non-smoker, osteoporosis, TAH 10 years ago.

Cues

1. What are your priorities with this patient?
2. What is the significance of cap refill?
3. What is the relationship between chest pain, cough and hypoxia?
4. What is the pathophysiological relationship between COPD and lung cancer?
5. What are some concerns in relation to respiratory presentation of this patient?
6. What is the relevance of the warmth to one calf?
7. What investigative or diagnostic procedures would you think would be relevant for this patient?

CONCEPT MAP 22.6 Nursing assessment for Janice

ASSESSMENT

Primary survey

A: Spontaneous, inc. WOB
B: RR 26
C: Poor perfusion
D: Alert
E: T 37.9 °C
F: HNPU
G: BGL 4.7 mmol/L

Secondary survey

CNS: E4 V5 M6 = 15 PEARLA 4 mm. T 37.9 °C
PAIN: c/o pain to chest 'tight' and shoulder pain – rated as 7/10, worse on deep inspiration
CVS: HR 110 bpm, regular. BP 150/90 mmHg. Centrally warm, centrally cyanotic and poorly perfused. cap refill >4 sec
RESP: RR 26 SpO$_2$ 88% RA, increased WOB, use of accessory muscles, pursed lip breathing, tripoding. Chest on auscultation, minimal air entry to bases, R=L, creps throughout midzones. Pt reports green sputum when able to expectorate.
GIT: SNT BS audible in all quadrants. BNO >3 days. BGL 4.7 mmol/L
RENAL (output): HNPU as yet
SKIN/INTEG: Poor integrity, poor peripheral perfusion. Nil skin tears. Clubbing. Left calf warmer than right.
MUSCULOSKELETAL (mobility): Strict RIB, with VTE prophylaxis – sit upright @ 45 degrees minimum
BMI: 22.4

Presentation

Janice is a 55-year-old female who has had a cough lasting longer than three weeks and associated fatigue. She has a family history of lung cancer (father) and has been a passive smoker for 30 years. She has also worked in a diesel fitters' business for the past 25 years as the office manager. Janice has a diagnosis of COPD (asthma and emphysema) which was confirmed seven years ago.

Concept map 22.6 further explores Janice's admission.

22.7 PLANNING CARE FOR LUNG CANCER

Planning for Janice will have a person-centred focus. Janice will require referrals to multidisciplinary team members and specialist oncology teams to assist in her care and treatment.

See **Concept Map 22.7** for an outline of Janice's care plan.

DIAGNOSIS

The diagnosis is **non-small cell lung cancer**

PLANNING

☑ Respiratory observations – at least hourly
☑ Monitor blood pressure closely (consider invasive monitoring)
☑ Vital signs
☑ Fluid balance chart
☑ Medication therapy
☑ Patient positioning
☑ Referrals to multidisciplinary team and specialist oncology team for non-small cell lung cancer
☑ Write a Nursing Prioritisation Planner

Further investigations:

☑ Staging of tumour/s
☑ Treatment plans

CONCEPT MAP 22.7 Diagnosis and planning for Janice

22.8 NURSING INTERVENTIONS TO SUPPORT HEALTH CARE FOR LUNG CANCER

Nursing interventions for Janice are explored in **Concept map 22.8**.

22.9 EVALUATION OF CARE FOR LUNG CANCER

As part of the further assessment of Janice's presentation, **Concept map 22.9** asks further questions in relation to her management.

22.10 DISCHARGE PLANNING AND COORDINATION OF CARE FOR LUNG CANCER

See further information for Janice's discharge planning in **Concept map 22.10**.

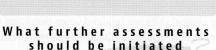

INTERVENTIONS

1 Assess pain, respiratory function, patient condition including psychosocial support.

2 ISBAR handover preparation for end-of-shift handover – what would you be handing over if your patient had increasing WOB and SOB? With SpO$_2$ <87%?

What further assessments should be initiated

Cues

1 What further questions or information would you like to know from Janice?

2 What is the deterioration here? How has the lung cancer been 'missed' for so long?

3 What possible reasons would there be for the patient to report pain in her chest and shoulder?

4 What could be the pathophysiological reason for pain and swelling to left calf?

CONCEPT MAP 22.8 Nursing interventions for Janice

EVALUATION

The medical team have been notified of Janice's increased WOB and SOB with associated hypoxia @ 86% SpO$_2$

Plan:

Medical officer has requested an arterial blood gas (ABG) analysis. While organising this test (it is not within RN scope at all facilities), Janice becomes anxious regarding her breathing, she is 'panicking' as she 'cannot breathe' and is worried 'that this will be my last few breaths'. She is only able to speak in words, not sentences.

Cues

1 What interventions need to be considered now for Janice? What is your priority here?

2 Does this newly diagnosed condition relate to the reason for presentation?

3 What do you think is the reason for this significant deterioration?

CONCEPT MAP 22.9 Evaluation and planning for Janice

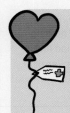

DISCHARGE PLANNING + COORDINATION OF CARE

How do the following areas of healthcare management **relate** to Janice's presentation? Which members of the healthcare team are **involved** in each area of management?

Non-small cell carcinoma/cancer

Medication

Oncology review and planning of care

Follow-up review with thoracic specialist or nurse practitioner – respiratory

Palliative care team if care is not curative

COPD

Medication

Physiotherapy

Occupational therapist to review home setting

Anxiety

Referral to psychologist and potentially psychiatrist, dependent upon patient's response

Patient education and 'coping' techniques

Breathing education and exercises

CONCEPT MAP 22.10 Discharge planning and coordination of care for Janice

SUMMARY

Cancer has a significant impact upon not only patients, but their families, significant others and communities. Cancer is a constant source of ongoing research due to the varying nature of patients presenting with cancer.

Cancer care, while a speciality in nursing, is an aspect you will come across in many departments or wards. For example, in surgical wards you will care for patients who are post-op bowel resections, such as Darby Fuller in the earlier concept maps.

CLINICAL SKILLS IN CANCER CARE

The following clinical skills are required when managing a person with cancer; consult your Clinical Skills resources, such as Tollefson and Hillman (2022), *Clinical Psychomotor Skills* (8th ed.).

PROBLEM-SOLVING SCENARIO

Using a concept map approach, how would you help Deborah Carson?

Deborah Carson is a 38-year-old patient who has returned to the ward (RTW) 30 minutes ago. She has undergone a total right mastectomy. Her post-op vitals are:

- HR 120, BP 90/40 mmHg, T 35.5, centrally and peripherally cool

- Wound – dressing dry and intact
- Drain – one in situ bellovac, has frank blood in chamber
- Pain to site, increasing and described as sharp.
1   With these vital signs and the other information, what are some pathophysiological processes in place that could affect her recovery?
2   What nursing considerations do you have for Deborah?

PORTFOLIO DEVELOPMENT

The useful websites below will assist in meeting continuing professional development activities to meet the NMBA yearly registration requirements for a Registered Nurse.
The Cancer Nurses Society of Australia is a resource for nurses and health professionals looking to develop specialised skills in cancer care and remain current in their practice. It provides ongoing continuing professional development and access to resources.

https://www.cnsa.org.au/about-us/about-us
The *Australian Journal of Cancer Nursing* is the official journal of the Cancer Nurses Society of Australia and contains evidence-based and peer-reviewed literature around cancer care.
https://journals.cambridgemedia.com.au/ajcn

USEFUL WEBSITES

Registered Nurse Standards for Practice
The Registered Nurse Standards for Practice consist of seven crucial standards that all nurses must follow. Download and review the standards at the following link. https://www.nursingmidwiferyboard.gov.au/Codes-Guidelines-Statements/Professional-standards/registered-nurse-standards-for-practice.aspx

Cancer Council Australia
A wealth of information for patients, carers, families and health professionals. https://www.cancer.org.au

The Lung Foundation Australia
A wealth of information for patients as well as healthcare professionals regarding lung cancer. https://lungfoundation.com.au/patients-carers/conditions/lung-cancer/overview
Australia and New Zealand Lung Cancer Nurses Forum (ANZ-LCNF)

'Representing and leading the thoracic oncology nursing community to increase the prominence, recognition and influence of nursing for better patient care.' https://anzlcnf.lungfoundation.com.au

AUSTRALIAN GOVERNMENT – DEPARTMENT OF HEALTH PUBLICATION

Investigating symptoms of lung cancer, a guide for all health professionals

https://www.canceraustralia.gov.au/ISLCguide

REFERENCES AND FURTHER READING

Australian Institute of Health and Welfare (AIHW). (2022). *Cancer data in Australia*. https://www.aihw.gov.au/reports/cancer/cancer-data-in-australia/contents/about

Brown, D., Edwards, H., Buckley, T., Aitken, R. L., Lewis, S. L., Bucher, L., McLean Heitkemper, M., Harding, M. M., Kwong, J., & Roberts, D. (2019). *Lewis's medical-surgical nursing ANZ* (5th ed.). Elsevier.

Craft, J., & Gordon, C. (2019). *Understanding pathophysiology* (3rd ed.). Elsevier Australia.

DeLaune, S., Ladner, P., McTier, L., Tollefson, J., & Lawrence, J. (2024). *Fundamentals of nursing* (3rd ed.). Cengage Learning Australia.

Derrickson, B. H., Burkett, B., Tortora, G. J., Peoples, G., Dye, D., Cooke, J., Diversi, T., McKean, M., Summers, S., Di Pietro, F., Engel, A., Macartney, M., & Green, H. (2021). *Principles of anatomy and physiology* (3rd ed.). Wiley and Son.

Edwards, H., Brown, D., Buckley, T., Aitken, R., & Plowman, E. (2019). *Lewis's medical-surgical nursing* (5th ANZ ed.). Elsevier.

Lung Foundation Australia. (2022). *Overview: lung cancer*. https://lungfoundation.com.au/health-professionals/conditions/lung-cancer/overview/

Rizzo, D. C. (2015). *Fundamentals of anatomy and physiology* (4th ed.). Cengage Learning.

CHAPTER 23

CHRONIC DISEASE MANAGEMENT

Chronic obstructive pulmonary disease (COPD) is a chronic lung disease which is life limiting. The occurrence of COPD among Aboriginal and Torres Strait Islander peoples is nearly five times that of the general population in Australia. One of the main causes of COPD is smoking and the classic symptoms are breathlessness and coughing. Exacerbations in COPD are usually caused by lung infections, and quite often require hospitalisation (Australian Commission on Safety and Quality in Health Care, 2021).

LEARNING OBJECTIVES

After reading this chapter, you should have an understanding of the:

1 assessment required for a person with a chronic condition/s.
2 prioritisation of key components in the development of plans of care for a person with the chronic condition of:
   – heart failure and portal hypertension
   – cancer of the larynx
   – chronic obstructive pulmonary disease (COPD)
3 prioritised and targeted nursing interventions required to promote recovery or prevent further deterioration of people presenting with the chronic conditions of heart failure and portal hypertension, cancer of the larynx, and COPD
4 evaluation phase and how the prioritised and targeted nursing interventions inform further assessment of the person, planning of care and collaboration with the healthcare team
5 discharge planning and coordination of care required in preparing the person for discharge and subsequent continuity of care between the person and their healthcare providers.

INTRODUCTION

Chronic diseases are conditions that have lasted for three months or more and require ongoing health care which impacts on a person's activities of daily living (ADL) and quality of life. Chronic conditions are long lasting and have significant social and economic consequences. Often people with a chronic disease have more than one predominant health condition, two or more chronic conditions are referred to as multimorbidity. In Australia the ten major chronic disease conditions are:

- arthritis
- asthma
- back pain
- cancer
- cardiovascular disease
- chronic obstructive pulmonary disease (COPD)
- diabetes
- chronic kidney disease
- mental health conditions
- osteoporosis.

One in two Australians have one or more of the ten major chronic disease conditions (Australian Institute of Health and Welfare [AIHW], 2022). Respiratory and heart disease and cancer are linked to tobacco use, poor nutrition, physical inactivity and alcohol consumption, and are the focus of this chapter.

23.1 ASSESSMENT OF RESPIRATORY, CARDIOVASCULAR AND ABDOMINAL PROBLEMS

In the collecting of subjective data, previous and current person-reported information is important in the determination of respiratory and cardiovascular symptoms (see **Box 23.1**).

BOX 23.1   SUBJECTIVE ASSESSMENT

- ➤ History of illness
- ➤ Past health history
- ➤ Family history
- ➤ Medications
- ➤ Surgery

Functional health patterns:
- – Health perception and management
- – Nutritional and metabolic
- – Elimination
- – Activity and exercise
- – Sleep and rest
- – Cognitive and perceptual
- – Self perception and concept
- – Role relationship
- – Sexuality and reproductive
- – Coping and stress
- – Values and beliefs
- ➤ Risk calculation

The collection of objective data is informed by the health history data and is highlighted in the physical assessment and diagnostic studies (see **Box 23.2**). In chronic disease management, multiple body systems will be part of the physical assessment, with respiratory, cardiovascular and gastrointestinal body systems being a prominent group.

23.2 ASSESSMENT FOR HEART FAILURE AND PORTAL HYPERTENSION

When undertaking a health assessment for heart failure and portal hypertension, refer to **Box 23.1** and **Box 23.2** for subjective and objective data collection.

Presentation

George Bouzounis is a 71-year-old retired builder that has been admitted to the emergency department (ED) with breathlessness for the last two hours. George has an audible wheeze and is producing frothy sputum. He has a history of hypertension, acute myocardial infarction, worsening heart failure and fatty liver disease.

Concept map 23.1 further explores George's initial care in the emergency department.

23.3 PLANNING CARE FOR HEART FAILURE AND PORTAL HYPERTENSION

Planning for the nursing care for acute heart failure and portal hypertension has the goals of:
- ■ increasing airway patency and oxygenation
- ■ patient education and consent to surgery

BOX 23.2   OBJECTIVE ASSESSMENT

- ➤ Inspect nose and nasal cavity
- ➤ Palpate frontal and maxillary sinuses
- ➤ Respiratory rate
- ➤ Inspection of the thorax
- ➤ Palpation of the thorax
- ➤ Percussion of the thorax
- ➤ Auscultation of the lungs
- ➤ Diagnostic tests – pulse oximetry, sputum, arterial blood gases, chest x-ray, computed tomography, magnetic resonance imaging, pulmonary ventilation-perfusion scan, bronchoscopy, thoracentesis
- ➤ Peripheral vascular system
  - – Vital signs
  - – Inspect skin, hair, venous pattern and oedema
  - – Palpate upper and lower extremities for temperature, moisture, pulses and capillary refill
  - – Auscultation of the arteries

- ➤ Thorax
  - – Inspection of bony structures, heart valves, epigastric area and PMI
  - – Palpation of bony structures, heart valves, epigastric area and PMI
  - – Auscultate heart sounds
  - – Diagnostic tests – cardiac biomarkers, biochemistry, blood glucose measurement, C-reactive protein, full blood count, clotting profile, cardiac natriuretic peptide markers, serum lipids, homocysteine, chest x-ray, electrocardiogram, exercise testing, echocardiogram, nuclear cardiology, cardiovascular magnetic resonance imaging, cardiac computed tomography, cardiac catheterisation
- ➤ Abdomen
  - – Inspection
  - – Auscultation
  - – Percussion
  - – Palpation

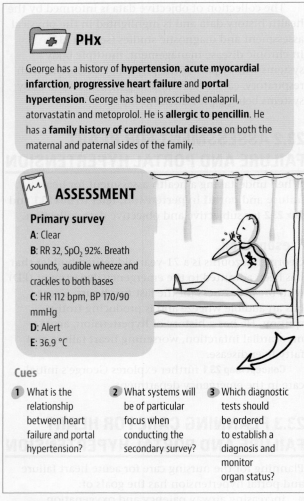

PHx

George has a history of **hypertension**, **acute myocardial infarction**, **progressive heart failure** and **portal hypertension**. George has been prescribed enalapril, atorvastatin and metoprolol. He is **allergic to pencillin**. He has a **family history of cardiovascular disease** on both the maternal and paternal sides of the family.

ASSESSMENT

Primary survey

A: Clear
B: RR 32, SpO₂ 92%. Breath sounds, audible wheeze and crackles to both bases
C: HR 112 bpm, BP 170/90 mmHg
D: Alert
E: 36.9 °C

Cues

1. What is the relationship between heart failure and portal hypertension?

2. What systems will be of particular focus when conducting the secondary survey?

3. Which diagnostic tests should be ordered to establish a diagnosis and monitor organ status?

CONCEPT MAP 23.1 Nursing assessment for George

- self-care in relation to physical activity for the first week
- ensuring a safe home environment and no adverse effects of therapy.

George is a partner in his care plan and contributes to his health care by following his plan of care and managing his condition in the home environment. **Box 23.3** lists the areas that are targeted in the planning stage of acute heart failure and portal hypertension management.

BOX 23.3   PLANNING FOR HEART FAILURE AND PORTAL HYPERTENSION

- Cardiac monitoring
- Daily weight
- Medication
- Blood tests
- Chest x-ray
- Monitor blood pressure and weight gain

- Sodium-restricted diet
- Fowler's position
- Vital signs
- Fluid balance chart
- Medication therapy
- Health education and home care:
  - Lifestyle modifications
  - Self-care
  - Physical activity
  - Medication.

Concept map 23.2 outlines a plan for George's care.

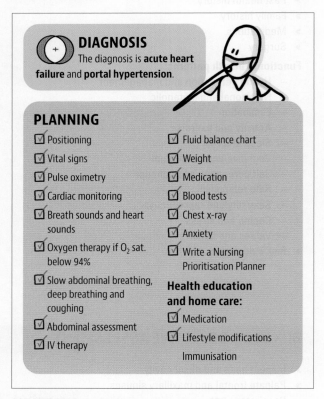

DIAGNOSIS
The diagnosis is **acute heart failure** and **portal hypertension**.

PLANNING

☑ Positioning
☑ Vital signs
☑ Pulse oximetry
☑ Cardiac monitoring
☑ Breath sounds and heart sounds
☑ Oxygen therapy if O₂ sat. below 94%
☑ Slow abdominal breathing, deep breathing and coughing
☑ Abdominal assessment
☑ IV therapy

☑ Fluid balance chart
☑ Weight
☑ Medication
☑ Blood tests
☑ Chest x-ray
☑ Anxiety
☑ Write a Nursing Prioritisation Planner

Health education and home care:

☑ Medication
☑ Lifestyle modifications
   Immunisation

CONCEPT MAP 23.2 Diagnosis and planning for George

23.4 NURSING INTERVENTIONS TO SUPPORT HEALTH CARE FOR HEART FAILURE AND PORTAL HYPERTENSION

Nursing interventions are implemented as part of person-centred care to reduce signs and symptoms and the progression of heart failure and portal hypertension. Medication therapy using various drug groups that are represented, for example by enalapril, atorvastatin, metoprolol, digoxin, frusemide and potassium (Broyles et al., 2023), all have a role in heart failure management.

Concept map 23.3 explores George's journey in the ED, before admission to the cardiac ward.

INTERVENTIONS

1 Positioning – Fowlers

2 Vital signs 4-hourly

3 Pulse oximetry 4-hourly

4 Cardiac monitor for arrhythmia detection

5 Breath and lung sounds assessment 4-hourly

6 Oxygen therapy if O$_2$ sat. below 94%

7 Slow abdominal breathing, deep breathing and coughing

8 IV therapy 0.9% sodium chloride 8/24

9 Fluid balance chart hourly

10 Medication enalapril, atorvastatin, metoprolol, digoxin, frusemide and potassium

11 Low fat and sodium diet

12 Relieve anxiety

13 Abdominal assessment

Health education and home care:

- Medication – enalapril, atorvastatin, metoprolol, digoxin, frusemide and potassium

- Lifestyle modification

What further assessments should be initiated

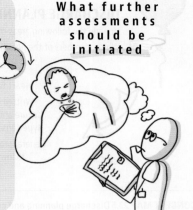

CONCEPT MAP 23.3 Nursing interventions for George

EVIDENCE-BASED PRACTICE

Pulmonary oedema presents as dyspnoea, tachypnoea, severe orthopnoea, large amounts of pink frothy sputum and the person feeling panicked. Report as an emergency.

23.5 EVALUATION OF CARE FOR HEART FAILURE AND PORTAL HYPERTENSION

As part of the further assessment of George's presentation, **Concept map 23.4** asks further questions in relation to George's management.

EVALUATION

George is responding to the treatment protocol for heart failure and portal hypertension in the cardiac ward.

Plan:

George's heart failure and portal hypertension will continue to be monitored and managed.

Cues

1 How is George's fatty liver disease related to portal hypertension?

2 Why does George require digoxin, frusemide and potassium?

3 What is the role of anticoagulants in treating heart failure?

CONCEPT MAP 23.4 Evaluation and planning for George

23.6 DISCHARGE PLANNING AND COORDINATION OF CARE FOR HEART FAILURE AND PORTAL HYPERTENSION

George's heart failure and portal hypertension requires discharge planning and further management at home – see **Concept map 23.5**.

23.7 ASSESSMENT FOR CANCER OF THE LARYNX

Presentation

Chun Wong is a 49-year-old man who has been admitted to the respiratory ward for a laryngectomy and modified neck dissection. He has been a smoker for 25 years and developed hoarseness in the last three months. He has been diagnosed with cancer of the larynx and the cancer lesions are advanced so a total laryngectomy is required, but with a modified neck dissection. After Chun recovers from surgery, he will commence chemotherapy. Chun's wife is with him while you conduct his admission to the ward.

As part of Chun's health assessment, refer to **Box 23.1** and **Box 23.2** assessment areas, with a specific focus on respiratory assessment areas.

Concept map 23.6 further explores Chun's care in the respiratory ward.

23.8 PLANNING CARE FOR CANCER OF THE LARYNX

Planning person-centred care for a person with cancer of the larynx has the goals of:

- oxygenation
- airway clearance
- consent to surgery
- preoperative and postoperative care.

Chun and his wife are partners in his care and contribute by discussing the plan of care and managing his recovery in the home environment. **Box 23.4** lists the areas that are targeted in the planning stage of caring for the person with cancer of the larynx.

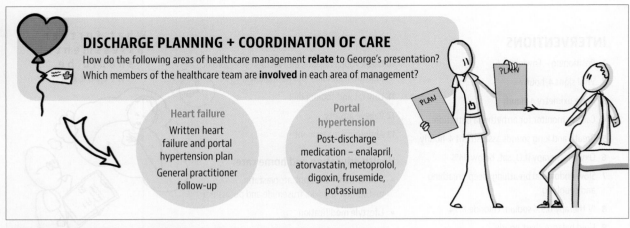

DISCHARGE PLANNING + COORDINATION OF CARE

How do the following areas of healthcare management **relate** to George's presentation? Which members of the healthcare team are **involved** in each area of management?

Heart failure
Written heart failure and portal hypertension plan
General practitioner follow-up

Portal hypertension
Post-discharge medication – enalapril, atorvastatin, metoprolol, digoxin, frusemide, potassium

CONCEPT MAP 23.5 Discharge planning and coordination of care for George

PHx

Chun has enjoyed good health until recently. He has been a smoker for the last 25 years.

ASSESSMENT

Primary survey
A: Patent
B: RR 24
C: Warm
D: Alert
E: T 36.6 °C
F: Voided, nil in
G: BGL 6.7 mmol/L

Secondary survey
CNS: alert and orientated
CVS: BP 145/80 bpm, HR 88 mmHg, T 36.6 °C, peripherally perfused

Resp: Hoarse voice, productive cough, scattered fine crackles at the base of the lungs. RR 24, SpO₂ 97%
GIT: Bowel sounds present with a non-tender abdomen
Renal: Urine concentrated but no abnormalities detected
Metabolic: BGL 6.7 mmol/L
Integumentary: Warm dry skin
Musculoskeletal: Equal limb strength
Chest x-ray to be reviewed.

CONCEPT MAP 23.6 Nursing assessment for Chun

BOX 23.4   PLANNING FOR CANCER OF THE LARYNX

- Preoperative and postoperative care
- Airway maintenance
- Oxygenation
- Surgery
- Pain management
- Diagnostic tests – chest x-ray, arterial blood gases (ABGs), full blood count, liver function, renal function
- Antibiotics

➤ Health education and home care:
- Self-care
- Physical activity
- Medication.

Concept map 23.7 outlines a plan for Chun's care.

DIAGNOSIS
Cancer of the larynx, with admission to the respiratory ward.

PLANNING

☑ Preoperative care
☑ Postoperative care
☑ Positioning
☑ Vital signs
☑ Pulse oximetry
☑ Breath sounds, cough, sputum assessments
☑ Stoma care and suctioning
☑ Oxygen therapy
☑ IV therapy 0.9% sodium chloride
☑ IV benzylpenicillin
☑ IV morphine and paracetamol for pain
☑ Slow abdominal breathing, deep breathing and coughing
☑ Nasogastric tube
☑ Fluid balance chart

☑ Psychosocial care
☑ Speech therapy
☑ Write a Nursing Prioritisation Planner

Health education and home care:

☑ Tracheostomy care
☑ Medication – oral antibiotics and oral paracetamol
☑ Fluids and nutrition

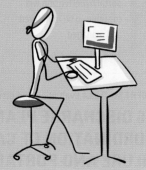

CONCEPT MAP 23.7 Diagnosis and planning for Chun

23.9 NURSING INTERVENTIONS TO SUPPORT HEALTH CARE FOR CANCER OF THE LARYNX

Nursing interventions are implemented as part of person-centred care to prevent the progression of cancer of the larynx.

Concept map 23.8 explores Chun's journey in the respiratory ward, which includes preoperative and postoperative care.

INTERVENTIONS

Preoperative and postoperative care including:

1 Positioning – Fowlers

2 Vital signs – postoperative and then 4 hourly

3 Pulse oximetry 4 hourly

4 Breath sounds, cough, sputum assessments 4 hourly

5 Oxygen therapy – nasal prongs 4 L/min

6 Stoma suctioning hourly

7 Stoma dressing 4 hourly

8 IV therapy 0.9% sodium chloride 8/24

9 Benzylpenicillin 1.2 g QID IV

10 Morphine 1 mg/hr via PCA and paracetamol 1 g QID IV oral for pain

11 Slow abdominal breathing, deep breathing and coughing hourly while awake

12 Nasogastric tube

13 Fluid balance chart

14 Monitor for anxiety and depression

15 Liaise with speech therapy

Health education and home care:

• Tracheostomy care

• Medication – oral antibiotics and paracetamol 1 g prn

• Fluids and nutrition

What further assessments should be initiated

CONCEPT MAP 23.8 Nursing interventions for Chun

23.10 EVALUATION OF CARE FOR CANCER OF THE LARYNX

As part of the further assessment of Chun's presentation, Concept map 23.9 asks further questions in relation to Chun's management.

EVALUATION

Chun had a disturbed sleep as the stoma required frequent suctioning during the night.

Plan:
Consult with the respiratory surgeon today.

Cue

1 Why does Chun have respiratory secretions via the tracheostomy tube?

CONCEPT MAP 23.9 Evaluation and planning for Chun

23.11 DISCHARGE PLANNING AND COORDINATION OF CARE FOR CANCER OF THE LARYNX

The discharge planning for Chun's cancer of the larynx has the foci of further management at home and a follow-up appointment with his general practitioner – see Concept map 23.10. Once his stoma has healed around the tracheostomy tube, chemotherapy will commence.

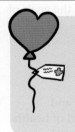

DISCHARGE PLANNING + COORDINATION OF CARE

How do the following areas of healthcare management **relate** to Chun's presentation? Which members of the healthcare team are **involved** in each area of management?

Written home care instructions

Tracheostomy care

Medication

Nutrition

Chemotherapy

CONCEPT MAP 23.10 Discharge planning and coordination of care for Chun

23.12 ASSESSMENT FOR CHRONIC OBSTRUCTIVE PULMONARY DISEASE (COPD)

Presentation

Victor Kostenko, a 71-year-old man, arrives via ambulance to the ED. His wife called for an ambulance as he became short of breath and restless. He has a barrel-shaped chest. He states that his sputum is green and the salbutamol has stopped working.

In the health assessment for Victor, refer to **Box 23.1** and **Box 23.2**, and as he has a known respiratory condition, the respiratory components of the assessment are important.

Concept map 23.11 further explores Victor's initial care in the ED.

 PHx

Victor, a 71-year-old male, is a long-term smoker. He has smoked cigarettes for the last 52 years, and is only smoking occasionally now as he finds it hard to completely give up smoking. Recently he has noticed that he has a cough mainly in the morning. While working in his shed he sometimes has to sit down and catch his breath. He has noticed that he has lost weight especially around his waistline. His GP diagnosed emphysema 12 months ago, and prescribed salbutamol.

 ASSESSMENT

Primary survey
A: Clear
B: RR 28, accessory muscle use, breath sounds diminished with widespread crackles, percussion hyper-resonant
C: HR 118 bpm, BP 162/88 mmHg. Breath sounds diminished, O_2 sat 92%
D: Alert and orientated
E: 37.9 °C

Secondary survey significant findings:
Chest x-ray reveals flat low diaphragm with lung hyperinflation

Pulmonary function tests show decreased tidal volume and vital capacity
Increased total lung capacity
Prolonged forced expiratory volume
Arterial blood gas reveals compensated chronic respiratory alkalosis – pH 7.26, PaO_2 79, $PaCO_2$ 57, HCO_3 – 27, O_2 sat 90%
Increased RBC and WBC count

CONCEPT MAP 23.11 Nursing assessment for Victor

23.13 PLANNING CARE FOR COPD

The planning of person-centred nursing care for the patient with life-limiting COPD will have the goals of:
- relieving breathlessness
- reversing lung infection
- minimising airway obstruction
- slowing the progression of the disease
- promoting quality of life.

Slowing the progression of the disease and promoting quality of life are particular foci of health education for the home environment. **Box 23.5** indicates the areas that are targeted in the planning stage for relieving an acute exacerbation of COPD.

BOX 23.5   PLANNING CARE FOR COPD

➤ Relieving symptoms
➤ Tests
➤ Medication
➤ Health education and home care

Concept map 23.12 outlines a plan for Victor's care.

REFLECTIVE PRACTICE

In COPD $PaCO_2$ is chronically elevated due to desensitised medullary chemoreceptors, which means breathing is driven by hypoxic stimulation of the peripheral chemoreceptors. With COPD being exacerbated, oxygen levels are very low and supplemental oxygen therapy is required. Increasing oxygen levels means that hypoxic stimulus to breathe is reduced. This in turn reduces the respiratory rate, increases $PaCO_2$ and may produce a respiratory arrest. Supplemental oxygen therapy is ideally low flow at 2–3 L/min via nasal prongs or 24–28% via an oxygen mask.

23.14 NURSING INTERVENTIONS TO SUPPORT HEALTH CARE FOR COPD

Nursing interventions are implemented as part of person-centred care, and to slow the progression of

DIAGNOSIS

Emphysema. In short stay unit attached to the emergency department until respiratory ward bed available.

PLANNING

- ☑ Positioning
- ☑ Oxygen
- ☑ Vital signs
- ☑ Pulse oximetry
- ☑ Salbutamol 5 mg nebulised
- ☑ Prednisolone 40 mg oral daily
- ☑ Ceftriaxone 1 g daily IV
- ☑ Roxithromycin 300 mg daily oral
- ☑ Huffing
- ☑ Percussion and postural drainage every 8 hours
- ☑ Pursed lip breathing and abdominal breathing hourly
- ☑ Breath sounds
- ☑ Tests – Arterial blood gases and sputum
- ☑ Fluid balance chart
- ☑ Weigh daily
- ☑ Increasing mobility
- ☑ Family coping
- ☑ Write a Nursing Prioritisation Planner

CONCEPT MAP 23.12 Diagnosis and planning for Victor

COPD. Medication therapy using a bronchodilator, steroid and antibiotics (Broyles et al., 2023) are essential components of care.

Concept map 23.13 explores Victor's journey in the ED and the attached short stay unit before transfer to the respiratory ward.

23.15 EVALUATION OF CARE FOR COPD

As part of the further assessment of Victor's presentation, **Concept map 23.14** asks further questions in relation to the support of Victor.

23.16 DISCHARGE PLANNING AND COORDINATION OF CARE FOR COPD

Victor and his wife are central in developing discharge planning and further coordination of care in the home environment, as Victor's COPD is a chronic condition that will require an increasing level of care in the future – see **Concept map 23.15**.

INTERVENTIONS

1. Positioning: high Fowlers
2. Oxygen 2 L/min nasal prongs
3. Vital signs hourly
4. Pulse oximetry hourly
5. 5 mg salbutamol nebulised, reassessed at 20 minutes then hourly
6. Prednisolone 40 mg daily oral for 5 days
7. Ceftriaxone 1 g daily IV for 7 days
8. Roxithromycin 300 mg daily oral for 10 days
9. Huffing
10. Percussion and postural drainage every 8 hours
11. Pursed lip breathing and abdominal breathing hourly while awake
12. Breath sounds 8 hourly
13. Tests – arterial blood gases and sputum as needed
14. Fluid balance chart
15. Weigh daily
16. Increasing mobility
17. Family coping

What further assessments should be initiated

CONCEPT MAP 23.13 Nursing interventions for Victor

EVALUATION

Victor's response to therapy was noted by decreased breathlessness, decreased work of breathing and improved oxygen saturation.

Plan:
Transfer to the respiratory ward when a bed becomes available.

Cue

1. What additional information can be given to Victor and his wife to provide health education while in the short stay unit to prepare them for transfer to the respiratory ward and then discharge to the home environment?

CONCEPT MAP 23.14 Evaluation and planning for Victor

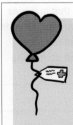

DISCHARGE PLANNING + COORDINATION OF CARE

How do the following areas of healthcare management **relate** to Victor's presentation? Which members of the healthcare team are **involved** in each area of management?

Medication – salbutamol puffer

Nutrition and hydration

Prevention – reduce respiratory tract infections, activity strengthening and respiratory hygiene

CONCEPT MAP 23.15 Discharge planning and coordination of care for Victor

SUMMARY

Chronic disease management is a challenging but rewarding component of providing person-centred nursing care. The focus of chronic disease management is a multidisciplinary approach to empower the individual to manage their chronic condition/s in the home environment. With the provision of a health management plan, including a healthy lifestyle, medication and carer support, the multidisciplinary team can assist the individual to maintain independence as much as possible with activities of daily living, and maintain the best possible quality of life while living with a chronic condition/s.

CLINICAL SKILLS IN RESPIRATORY, CARDIOVASCULAR AND LIVER HEALTH

The following clinical skills are required when managing a person with chronic disease; consult your Clinical Skills resources, such as Tollefson and Hillman (2022), *Clinical Psychomotor Skills* (8th ed.).

- Temperature, pulse and respiration
- Blood pressure
- Pulse oximetry
- Pain assessment
- Height, weight and waist circumference measurements
- Blood glucose measurement
- Focused respiratory health history and physical assessment
- Focused cardiovascular health history and physical assessment
- Focused gastrointestinal health history and abdominal physical assessment
- Preoperative care
- Postoperative care
- 12-lead electrocardiogram
- Inhaled medication
- Oral medication
- Intravenous medication
- Oxygen therapy via nasal cannula or various masks
- Oropharyngeal and nasopharyngeal suctioning
- Artificial airway suctioning
- Tracheostomy care
- Nasogastric tube insertion

PROBLEM-SOLVING SCENARIO

Using a concept map approach, how would you assist Clive Millman?

Clive Millman is a 72-year-old man. He has a history of smoking for 30 years which he gave up 12 years ago, when he was diagnosed with hypertension and hypercholesterolaemia by his general practitioner. Clive has developed a niggling pain near his umbilicus and he can feel his 'belly button beat'. As Clive's general practitioner is sick with COVID-19, Clive has come to the ED for care. An abdominal ultrasound reveals an **abdominal aortic aneurysm** (AAA). The size of the aneurysm is 5.4 cm and just below the threshold size for surgical repair.

1   What are the risk factors for an AAA?
2   What are the associated signs and symptoms of an AAA?
3   What is the management of an AAA in the community?
4   When should an AAA be surgically repaired?
5   What is the postoperative management for an AAA repair?

PORTFOLIO DEVELOPMENT

Wherever you practise nursing, you will need ongoing continuing professional development to ensure that you are delivering current evidence-based nursing care that provides the best possible outcomes for the patient. As care for patients with chronic disease is based on evidence-based practice and ongoing clinical-based research, engaging in continuing professional development activities will enable the nurse to provide contemporary healthcare practice for patients with chronic conditions.

The useful websites below will assist in meeting continuing professional development activities to meet the NMBA yearly registration requirements for a Registered Nurse.

USEFUL WEBSITES

Cardiac Society of Australia and New Zealand https://www.csanz.edu.au/for-professionals/position-statements-and-practice-guidelines

Heart Foundation https://www.heartfoundation.org.au

Lung Foundation Australia https://lungfoundation.com.au/about/who-we-are

The Thoracic Society of Australia and New Zealand https://www.thoracic.org.au/about-us/about-us

Nursing and Midwifery Board of Australia, Decision-making framework for nursing and midwifery (2020) https://www.nursingmidwiferyboard.gov.au/codes-guidelines-statements/frameworks.aspx

REFERENCES AND FURTHER READING

Amakali, K. (2015). Clinical care for the patient with heart failure: A nursing care perspective. *Cardiovascular Pharmacology Open Access*, *4*(2). 5 pages. DOI: 10.4172/2329-6607.1000142

Australian Commission on Safety and Quality in Health Care. (2021). *2.1 Chronic obstructive pulmonary disease (COPD)*. https://www.safetyandquality. gov.au/our-work/healthcare-variation/ fourth-atlas-2021/chronic-disease- and-infection-potentially-preventable- hospitalisations/21-chronic-obstructive- pulmonary-disease-copd

Australian Institute of Health and Welfare (AIHW). (2022). *Chronic disease*. https:// www.aihw.gov.au/reports-data/health- conditions-disability-deaths/chronic- disease/overview

Awoke, M., Baptiste, D-L., Davidson, P., Roberts, A., & Dennison-Himmelfarb, C. (2019). A quasi-experimental study examining a nurse-led education program to improve knowledge, self-care, and reduce readmission for individuals with heart failure. *Contemporary Nurse*, *55*(1),

15–26. https://doi.org/10.1080/10376178. 2019.1568198

Billington, J., & Luckett, A. (2019). Care of the critically ill patient with a tracheostomy. *Nursing Standard*, *34*(9), 59–65. DOI: 10.7748/ns.2018.e11297

Broyles, B., Reiss, B., Evans, M., Pleunik, S., Page, R., & Badoer, E. (2023). *Pharmacology in nursing* (4th ANZ ed.). Cengage Learning Australia.

DeLaune, S., Ladner, P., McTier, L., Tollefson, J., & Lawrence, J. (2024). *Fundamentals of nursing* (3rd ed.). Cengage Learning Australia.

Heo, S., Moser, D., Lennie, T., Grudnowski, S., Kim, J. S., & Turrise, S. (2019). Patients' beliefs about causes and consequences of heart failure symptoms. *Western Journal of Nursing Research*, *41*(11), 1623–1641. DOI: 10.1177/0193945918823786

Hodson, M., & Sherrington, R. (2014). Treating patients with chronic obstructive pulmonary disease. *Nursing Standard*, *29*(9), 50–58. DOI: 10.7748/ns.29.9.50.e9061

Mechler, K., & Liantonio, J. (2019). Palliative care approach to chronic diseases.

Primary Care: Clinics in Office Practice, *46*(3), 415–432.

Moller, S., & Bendsten, F. (2018). The pathophysiology of arterial vasodilatation and hyperdynamic circulation in cirrhosis. *Liver International*, *38*(4), 570–580. https:// doi/epdf/10.1111/liv.13589

Neighbors, M., & Tannehill-Jones, R. (2023). *Human diseases* (6th ed.). Cengage.

Pettersson, M., & Bergbom, I. (2019). Life is about so much more: Patients' experiences of health, well-being, and recovery after operation of abdominal aortic aneurysm with open and endovascular treatment – A prospective study. *Journal of Vascular Nursing*, *37*(3), 160–168. https://doi.org/ 10.1016/j.jvn.2019.06.002

Riley, J. (2015). The key roles for the nurse in acute heart failure management. *Cardiac Failure Review*, *1*(2), 123–127. DOI: 10.15420/cfr.2015.1.2.123

Schreiber, M. (2018). Abdominal aortic aneurysm. *Medsurg Nursing*, *27*(4), 254–256.

Tollefson, J., & Hillman, E. (2022). *Clinical psychomotor skills: Assessment tools for nurses* (8th ed.). Cengage Learning Australia.

CHAPTER 24

PRIMARY HEALTH CARE

Primary health care is the 'entry level' into the health system within Australia and is usually a person's first experience or encounter with the healthcare system. Primary health care includes a broad range of services which range from health promotion and prevention to treatment and management of chronic conditions. Statistics from the Australian Institute of Health and Welfare show that:

- more than 33 per cent of Australians visit a general practitioner (GP) 2–3 times per year, and 12 per cent saw their GP 12 times or more in 2018
- there were 158 million GP attendances in 2018–2019
- there was A$66.9 billion spent on primary health care in 2019–2020 (33.1% of the health budget).

As you can see, primary health care makes up a very large part of all health care encounters (Australian Institute of Health and Welfare [AIHW], 2016, 2022b).

LEARNING OBJECTIVES

After reading this chapter, you should have an understanding of the:

1. primary healthcare services that are available in Australia
2. prioritisation of key components in the development of a plan of care
3. prioritised and targeted nursing interventions required to promote recovery and ongoing care provision
4. evaluation phase and how the prioritised and targeted nursing interventions inform further assessment, planning and collaboration with the healthcare team
5. discharge planning and subsequent continuity of care between the person and their healthcare providers.

INTRODUCTION

Primary health care is essentially 'the first step' in a patient's care and it is practised commonly in nursing and allied health. Primary health care is focused on health promotion, illness prevention, care of the sick, advocacy and community development.

A dynamic improvement in health and life expectancy has occurred in the last century – notably due to advances in medical research and in living conditions. The World Health Organization (WHO) embarked upon 'health for all by the year 2000' to address the issues of inequality within healthcare systems. The WHO Declaration of Alma-Ata in 1978 called for:

- equity
- fundamental human rights
- community participation and maximal community self-reliance
- use of socially acceptable technology
- health promotion and disease prevention
- involvement of government departments other than health departments
- political action
- cooperation between countries
- reduction of money spent on armaments (the process of preparing for war), to increase funds for 'Primary Health Care'
- world peace (Edwards et al., 2019).

These principles from the WHO declaration underpin what is known today as 'primary health care' (WHO, 2021). Primary health care 'focuses on social justice, equity, community participation, socially acceptable and affordable technology, the provision of services on the basis of the needs of the population, health education and work to improve the root causes of ill-health' (DeLaune et al., 2024). Primary care is focused on working with people to enable them to make their own decisions about their healthcare needs. It provides means and educational resources to enable the person to better care for themselves (Edwards et al., 2019).

Primary health care is practised in all aspects of nursing. The phrase 'discharge planning begins on admission' addresses many components of primary health care as within the hospital system most patients will require ongoing treatment or follow-up after discharge. This is where primary health care comes into the patient's holistic and person-centred care requirements.

24.1 PRIMARY HEALTHCARE SERVICES

Primary health care is an ever-changing field within Australia – and is particularly relevant in health care in rural and regional areas. Primary health care is incredibly diverse in its application, mostly due to the very geographical constraints that makes up Australia. Primary health care is based upon demand and need; and this is continuing to change due to many factors such as:

- The ageing population
- Chronic disease management
- Increase in kidney dialysis requirements of Australians
- Availability of mental health resources
- Dementia
- Access to services and specialists' clinics for all Australians.

Think about how many community-based healthcare teams there are in your local area (available services may differ in rural or remote areas); however, primary health care looks at ensuring healthcare needs are met for every Australian, regardless of their postcode (AIHW, 2022a).

As with all healthcare concerns in any country, cost is a driving factor. The cost of hospitalisation far outweighs the cost of a patient being reviewed by their GP and practice nurse. Primary health care aims to keep people out of hospital and managed in the community for treatments that can be arranged elsewhere or as an outpatient. For example, regular screening for cardiovascular disease by GPs establishes care for raised cholesterol levels, rather than waiting for the patient to have an ischaemic event. Primary health care aims to *manage and prevent* rather than *cure*. Primary health care is about making sure everyone has access to health and

medical facilities to manage their health conditions, and to perform screening and testing to ensure health and wellbeing (AIHW, 2016, 2020).

Stratification or management of risk factors is undertaken in primary health care. Often, in rurally isolated areas, the management will be provided by the GP. Risk factor management or intervention is undertaken by different healthcare professionals, dependent upon where the patient is geographically within Australia. Nursing intervention/s can come

SAFETY IN NURSING ⚠

PATIENT SAFETY IN PRIMARY HEALTH CARE

The Australian Commission on Safety and Quality in Health Care (2015) established a comprehensive literature review to ascertain potential gaps in healthcare delivery in primary health.

From this report, three factors were identified as associated with an increase in patient safety risks:

1 older age, more co-morbidities, and more frequent emergency department visits

2 diagnostic errors have been commonly associated with moderate to severe health outcomes

3 lack of consistent medical record storage (electronic vs paper based).

The findings of this significant study indicated that although there are many deficits, there are far more strengths in our existing system. The report also highlights that early warning systems, or incident management systems, are a key factor in establishing safety for all patients. The report can be accessed here: https://www.safetyandquality.gov.au/sites/default/files/migrated/Patient-safety-in-primary-healthcare-a-review-of-the-literature-August-2015.pdf from community nursing teams or from practice or outpatient clinics or departments. Emergency department presentations can also refer and aim to minimise risk factors through effective treatment and, perhaps more importantly, ongoing management (AIHW, 2019; Australian Government, 2021).

24.2 DEVELOPING A PLAN OF CARE

With any chronic condition a very large component of nursing care is monitoring the patient's progress or deterioration. For example, if a patient has a clinic visit or calls from their home to report dizziness, increased fatigue or foul breath – these are all side effects or complications of chronic kidney disease (CKD) which is one of the most commonly managed conditions in the primary healthcare arena in Australia. A primary healthcare team will be made up of a variety of healthcare professionals, depending on the specifics of the location and the patient's requirements. As part of a primary healthcare team, your role is to report findings or significant changes to a patient's status to healthcare team members.

Documentation of health status is essential as this is vital information concerning your patient – imagine not documenting observations after you performed them? While reporting seems logical, it becomes even more crucial in primary health care as multiple healthcare professionals will be involved in the patient's care. A person cannot *not* communicate! Communication in nursing, as you would be aware, is an essential and integral component of our daily roles. The way in which we communicate depends greatly on our life experiences, our understanding of the message being conveyed, and countless other factors (DeLaune et al., 2024; Edwards et al., 2019).

Communication with not only our patient and their family, but members of the multidisciplinary healthcare team, is the quintessential component in the whole mechanism of ongoing care, health promotion and wellness – and hence monitoring of health status in primary health care. If we do not address our patient's concerns and refer them to appropriate members of the multidisciplinary healthcare team, the patient will not be receiving holistic person-centred care.

Finally, a component of primary health care based on holistic nursing care, is to ensure that patients have access to

- accommodation (if required for appointments; e.g. rural patients)
- transport to and from appointments
- family support, if available
- Centrelink or social security payments (you may need to access a social worker)
- review of home environment; i.e. Does the patient require home help? How are they coping with activities of daily living (ADLs)?

EVIDENCE-BASED PRACTICE

Primary health care – chronic disease management

The Queensland Government – Office of Rural and Remote Health Clinical Support Unit have managed the ongoing evidence-based practice requirements of primary health care through the development of the *Primary Clinical Care Manual* (now in its 11th edition, 2022) that provides management and treatment flowcharts for use across Australia. It is the principal clinical reference in rural, remote and isolated practices throughout Queensland, Victoria and the Australian Defence Force.

The manual is free to access and can be found here: https://www.health.qld.gov.au/rrcsu/clinical-manuals/ primary-clinical-care-manual-pccm

- grocery/shopping needs and associated social needs
- religious input, if appropriate
- translation or interpreter services
- ongoing counselling or psychological support, if required
- review of pathology and explanation of results
- identification of further complications of their health; for example, side effects from medications, progression of disease, etc.
- vaccination status.

24.3 NURSING INTERVENTIONS

To 'recap', all nursing interventions across the scope of this text start with effective and adequate care management involving:

- interpersonal skills
- communication skills
- assessment skills
- documentation skills.

We have already attested that each and every patient is unique, and likewise for their chronic disease/s progression, or recovery from illness, injury or trauma. In order to provide holistic patient care and excellent education and healthcare provision, we need to utilise the myriad healthcare professionals at our disposal. Social workers, community nurses, wound care specialists, psychologists, psychiatrists, dieticians, physiotherapists, doctors and our nursing colleagues – all have different exposure and experience in healthcare delivery.

Regardless of the patient's needs, the nursing process of primary survey and rapid assessment is always going to be required when someone is unwell or requires escalation in primary health care. **Figure 24.1** shows an example of rapid assessment and escalation guidelines from the *Primary Clinical Care Manual* of Queensland Health.

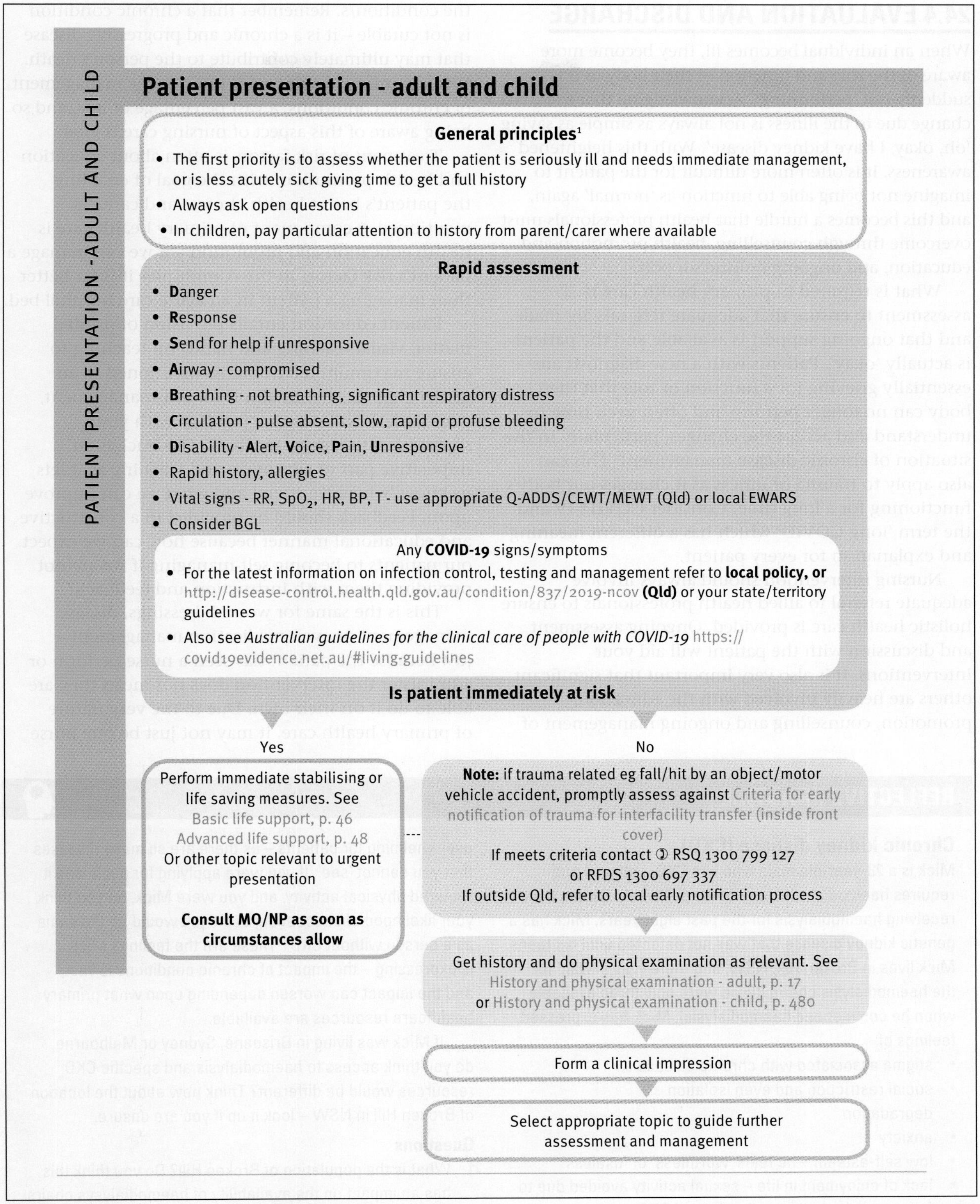

PATIENT PRESENTATION - ADULT AND CHILD

Patient presentation - adult and child

General principles[1]

- The first priority is to assess whether the patient is seriously ill and needs immediate management, or is less acutely sick giving time to get a full history
- Always ask open questions
- In children, pay particular attention to history from parent/carer where available

Rapid assessment

- **D**anger
- **R**esponse
- **S**end for help if unresponsive
- **A**irway - compromised
- **B**reathing - not breathing, significant respiratory distress
- **C**irculation - pulse absent, slow, rapid or profuse bleeding
- **D**isability - **A**lert, **V**oice, **P**ain, **U**nresponsive
- Rapid history, allergies
- Vital signs - RR, SpO$_2$, HR, BP, T - use appropriate Q-ADDS/CEWT/MEWT (Qld) or local EWARS
- Consider BGL

Any **COVID-19** signs/symptoms

- For the latest information on infection control, testing and management refer to **local policy, or** http://disease-control.health.qld.gov.au/condition/837/2019-ncov **(Qld)** or your state/territory guidelines
- Also see *Australian guidelines for the clinical care of people with COVID-19* https://covid19evidence.net.au/#living-guidelines

Is patient immediately at risk

Yes

Perform immediate stabilising or life saving measures. See
Basic life support, p. 46
Advanced life support, p. 48
Or other topic relevant to urgent presentation

Consult MO/NP as soon as circumstances allow

No

Note: if trauma related eg fall/hit by an object/motor vehicle accident, promptly assess against Criteria for early notification of trauma for interfacility transfer (inside front cover)
If meets criteria contact ☏ RSQ 1300 799 127
or RFDS 1300 697 337
If outside Qld, refer to local early notification process

Get history and do physical examination as relevant. See
History and physical examination - adult, p. 17
or History and physical examination - child, p. 480

Form a clinical impression

Select appropriate topic to guide further assessment and management

FIGURE 24.1 Patient presentation and rapid assessment

SOURCE: STATE OF QUEENSLAND (QUEENSLAND HEALTH)

24.4 EVALUATION AND DISCHARGE

When an individual becomes ill, they become more aware of the role and function of their body as it is suddenly not 'performing'. Acknowledging that there is a change due to the illness is not always as simple as saying 'oh, okay, I have kidney disease'. With this heightened awareness, it is often more difficult for the patient to imagine not being able to function as 'normal' again, and this becomes a hurdle that health professionals must overcome through counselling, health promotion and education, and ongoing holistic support.

What is required in primary health care is assessment to ensure that adequate referrals are made, and that ongoing support is available and the patient is actually 'okay'. Patients with a new diagnosis are essentially grieving for a function or role that their body can no longer perform and often need time to understand and accept the changes, particularly in the situation of chronic disease management. This can also apply to trauma or illness as it changes our body's functioning for a long time. Consider COVID-19 and the term 'long COVID' which has a different meaning and explanation for every patient.

Nursing intervention should always involve adequate referral to allied health professionals to ensure holistic health care is provided. Ongoing assessment and discussion with the patient will aid your interventions. It is also very important that significant others are heavily involved with the education, promotion, counselling and ongoing management of

the condition/s. Remember that a chronic condition is not curable – it is a chronic and progressive disease that may ultimately contribute to the person's death. While primary health care is not just the management of chronic conditions, a vast percentage of it is, and so being aware of this aspect of nursing care is vital.

Treatment of risk factors is often about education and health promotion, with the goal of enabling the patient's better health choices and care. As mentioned, a component of primary health care is health education and promotion – if we can manage a patient's risk factors in the community it is far better than managing a patient in an acute care hospital bed.

Patient education entails provision of printed matter, visual teaching and hands-on teaching to ensure maximum retention. As mentioned in an earlier chapter, if your aim is for self-management, your patient will need to 'practise' with your supervision to receive feedback. Feedback is an imperative part of education and teaching as it lets us know 'where we stand' and what we can improve upon. Feedback should be provided in a constructive and educational manner because how can we expect our patients to become self-managing if we are not providing them with instruction and feedback?

This is the same for wound dressings, disease management or even medication management – just because the patient has seen a nurse perform or administer the intervention does not mean they are able to do it on their own. Due to the very nature of primary health care, it may not just be one nurse

REFLECTIVE PRACTICE

Chronic kidney disease (CKD)

Mick is a 28-year-old male who has CKD – stage 4 and requires haemodialysis three times per week. He has been receiving haemodialysis for the past eight years. Mick has a genetic kidney disease that was not detected until his teens. Mick lives in Broken Hill, NSW, and there was a 'wait' for the haemodialysis chairs (there were only three available when he commenced haemodialysis). Mick has expressed feelings of:

- stigma associated with chronic disease
- social restriction and even isolation
- degradation
- anxiety
- low self-esteem – he feels 'worthless' or 'useless'
- lack of enjoyment in life – sexual activity avoided due to fatigue, and other complications of CKD
- loss of control.

Chronic disease is a different experience for every person. Stigma around chronic conditions can be

overwhelming for patients – as there are so many diseases that you cannot 'see'. If you were applying for a job, and it required physical activity, and you were Mick, do you think your likelihood of succeeding in the job would be the same as a person without CKD? These are the feelings Mick is expressing – the impact of chronic conditions is vast, and the impact can worsen depending upon what primary healthcare resources are available.

If Mick was living in Brisbane, Sydney or Melbourne, do you think access to haemodialysis and specific CKD resources would be different? Think now about the location of Broken Hill in NSW – look it up if you are unsure.

Questions

1   What is the population of Broken Hill? Do you think this has an impact on the availability of haemodialysys chairs for treatment?
2   With respect to Mick's feelings, what could you do if you were evaluating his care? What would the role of the primary healthcare nurse be here?

providing the ongoing education and teaching to the patient. Therefore, it is incredibly important to document your teaching and the patient's response.

Regardless of where your patient lives and what services they can access, they will be able to make informed health decisions and direct their own health care if given the appropriate information. It is important to remember that the multidisciplinary healthcare team approach is not severed upon discharge, but essentially strengthened.

SUMMARY

Primary health care is care that is not related to a hospital visit. It includes health promotion, health prevention, early intervention, treatment of acute conditions and chronic disease management.

Primary health care is generally delivered in community centres, general practices, allied health practices and via telehealth facilities (such as Zoom, Skype, etc.). The healthcare professionals who make up primary health care are:
- nurses
- general practitioners
- nurse practitioners
- midwives
- allied health professionals
- pharmacists
- dentists
- Aboriginal and Torres Strait Islander health practitioners.

Around 35 per cent of the total health expenditure is for primary health care; in comparison, hospitals receive approximately 39 per cent of health expenditure funding (AIHW, 2016).

CRITICAL THINKING QUESTIONS

1 What are the national priority areas for health within Australia? How do they relate to primary health care?

2 How has primary health care expanded its role due to COVID-19?

PORTFOLIO DEVELOPMENT

A good starting point for developing your professional portfolio in primary health care is this AIHW link: https://www.aihw.gov.au/reports-data/health-welfare-services/primary-health-care/overview.

This website outlines the current primary healthcare goals and looks at the development of primary health care and patient needs. The Australian Government also has Primary Health Networks (PHN's) contacts for each state within Australia at: https://www.health.gov.au/initiatives-and-programs/phn/contacts.

USEFUL WEBSITES

Registered Nurse Standards for Practice
The Registered Nurse Standards for Practice consist of seven crucial standards that all nurses must follow. Download and review the standards at the following link. https://www.nursingmidwiferyboard.gov.au/Codes-Guidelines-Statements/Professional-standards/registered-nurse-standards-for-practice.aspx

Australian Primary Health Care Nurses Association (APNA)
The APNA is the peak professional body for nurses working in primary health care. https://www.apna.asn.au

Primary Health Care – Australian Medical Association
The AMA provides a position statement on the role of general practice for the delivery of primary health services in Australia. https://www.ama.com.au/articles/primary-health-care-2021

Primary Care
The Department of Health and Aged Care has an overview for consumers and health professionals regarding primary health care within Australia. https://www1.health.gov.au/internet/main/publishing.nsf/Content/primarycare

REFERENCES AND FURTHER READING

Australian Commission on Safety and Quality in Health Care. (2015). *Patient safety in primary healthcare*. https://www.safetyandquality.gov.au/sites/default/files/migrated/Patient-safety-in-primary-healthcare-a-review-of-the-literature-August-2015.pdf

Australian Government. (2021). *About Medicare*. https://www.servicesaustralia.gov.au/about-medicare?context=60092

Australian Institute of Health and Welfare (AIHW). (2016). *Primary health care in Australia*. https://www.aihw.gov.au/reports/primary-health-care/primary-health-care-in-australia/contents/about-primary-health-care

Australian Institute of Health and Welfare (AIHW). (2019). *Rural and remote health*. https://www.aihw.gov.au/reports/rural-remote-australians/rural-remote-health/contents/summary

Australian Institute of Health and Welfare (AIHW). (2020). *Rural and remote health*. https://www.aihw.gov.au/reports/australias-health/rural-and-remote-health

Australian Institute of Health and Welfare (AIHW). (2022a). *Health expenditure*. https://www.aihw.gov.au/reports/health-welfare-expenditure/health-expenditure

Australian Institute of Health and Welfare (AIHW). (2022b). *Primary health care*: Overview. https://www.aihw.gov.au/reports-data/health-welfare-services/primary-health-care/overview

DeLaune, S., Ladner, P., McTier, L., Tollefson, J., & Lawrence, J. (2024). *Fundamentals of nursing* (3rd ed.). Cengage Learning Australia.

Edwards, H., Brown, D., Buckley, T., Aitken, R., & Plowman, E. (2019). *Lewis's medical-surgical nursing* (5th ANZ ed.). Elsevier.

Queensland Health. (2022). *Primary clinical care manual (11th ed.)*. www.health.qld.gov.au/orrh/clinical-manuals/primary-clinical-care-manual-pccm/view-current-edition

World Health Organization (WHO). (2021). *Universal health coverage (UHC)*. https://www.who.int/news-room/fact-sheets/detail/universal-health-coverage-(uhc)

CHAPTER 25

RURAL AND REMOTE HEALTH CARE

Twenty-eight per cent of the Australian population live in areas that are classified as rural or remote. These Australians face many challenges when accessing medical services and often have poorer health outcomes compared to people living in metropolitan and regional areas. Data demonstrates that those living in rural and remote areas have significantly higher rates of deaths, injury, hospitalisations and have poorer access to health and primary healthcare services.

There are five classes of relative remoteness that define 'rural and remote':
1. major cities
2. inner regional
3. outer regional
4. remote
5. very remote.

There are other significant barriers to social services such as education, employment and housing for those who live in rural and remote areas (Australian Institute of Health and Welfare [AIHW], 2022).

The healthcare needs of this large population of Australians are as diverse as their locations.

LEARNING OBJECTIVES

After reading this chapter, you should have an understanding of the:
1. rural and remote healthcare services in Australia
2. prioritisation of key components in the development of a plan of care
3. prioritised and targeted nursing interventions required to promote recovery and ongoing care provision
4. evaluation phase and how the prioritised and targeted nursing interventions inform further assessment, planning and collaboration with the healthcare team
5. discharge planning and coordination of care, including patient education and management.

INTRODUCTION

Australia is a highly urbanised society with around 70 per cent of our population living in capital cities or major cities. The remaining population live in either regional cities or large country towns and remote areas (AIHW, 2022).

There are many ways to describe rural and remote areas: 'isolated', 'the country', 'the bush' or 'the outback'. No matter the term, it is evident that rural or remote towns do not have all the facilities that a city or regional centre does. Hospitals are smaller or are deemed as multipurpose clinics with only a small number of acute care beds and an emergency department that is only open during office hours. These towns or villages are generally supported by the Royal Flying Doctor Service or the Air Ambulance service of the state or territory.

The role of the nurse is often extended within the rural or remote setting as there is often limited or no medical cover. With this in mind, many states and territories have provided guidelines for nursing staff to utilise in emergency care.

Rural health funding is constantly evolving to meet the ever-changing needs of rural Australians. Rural health focuses on primary health care and health promotion as both an interventional form of health care and a positive and empowering message. A large number of rural Australians access health care through their general practitioners (GPs) and rely on referrals from their GPs for ongoing health care and management. Most rural GP clinics have practice nurses who will discuss medical management and health promotion with patients in an attempt to prevent the consequences of chronic illness or disease.

25.1 RURAL AND REMOTE HEALTHCARE SERVICES

When patients present to hospital they are often confronted with a multitude of nurses, doctors, allied health professionals and auxiliary staff. Patients and their families may not know 'who does what' and are often too afraid to ask questions since they are not sure 'who' to ask. In rural and remote health care, this is often far from the case, with reduced staffing, accessibility of services and resources (Edwards et al., 2019).

Multidisciplinary care is an integrated team approach to health care for patients, where medical, nursing and allied healthcare professionals consider all aspects of patient care and collaboratively design an individual care plan for each patient. Therefore, an essential skill in multidisciplinary care is effective communication.

Multidisciplinary care encompasses:

- a shared, collaborative and group decision-making approach
- a focus on continuity of care
- development of pathways and protocols for treatment and care
- development of appropriate referral networks, including appropriate referral pathways to meet psychosocial needs
- development of team protocols and guidance.

Access to health care is an important factor in the health and wellbeing of Australians. If you lived 500 km from an orthopaedic surgeon, how do you think this would impact your treatment? How difficult do you think it would be to organise your family and your treatment if you had to leave home and travel this distance? This is a very real situation for Australians living in rural and remote areas. Many rural hospitals provide some surgical intervention but do not have facilities to perform orthopaedic surgery. The patient must then be transferred to a facility that can perform the surgery and that means they will need to find their own way home at their own expense, then organise their family and life again for any subsequent follow-up.

It would be a large task to identify all the different types of services within Australian rural health. Each town or settlement has different facilities. Within the realm of rural and remote health care, often the communities themselves strive to achieve access to what they require. For example, if a town has a large population of diabetics, fundraising and so on would occur to ensure there was a diabetic educator or some form of community/primary healthcare worker available to enable better health outcomes for that community.

Rural and remote areas are often crippled by the availability of staff. It is common to not have a pharmacist on staff in a base hospital as there is not enough incentive for healthcare professionals to travel outside of metropolitan areas to seek employment. Having said that, it is not just a shortage of allied health professional staff, it is nursing, medical and diagnostic staff as well. This leads to many people needing to travel to metropolitan areas for their healthcare needs.

Health professionals that are available in rural and remote settings are the Royal Flying Doctor Service and/or Air Ambulance service for that state or territory, and a retrieval team usually from a tertiary hospital facility. Knowing who to contact is an essential component of rural and remote nursing.

As a nurse, other personnel you can expect to liaise with include:

- emergency services (ambulance officers, firemen/women and police officers)
- referral agencies (home care, Meals on Wheels)
- other hospital staff (nurses, cleaners, doctors, supervisors)
- community agencies (domiciliary nurses, community mental health)
- healthcare team (medical, nursing, allied health and family members)
- volunteers – quite common in rural and remote hospitals. Volunteers play an important part in fundraising and ensuring that patients have basic toiletries and phone cards to contact family that may be several hundred kilometres away on a station.

In some communities, the nurse is the only healthcare professional available. It is important that nurses in rural and remote areas can access support and back-up for managing patient care. Rural and remote nursing is different to nursing in a metropolitan or regional hospital. Environments consist of limited to no medical support, including specialists, and this requires nursing staff to be resourceful and assume higher levels of responsibility than their urban counterparts. Rural and remote nurses need to be multiskilled and are seen as 'generalised' rather than 'specialised' due to the nature of patient care provided every day.

Access to equitable health care within Australia is a key issue in rural health. Imagine having to drive five hours to see a doctor or to obtain prescriptions? As mentioned, it is difficult to discuss what is available in every rural and remote setting within Australia as it will be specific to that area and surrounding community.

CONFIDENTIALITY

Confidentiality and privacy are key principles for healthcare professionals. Maintenance of healthcare records and providing information and/or interventions is even more important in rural areas. Access to information needs to be restricted in all circumstances as there is a high probability that the patient is known to the healthcare team member. Acknowledging your professional and personal standards is also important. You cannot, ethically, provide care and nursing interventions for a close friend or relative; however, in an emergency situation you may not have an option.

One of the difficulties in seeking treatment that exists in rural and remote communities is courtesy of the 'bush telegraph'. Patients fear that seeking treatment for illnesses such as mental health or drug and alcohol addiction will be broadcast to the whole town. In essence, it is difficult to seek care for highly personal reasons if you know the person providing care for you and you do not like or trust them.

Clinical Education Skills Australia provides information regarding rural and remote placements and while it is aligned to clinical placement, it is very relevant to nursing practice. The information can be found here: https://www.clinedaus.org.au/topics-category/confidentiality-and-professional-boundaries-on-a-170.

25.2 DEVELOPING A PLAN OF CARE

A very large component of nursing care is derived from nursing care plans. Nursing care plans can be generic (e.g. 'day 5 post hip replacement') or very specific. The aim of nursing care plans is to guide care and enable nurses to effectively manage their time and the patient's needs. The application of concept maps further addresses the nursing care plan and incorporates all aspects of the nursing process.

Another aim of nursing care plans is *individualised* nursing care, as opposed to the same care for all of our patients. Tailoring nursing care to the patient results in happier families and patients, as they feel like a 'person' not a bed number or 'patient in bed 7'.

Nursing care plans contain the following information:

- activities of daily living (ADLs)
- vital signs – frequency
- feeding – assistance required, diet, tolerance
- mobility
- rehabilitation
- psychosocial factors
- referrals.

Nursing care plans enable nurses to analyse their patient's needs. From assessment tools to diagnostic tools, nursing care plans provide up-to-date information and are the documents that justify our interventions and nursing cares.

The use of care plans or clinical pathways is an effort to streamline nursing documentation. At a glance we can see what our patients require and when. Specialised care plans (e.g. for stomas, myocardial infarctions or post total knee replacement) allow patient care to be looked at from a specific focus as well as a multidisciplinary approach. Furthermore, they ensure that each patient receives necessary interventions as deemed appropriate by the pathway. Some pathways have been generated as a result of a sentinel event, and the cares to be provided and in what order need to be signed for and highlighted for each shift to ensure cares or interventions are not forgotten or missed. Within rural and remote nursing, care plans will often detail if a patient is for transfer to a tertiary hospital, has just returned, or what services the patient may need to be transferred for.

Knowing how to carry out an accurate health assessment – from taking the health history through to performing a physical examination – will help you uncover significant problems and assist in planning your care appropriately. Assessment involves collecting two kinds of data – objective and subjective.

Objective data is obtained through observation and is verifiable; for instance, if we document a patient is febrile, a temperature is recorded on observation charts that correlates and verifies this. Subjective data is provided by the patient and is based on what they say; for instance, there is no way to confirm that the patient has a headache, we merely act upon what our patient tells us.

The focus of health care in the twenty-first century has shifted from a medical model of ill health to a person-centred holistic care and health promotion model, using theory, research and evidence-based practice as basis for practice. Nursing has moved from being focused on disease to caring for the whole person with an illness, with emphasis on the preservation and maintenance of good health through extensive patient education and health promotion.

A health history is used to gather subjective data about the patient and to explore past and present problems. First, ask the patient about their general physical and emotional health, and then move onto specific body systems. The accuracy and amount of information you obtain from your interviewing will depend largely on your skill as an interviewer (DeLaune et al., 2024; Edwards et al., 2019).

As mentioned, in some communities a nurse is the only healthcare professional available and so the nurse is reliant upon services such as the Royal Flying Doctor Service for medical advice. It is important that nurses in rural and remote communities can access support for managing patient care in diverse situations. Other sources of support include telemedicine or telehealth, eMedicine and phone calls to tertiary referral hospitals or retrieval services.

We have already established that rural and remote nursing is different to nursing in regional and metropolitan areas. Environments with limited medical support, including specialists and the availability of allied health services, require nurses to be resourceful and assume high levels of responsibility. Rural and remote nurses need to be multiskilled and adaptable to rapid change.

Rural and remote nurses have to be competent to work in various situations and be able to recommend practical treatment strategies that meet a patient's needs. Nurses must be able to access the most up-to-date information for evidence-based practice, protocols, procedures and/or standards for practice. This means having hard copies of the most recent and referred-to documents in case the internet is not reliable. It also involves thinking of all the 'what ifs'. Think of a massive dust storm – often wind speeds are so high that internet connections and mobile phone services are down for the duration. Power is also often cut, so the town will need to rely on generators (if they have them). Ensuring that you have access to information offline or via hard copy is crucial to management of patients and their needs.

Entwined with all of this, the nurse must know when, for that community or hospital, the patient needs to be referred to a tertiary hospital or for transfer by the Royal Flying Doctor Service or Air Ambulance.

There is a lot of information to maintain and keep up to date with and the only way to ensure you can do this is via ongoing education and training.

25.3 NURSING INTERVENTIONS
Utilising assessment tools identified in nursing care plans, standards for practice or clinical pathways enable the nurse to systematically assess the patient, bearing in mind that it may have been months since the last patient presentation with similar circumstances. These policies, procedures or care plans are very useful in a setting where, for example, you may only receive limited numbers of critically ill patients or patients suffering a compound fracture.

A point that cannot be stressed enough is that no matter where you work, you must ensure that you are acting within your scope of practice. In rural and remote nursing it is quite common to have an expanded scope of practice, provided that there are policies, procedures, standards for practice or guidelines to support this addition to your role.

The arrival of a trauma patient is not uncommon in rural and remote nursing. The trauma can range from mechanical and high-speed injuries to envenomation to obstetric and paediatric emergencies. Trauma in rural areas means that patients are located large distances from tertiary or metropolitan hospitals, and this impacts the level of medical care available. In New South Wales alone, more than 25 per cent of seriously injured patients are initially managed in rural and remote settings (Curtis et al., 2019). For the major trauma patient, this can adversely affect life expectancy. A person suffering a major injury in rural Australia is twice as likely to die than if the same accident had occurred near a metropolitan hospital.

Curtis et al. (2019) have identified characteristics of, and problems associated with, rural trauma – in comparison with metropolitan areas, rural trauma involves:

- greater distances travelled
- higher speeds of travel leading to more severe injuries
- poor quality roads
- older vehicles in poorer condition
- poor seatbelt compliance
- fatigue and alcohol
- delays in discovery times as a result of remoteness/ longer transport times
- rural ambulances being less well equipped to deal with multi-trauma
- rural practitioner levels of trauma experience less frequent
- hospitals being less well equipped to deal with major road crashes and multiple patients.

When working in rural and remote areas, there will be modifications to clinical pathways due to the limited resources and facilities. For example, NSW Health has created a pathway to outline how to assess and manage patients with suspected acute coronary syndromes (ACS). This pathway standardises practice across all health services operating in NSW, including rural, remote and metropolitan areas and identifies the process for patients to be transferred or retrieved regardless of differences in facilities to ensure the same treatment is available to all patients regardless of their location (see **Figure 25.1**).

25.4 EVALUATION AND DISCHARGE

Hospitals in rural and remote settings will have protocols documenting allocation of patients to specific areas. Often there are several referral points for the one hospital, and it ultimately depends upon the care the patient needs. If the patient requires transfer to another healthcare facility, there will be relevant documentation and procedures in place to ensure patient transfers occur consistently and safely.

Alongside the difficulties of long distances comes the inevitable weather restrictions that are not really a consideration in metropolitan areas. If there is a massive dust storm (a common occurrence in many outback towns), pilots do not have safe or adequate vision and cannot land or take off. Conversely, in winter, frost, snow or poor visibility due to fog are other delaying factors. High wind speeds will also keep a plane landed, as will too many pilot hours, so another pilot will need to be flown out to fly the plane. Other delays in retrievals can be due to a greater need for the service elsewhere in the state or territory and this means that your patient will remain in the rural hospital, sometimes for days, until transport can be arranged.

Any hospital in a rural and remote setting will have a trauma set-up, usually a bed area in the emergency department with appropriate space and supplies to attend to almost any emergency to the full potential of that health service. It is difficult to grasp that in rural and remote hospitals there is not always a doctor onsite, especially overnight, and other services are limited outside business hours. It is a good idea to familiarise yourself with the trauma or 'resus' bay and the emergency trolley to ensure you are aware of the location of vital pieces of equipment and medication. There are always checks performed on this equipment and this is vital to ensure that when it is needed everything is available.

Patient education and management

A very large part of our role is to empower patients through education and ongoing support and management. Enabling patients to take care of themselves empowers them and their significant others and gives them the right to have a say in their healthcare decisions. Many elderly patients now will still agree with a doctor as they believe doctors know best – even if it is something that the patient does not agree with.

The implementation of health promotion and patient education is highly individualised. While nurses are seen as possessing the knowledge, it is not always so. Never be afraid to tell a patient that you are not entirely sure – but make sure that you find out the information on the procedure or treatment so that you can both learn. It is also important to bear in mind that patient education and health promotion needs to be aimed at significant others. Also, the following factors must be considered:

- lay terms (avoid medical jargon)
- recognition of the patient's understanding and past experiences

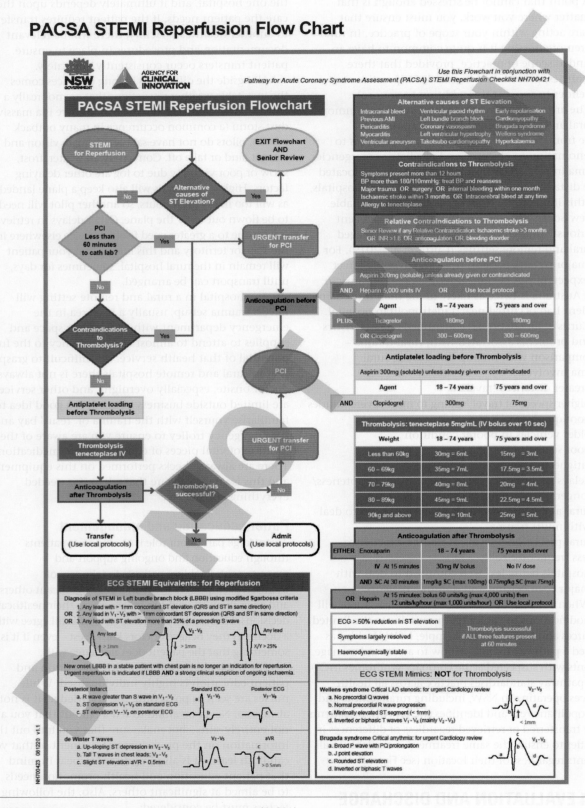

FIGURE 25.1 Pathway for acute coronary syndrome assessment (PACSA)

SOURCE: NSW AGENCY FOR CLINICAL INNOVATION, PACSA STEMI REPERFUSION FLOW CHART. SYDNEY, 2021. AVAILABLE FROM:
HTTPS://ACI.HEALTH.NSW.GOV.AU/__DATA/ASSETS/PDF_FILE/0019/824140/PACSA-STEMI-REPERFUSION-FLOW-CHART-SAMPLE.PDF

- learning mechanisms (visual, auditory, etc.)
- willingness of the patient to learn.

Almost daily in our nursing practice, we come across patients who are undergoing stressful events; for example, in the form of illness, death, birth or life-altering surgery. How a person responds to these stressful events has a lot to do with perception and their coping mechanisms. In providing nursing interventions in the form of health teaching and health promotion, we must understand how the patient is attempting to cope with the stressor. Some coping mechanisms involve keeping negative or uncomfortable feelings within, and often the patient will not acknowledge, or avoid, the situation, by, for example, simply not performing blood glucose levels or taking their prescribed medications.

Health promotion and education involves individualised patient assessment and relevant intervention. Identification of issues relating to specific healthcare problems for that patient enables the patient and the nurse to intervene and set in motion interventions to address these issues.

In providing health education, promotion and teaching for rural and remote Australians, the nurse must ensure that they are aware of facilities available and how to access them. Patients and their families need to be informed of when and where appointments will be and how to arrange them.

For example, Jane is a 36-year-old female with congenital kidney disease. Jane requires haemodialysis three times a week. Currently in her hometown of Lagoona, there are no available 'spots' for Jane to receive haemodialysis, so Jane must go to Trippet, the referral hospital 500 km away for treatment indefinitely as it is not known when a spot will be available for Jane to receive dialysis in her hometown. In Jane's situation, she will need to leave her job and travel to Trippet to receive necessary care. She will most likely be alone as her family run a station and cannot leave it unattended for long periods of time.

So, in order to provide holistic care for Jane, you would be involved in:

- arranging treatment at alternative hospital
- arranging accommodation for Jane
- handing over Jane's care – medical conditions, medications, renal disease, etc.
- ensuring that Jane and her family are aware of what is going on
- initiating the application process for rural and remote assistance (e.g. in NSW, IPTAAS)
- providing medical certificates for Jane's employer if she can maintain her employment on return
- contacting Centrelink and commencing procedures for payments for Jane and ensuring that she is receiving all that she should be
- answering any questions.

Jane's case is not uncommon in rural and remote areas as there are simply not enough facilities required

for meeting the needs of the residents. State governments have set up schemes whereby patients and their families can claim funds to assist them in their travels.

In rural and remote nursing there are multiple service providers that require contacting and communicating with, for example:

- referral hospitals – larger rural hospital (base hospital)
- tertiary hospitals
- retrieval teams
- Royal Flying Doctor Service
- Air Ambulance
- GPs
- other healthcare clinics within that cluster or area health service
- emergency personnel
- telemedicine providers
- outpatient departments for follow-up treatment
- private providers.

If a patient presented to emergency in a base hospital in a rural setting with chest pains, then this would be a fairly typical pathway:

1 Assessed and treatment initiated > let's presume the patient has ST elevation acute coronary syndrome
2 Thrombolysed – medical management as per cardiologist
3 Tertiary hospital contacted to arrange a coronary angiogram and to book a bed
4 Patient will remain in rural hospital until bed becomes available with tertiary hospital and this can take up to two weeks due to bed pressures
5 Patient is accepted and has a bed, Air Ambulance or Royal Flying Doctor Service contacted to arrange transport of patient to tertiary hospital
6 Patient is transferred, generally by air, to destination
7 Patient receives coronary angiography and follow-up treatment and assessment
8 Patient must find *own* way home
9 Patient is followed up by local medical officers and must attend outpatient clinic in tertiary hospital as specified by cardiologist.

All up, this process could take anywhere from days to weeks, and the patient must find their own way home from the destination. So, for example, Griffith NSW is home, the patient is flown from Griffith to Sydney but must arrange and pay for their own way home. Schemes such as IPTAAS cover some costs, but the reimbursement is not 100 per cent so there is always an out-of-pocket expense.

There is not an easy fix for rural and remote health, nor is there a guide for use in all hospitals. The foundation of rural and remote health care is on assessment of the patient and management of their needs/concerns/requirements in accordance with local policy. Geographic location will often determine what type of transport or retrieval service is required, and to which referral tertiary hospital.

SUMMARY

Rural and remote health care is a completely different nursing experience. It takes knowledge and practice to know 'who' to contact, what hospital does 'what' and the processes involved in transferring patients to tertiary or base hospitals for further intervention or management. It is essential that nursing staff are aware of the services provided in each referral hospital so that we can impart that knowledge to the patients and their families. Most patients know that if they break a bone in Broken Hill, for example, they will have to 'go to Adelaide' as the hospital in Broken Hill does not have the staff nor the facilities to provide orthopaedic services.

You cannot, however, group all rural healthcare facilities together as they are all inherently different, and provision of one service in one community may be specific to the needs of that community.

Familiarising yourself with the points of referral, methods of travel home, places for accommodation that offer discounts for rural and remote residents, and simple things like where to park are incredibly helpful for families going through an already stressful period.

Rural and remote nursing is a highly diverse speciality within Australian health care. Working and living in a small community comes with its own problems. For example, being known for your professional role and having no clear boundary between work and home, or caring for local community members and finding out more than you feel comfortable with as you are in direct care of the person. Confidentiality and privacy are underpinning principles for healthcare professionals, and in large urban areas, it is highly unlikely that you will ever need to provide care for someone that you actually *know*; however, in rural and remote communities this is very likely so boundaries need to be set and maintained.

Management of trauma and emergency situations in rural and remote settings will usually require transfer to a metropolitan or tertiary hospital. This is because many interventional treatments and surgeries cannot be performed in rural and remote locations due to shortage of staff, services and equipment. Ensuring that you are familiar with your role and scope of practice is essential in maintaining quality patient care. Utilising your excellent interpersonal skills is also necessary to ensure that retrieval teams and ambulances are fully aware of the patient's presenting problem, interventions already undertaken, medications given and so on.

PROBLEM-SOLVING SCENARIO

You are working in a multipurpose facility in western Queensland. You have access to a laboratory from 0800–1700 daily, with only point-of-care testing available outside of these hours.

You have a patient present at 2300 hours with central chest pain, crushing in nature, associated with ECG changes, nausea, diaphoresis and hypotension. Point-of-care testing provides the following values:

- Cardiac Troponin (CTnI)
- UEC
- ABG.

1 What equipment is available to you and how can you effectively assess and manage this patient's presentation?
2 Would point-of-care testing be sufficient to initially manage this patient?
3 If thrombolytic therapy was ordered, how could you safely manage this patient overnight with only point-of-care testing?
4 What diagnostic testing would this patient require?
5 How could you educate the patient on the need to be transferred to another hospital if they required an angiogram?

PORTFOLIO DEVELOPMENT

Australian Institute of Health and Welfare
A good starting point for developing your professional portfolio in rural health care is this AIHW website that outlines the current state of rural and remote health and looks at the risk factors and health status of Australians who live in these areas. https://www.aihw.gov.au/reports/rural-remote-australians/rural-and-remote-health

Other useful information around Aboriginal and Torres Strait Islander peoples' health and wellbeing can be found at the AIHW website here: https://www.aihw.gov.au/reports/aus/234/indigenous-health/indigenous-health-and-wellbeing

The other useful websites below will assist in meeting continuing professional development activities to meet the NMBA yearly registration requirements for a Registered Nurse.

USEFUL WEBSITES

Registered Nurse Standards for Practice
The Registered Nurse Standards for Practice consist of seven crucial standards that all nurses must follow. Download and review the standards at the following link.
https://www.nursingmidwiferyboard.gov.au/Codes-Guidelines-Statements/Professional-standards/registered-nurse-standards-for-practice.aspx

NSW Health Retrieval Handover Procedure
This is a policy to confirm the process and coordinate handover and transfer of care between hospital clinicians and medical retrieval teams. https://www1.health.nsw.gov.au/pds/ActivePDSDocuments/PD2012_019.pdf
Council of Remote Area Nurses of Australia

CRANAplus
CRANAplus is the peak professional body for the remote and isolated health workforce in Australia. https://crana.org.au

Rural Health Resources
The Department of Health and Aged Care has a website with resources for rural health. https://www1.health.gov.au/internet/main/publishing.nsf/Content/ruralhealth-overview

REFERENCES AND FURTHER READING

Australian Institute of Health and Welfare (AIHW). (2022). *Rural and remote health.* https://www.aihw.gov.au/reports/rural-remote-australians/rural-and-remote-health

Curtis, K., Ramsden, C., Shaban, R., Fry, M., & Considine, J. (2019). *Emergency and trauma care for nurses and paramedics* (3rd ed.). Elsevier.

DeLaune, S., Ladner, P., McTier, L., Tollefson, J., & Lawrence, J. (2024). *Fundamentals of nursing* (3rd ed.). Cengage Learning Australia.

Edwards, H., Brown, D., Buckley, T., Aitken, R., & Plowman, E. (2019). *Lewis's medical-surgical nursing* (5th ANZ ed.). Elsevier.

Queensland Health. (2022). *Primary clinical care manual* (11th ed.). www.health.qld.gov.au/orrh/clinical-manuals/primary-clinical-care-manual-pccm/view-current-edition

COLLATED CONCEPT MAPS

Chapter 3: Respiratory System

CONCEPT MAP SEQUENCE FOR ASTHMA

Presentation

Alicia Jones is an 18-year-old university student who has been admitted to the emergency department with breathlessness for the last two hours which is not responding to her salbutamol puffer. Alicia has an audible wheeze and she can only speak in short sentences. She has had a cold for the last five days, and it is now affecting her sinuses.

Concept maps 3.1–3.5 explore Alicia's initial care in the emergency department.

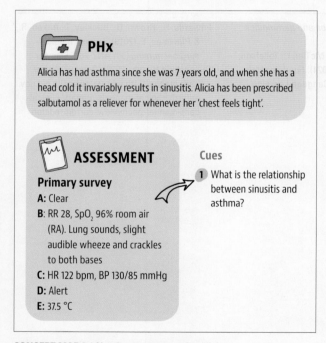

PHx

Alicia has had asthma since she was 7 years old, and when she has a head cold it invariably results in sinusitis. Alicia has been prescribed salbutamol as a reliever for whenever her 'chest feels tight'.

ASSESSMENT

Primary survey

A: Clear

B: RR 28, SpO$_2$ 96% room air (RA). Lung sounds, slight audible wheeze and crackles to both bases

C: HR 122 bpm, BP 130/85 mmHg

D: Alert

E: 37.5 °C

Cues

1 What is the relationship between sinusitis and asthma?

CONCEPT MAP 3.1 Nursing assessment for Alicia

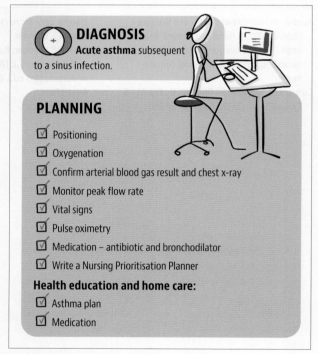

DIAGNOSIS

Acute asthma subsequent to a sinus infection.

PLANNING

- ☑ Positioning
- ☑ Oxygenation
- ☑ Confirm arterial blood gas result and chest x-ray
- ☑ Monitor peak flow rate
- ☑ Vital signs
- ☑ Pulse oximetry
- ☑ Medication – antibiotic and bronchodilator
- ☑ Write a Nursing Prioritisation Planner

Health education and home care:

- ☑ Asthma plan
- ☑ Medication

CONCEPT MAP 3.2 Diagnosis and planning for Alicia

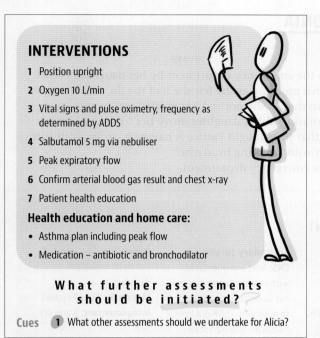

INTERVENTIONS

1 Position upright

2 Oxygen 10 L/min

3 Vital signs and pulse oximetry, frequency as determined by ADDS

4 Salbutamol 5 mg via nebuliser

5 Peak expiratory flow

6 Confirm arterial blood gas result and chest x-ray

7 Patient health education

Health education and home care:

• Asthma plan including peak flow

• Medication – antibiotic and bronchodilator

What further assessments should be initiated?

Cues   **1** What other assessments should we undertake for Alicia?

CONCEPT MAP 3.3 Nursing interventions for Alicia

DISCHARGE PLANNING + COORDINATION OF CARE

How do the following areas of healthcare management **relate** to Alicia's presentation? Which members of the healthcare team are **involved** in each area of management?

Sinusitis   Asthma

Develop a written asthma plan with information related to the current infection.

Develop an education plan for Alicia's medication.

Post-discharge medication – 250 mg cefuroxime BD orally for 10 days and salbutamol as required

CONCEPT MAP 3.5 Discharge planning and coordination of care for Alicia

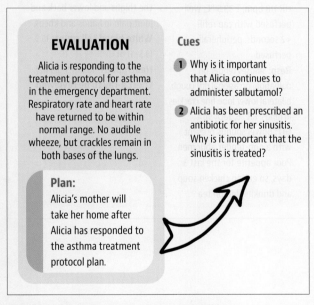

EVALUATION

Alicia is responding to the treatment protocol for asthma in the emergency department. Respiratory rate and heart rate have returned to be within normal range. No audible wheeze, but crackles remain in both bases of the lungs.

Plan:

Alicia's mother will take her home after Alicia has responded to the asthma treatment protocol plan.

Cues

1 Why is it important that Alicia continues to administer salbutamol?

2 Alicia has been prescribed an antibiotic for her sinusitis. Why is it important that the sinusitis is treated?

CONCEPT MAP 3.4 Evaluation and planning for Alicia

CONCEPT MAP SEQUENCE FOR PNEUMONIA

Presentation

Patrice Bell is a 62-year-old widow who was brought into the emergency department by her daughter. Patrice had an appointment with her general practitioner (GP) this morning as she felt she had the flu, and when her daughter arrived at the family home to take her mother to the GP she noticed her mother was being vague. While in the car Patrice appeared to have trouble concentrating so her daughter drove her to the emergency department. Patrice's daughter stated to the triage nurse that she thought Patrice is having a stroke, with Patrice stating 'it's the flu and not a stroke, as I'm aching all over with a roaring headache'.

Concept maps 3.6–3.10 explore Patrice's initial care in the emergency department.

PHx

Patrice has **enjoyed good health,** which she attributes to being a keen gardener. She had her **annual influenza injection** so cannot understand why she has the flu this year.

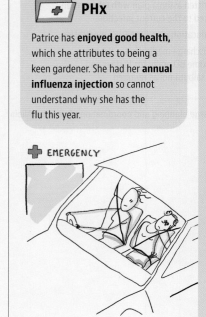

ASSESSMENT

Primary survey
A: Clear
B: RR 24, pulse oximetry 96% on room air, lung sounds reveal bilateral lower lobe fine crackles
C: Pulse 122 bpm, BP 140/80 mmHg, skin flushed, cap refill >2 seconds
D: Alert and orientated. Headache predominantly in sinuses but radiates into forehead, pain scale 5/10. Equal limb strength
E: 38.3 °C

Secondary survey
CNS: Alert and orientated, with patient stating that she has to concentrate to respond to questions. Still has a frontal headache, 5/10 pain scale unchanged
CVS: BP 135/90 mmHg, HR 118 bpm, T 38.6 °C, well perfused with cap refill <2 seconds, peripherally perfused
Resp: Sinuses tender on palpation, occasional dry cough, bilateral lower lobe fine crackles in lungs. RR 26, SaO₂ 96%.
GIT: Bowel sounds present with a non-tender abdomen. Poor appetite for the last 3 days, so eating chicken soup and drinking lemon tea.

Renal: Urine concentrated but no abnormalities detected.
Metabolic: BGL 5.7 mmol/L
Integumentary: Warm dry skin.
Musculoskeletal: Equal limb strength with muscle pain in the thighs and lower back and joint pain in hands and knees.
White blood cell count: 15.9 (3.5–11 nL)
Neutrophils: 10.6 (1.5–7.5 nL)
Chest x-ray to be reviewed

CONCEPT MAP 3.6 Nursing assessment for Patrice

DIAGNOSIS
Community acquired **pneumonia**, with admission to the respiratory ward.

PLANNING

☑ Positioning

☑ Vital signs

☑ Pulse oximetry

☑ Lung sounds, cough, sputum

☑ Oxygen therapy

☑ IV therapy 0.9% sodium chloride

☑ Fluid balance chart

☑ Initial antibiotic therapy regimen for unidentified microorganism – Benzylpenicillin and Azithromycin

☑ Paracetamol for temperature and also for pain management based on secondary assessment data

☑ Slow abdominal breathing, deep breathing and coughing

☑ Write a Nursing Prioritisation Planner

Health education and home care:

☑ Medication – oral antibiotics and oral paracetamol

☑ Fluids and nutrition

☑ Education about signs and symptoms of pneumonia, failure or decreased response to treatment (e.g. pyrexia, productive cough, shortness of breath etc.) and when to seek further medical care.

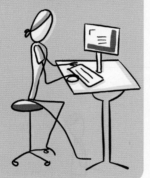

CONCEPT MAP 3.7 Diagnosis and planning for Patrice

INTERVENTIONS

1 Positioning: Fowlers

2 Vital signs 4-hourly

3 Pulse oximetry 4-hourly

4 Lung sounds, cough, sputum 4-hourly assessment

5 Oxygen therapy: nasal prongs 4 L/min

6 IV therapy 0.9% sodium chloride 8/24

7 Benzylpenicillin 1.2 g QID IV

8 Fluid balance chart

9 Azithromycin 500 mg daily IV over 1 hour

10 Paracetamol 1 g QID oral for temperature

11 Slow abdominal breathing, deep breathing and coughing

Health education and home care:

• Medication: oral antibiotics and oral paracetamol

• Fluids and nutrition

• Education about signs and symptoms of pneumonia, including failure or decreased response to treatment and when to seek further medical care.

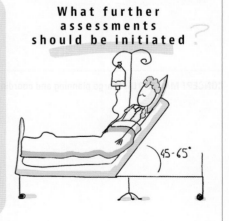

What further assessments should be initiated

45–65°

CONCEPT MAP 3.8 Nursing interventions for Patrice

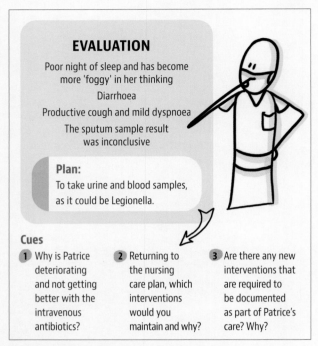

EVALUATION

Poor night of sleep and has become more 'foggy' in her thinking

Diarrhoea

Productive cough and mild dyspnoea

The sputum sample result was inconclusive

Plan:
To take urine and blood samples, as it could be Legionella.

Cues

1 Why is Patrice deteriorating and not getting better with the intravenous antibiotics?

2 Returning to the nursing care plan, which interventions would you maintain and why?

3 Are there any new interventions that are required to be documented as part of Patrice's care? Why?

CONCEPT MAP 3.9 Evaluation and planning for Patrice

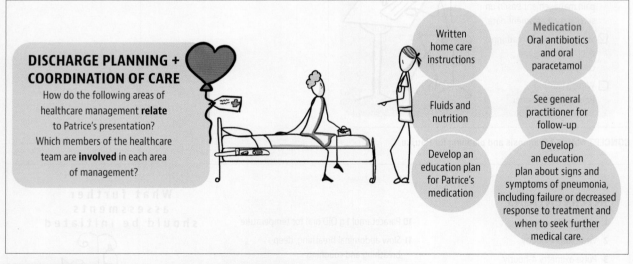

DISCHARGE PLANNING + COORDINATION OF CARE

How do the following areas of healthcare management **relate** to Patrice's presentation? Which members of the healthcare team are **involved** in each area of management?

Written home care instructions

Fluids and nutrition

Develop an education plan for Patrice's medication

Medication
Oral antibiotics and oral paracetamol

See general practitioner for follow-up

Develop an education plan about signs and symptoms of pneumonia, including failure or decreased response to treatment and when to seek further medical care.

CONCEPT MAP 3.10 Discharge planning and coordination of care for Patrice

CONCEPT MAP SEQUENCE FOR PNEUMOTHORAX

Presentation

Frank Musumeci is a 26-year-old builder who was brought to the emergency department by ambulance. Frank was driving his utility when he felt the sudden onset of severe retrosternal chest pain and acute difficulty breathing. He was unable to continue driving and pulled off the road. He called for an ambulance on his mobile phone.

On examination, Frank is a muscular young man who is experiencing acute respiratory distress and is gasping for air. His blood pressure is 140/80 mmHg, pulse 100 bpm, respiratory rate 35/minute and shallow and temperature 37.1 °C. His skin colour is pale, but not cyanotic. His lung sounds are diminished on the right side, without wheezing or crackles. His heart sounds are normal and abdominal examination is unremarkable. His extremities showed no clubbing or oedema.

Concept maps 3.11–3.15 explore Frank's initial care in the emergency department.

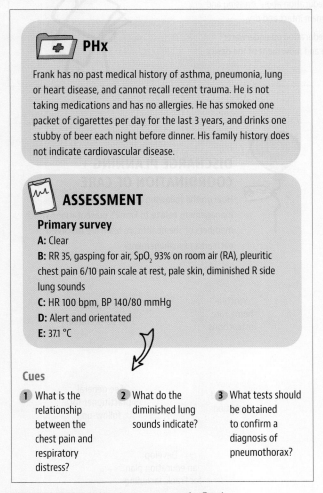

PHx

Frank has no past medical history of asthma, pneumonia, lung or heart disease, and cannot recall recent trauma. He is not taking medications and has no allergies. He has smoked one packet of cigarettes per day for the last 3 years, and drinks one stubby of beer each night before dinner. His family history does not indicate cardiovascular disease.

ASSESSMENT

Primary survey
A: Clear
B: RR 35, gasping for air, SpO₂ 93% on room air (RA), pleuritic chest pain 6/10 pain scale at rest, pale skin, diminished R side lung sounds
C: HR 100 bpm, BP 140/80 mmHg
D: Alert and orientated
E: 37.1 °C

Cues

1 What is the relationship between the chest pain and respiratory distress?

2 What do the diminished lung sounds indicate?

3 What tests should be obtained to confirm a diagnosis of pneumothorax?

CONCEPT MAP 3.11 Nursing assessment for Frank

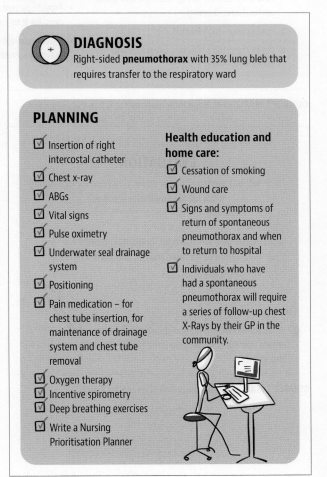

DIAGNOSIS

Right-sided **pneumothorax** with 35% lung bleb that requires transfer to the respiratory ward

PLANNING

- ☑ Insertion of right intercostal catheter
- ☑ Chest x-ray
- ☑ ABGs
- ☑ Vital signs
- ☑ Pulse oximetry
- ☑ Underwater seal drainage system
- ☑ Positioning
- ☑ Pain medication – for chest tube insertion, for maintenance of drainage system and chest tube removal
- ☑ Oxygen therapy
- ☑ Incentive spirometry
- ☑ Deep breathing exercises
- ☑ Write a Nursing Prioritisation Planner

Health education and home care:

- ☑ Cessation of smoking
- ☑ Wound care
- ☑ Signs and symptoms of return of spontaneous pneumothorax and when to return to hospital
- ☑ Individuals who have had a spontaneous pneumothorax will require a series of follow-up chest X-Rays by their GP in the community.

CONCEPT MAP 3.12 Diagnosis and planning for Frank

INTERVENTIONS

1 Insertion of right intercostal catheter and attachment of underwater drainage system

2 Chest x-ray

3 ABGs

4 Vital signs – every 15 minutes first hour, hourly for the next four hours, then 4 hourly

5 Pulse oximetry and lung sounds – as above with vital signs

6 Underwater seal drainage system – checked hourly for bubble, swing, drainage, and gauze and occlusive dressing

7 Positioning – high Fowlers

8 Check chest tube insertion site gauze and occlusive dressing 8 hourly

Pain management:

9 Chest tube insertion – 1% lignocaine + 1:10 000 adrenaline SC

10 Chest tube maintenance – for example, tramadol and diclofenac

11 Chest tube removal – for example, tramadol

Health education and home care:

- Cease smoking to reduce risk of reoccurrence
- Monitor catheter insertion site
- Provide patient education about dressing and need for it to remain intact and dry
- Provide patient education on underwater drainage system and movement of the device.

What further assessments should be initiated

CONCEPT MAP 3.13 Nursing interventions for Frank

EVALUATION

Frank will be transferred to the respiratory ward for monitoring while his pneumothorax resolves.

Plan:
Discharge Frank when his intercostal catheter has been removed for more than 24 hours without adverse effect.

Cues

1 What additional information should we obtain to ensure that Frank's right lung is reinflated? Why is this important?

CONCEPT MAP 3.14 Evaluation and planning for Frank

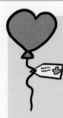

DISCHARGE PLANNING + COORDINATION OF CARE

How do the following areas of healthcare management **relate** to Frank's presentation? Which members of the healthcare team are **involved** in each area of management?

Written home care instructions

Medication
Oral paracetamol

Fluids and nutrition

See general practitioner for follow-up.

Develop an education plan for Frank, including:

- signs and symptoms of return of pneumothorax

- no heavy lifting, running, swimming, exposure to high altitudes for 4-6 weeks after resolution of pneumothorax

- ceasing smoking to reduce risk of recurrence.

CONCEPT MAP 3.15 Discharge planning and coordination of care for Frank

Chapter 4: Cardiovascular system

CONCEPT MAP SEQUENCE FOR ACUTE MYOCARDIAL INFARCTION

Presentation

Wesley Shapiro is a 58-year-old man who was assisting his friend in the launching of a small boat from a boat trailer when he started to feel sore in the chest. He thought the soreness was due to pulling a muscle, but this pain spread to down his left arm and upper jaw. He mentioned the pain to his friend who then decided to put the boat back on the trailer and drive Wesley to the local hospital.

Concept maps 4.1–4.5 explore Wesley's initial care in the emergency department.

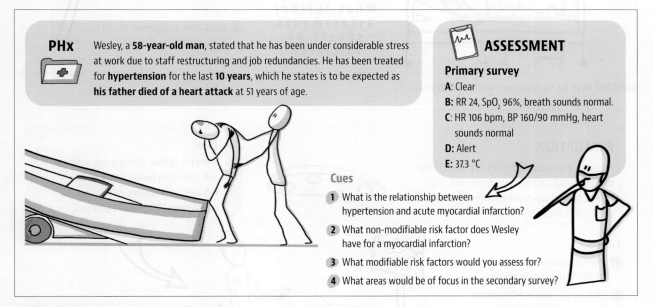

PHx Wesley, a **58-year-old man**, stated that he has been under considerable stress at work due to staff restructuring and job redundancies. He has been treated for **hypertension** for the last **10 years**, which he states is to be expected as **his father died of a heart attack** at 51 years of age.

ASSESSMENT

Primary survey
A: Clear
B: RR 24, SpO$_2$ 96%, breath sounds normal.
C: HR 106 bpm, BP 160/90 mmHg, heart sounds normal
D: Alert
E: 37.3 °C

Cues

1. What is the relationship between hypertension and acute myocardial infarction?

2. What non-modifiable risk factor does Wesley have for a myocardial infarction?

3. What modifiable risk factors would you assess for?

4. What areas would be of focus in the secondary survey?

CONCEPT MAP 4.1 Nursing assessment for Wesley

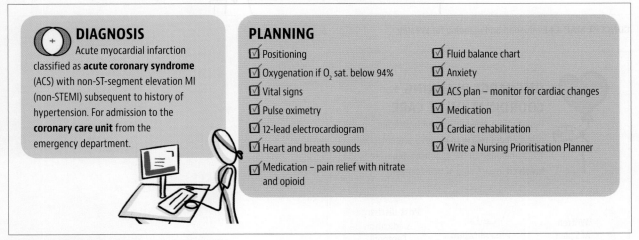

DIAGNOSIS
Acute myocardial infarction classified as **acute coronary syndrome** (ACS) with non-ST-segment elevation MI (non-STEMI) subsequent to history of hypertension. For admission to the **coronary care unit** from the emergency department.

PLANNING
- ☑ Positioning
- ☑ Oxygenation if O$_2$ sat. below 94%
- ☑ Vital signs
- ☑ Pulse oximetry
- ☑ 12-lead electrocardiogram
- ☑ Heart and breath sounds
- ☑ Medication – pain relief with nitrate and opioid
- ☑ Fluid balance chart
- ☑ Anxiety
- ☑ ACS plan – monitor for cardiac changes
- ☑ Medication
- ☑ Cardiac rehabilitation
- ☑ Write a Nursing Prioritisation Planner

CONCEPT MAP 4.2 Diagnosis and planning for Wesley

INTERVENTIONS

1 Position upright
2 Oxygen if O$_2$ sat. below 94%
3 Vital signs and pulse oximetry, frequency as determined by ADDS
4 Continuous cardiac monitoring
5 Sublingual glyceryl trinitrate

6 Morphine
7 Fluid balance chart
8 Heart and breath sounds
9 Blood tests
10 12-lead ECG

11 Monitor for stress and anxiety
12 Psychosocial support
13 Medication – aspirin, heparin and captopril

Health education and home care:
• Cardiac rehabilitation plan

What further assessments should be initiated

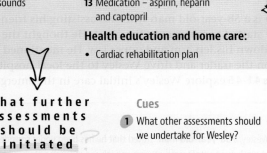

Cues
1 What other assessments should we undertake for Wesley?

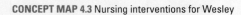

CONCEPT MAP 4.3 Nursing interventions for Wesley

EVALUATION

Wesley is responding fairly well to the treatment protocol for ACS in the coronary care unit, but cardiac markers are elevated and intermittent chest pain is occurring.

Plan:
Wesley is to have coronary angiography and if coronary revascularisation is required, a percutaneous coronary intervention (PCI) will be performed.

Cues
1 Why is it important that Wesley has his chest pain fully relieved?

2 What are the nursing interventions for pre coronary angiography and why?

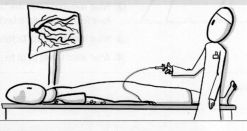

3 What are the nursing interventions for post-PCI and why?

CONCEPT MAP 4.4 Evaluation and planning for Wesley

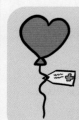

DISCHARGE PLANNING + COORDINATION OF CARE

How do the following areas of healthcare management **relate** to Wesley's presentation? Which members of the healthcare team are **involved** in each area of management?

Written ACS plan

Cardiac rehabilitation

Post-discharge medication Captopril and GTN

CONCEPT MAP 4.5 Discharge planning and coordination of care for Wesley

CONCEPT MAP SEQUENCE FOR ATRIAL FIBRILLATION AND DEEP VEIN THROMBOSIS

Presentation

Margaret Dungala Pierce is a 65-year-old widow and a proud Yorta Yorta woman and was admitted to the emergency department (ED) with a past history of an anterior acute myocardial infarction (AMI) six years ago and mild heart failure controlled by enalapril with atorvastatin. She has had dyspnoea on exertion for the past two weeks, and her general practitioner (GP) ordered a 12-lead electrocardiogram which displayed atrial fibrillation (AF) with a ventricular rate of 80 beats per minute.

Concept maps 4.6–4.10 explore Margaret's initial care in the emergency department, before transfer to the coronary care unit for further care.

 PHx

Margaret has a past history of an anterior acute myocardial infarction six years ago and mild heart failure controlled by enalapril and atorvastatin. She has had dyspnoea on exertion for the past two weeks, and a 12-lead electrocardiogram taken at the general practice today revealed atrial fibrillation with a ventricular rate of 80 beats per minute.

Cues

1. What is the relationship between acute myocardial infarction and heart failure?
2. What is the relationship between dyspnoea and heart failure?
3. What is the relationship between dyspnoea and atrial fibrillation?
4. What is the relationship between heart failure and reduced peripheral circulation?

 ASSESSMENT

Primary survey

A: Clear
B: RR 24, dyspnoea on exertion, SaO$_2$ 96% on room air, chest x-ray shows enlarged heart with clear lungs
C: HR 90 bpm, BP 150/95 mmHg, pedal pulses present but weak to palpate. A 12-lead electrocardiogram showed an old anterior AMI, atrial fibrillation and no pulmonary hypertension
D: Alert and orientated. No pain
E: 36.8 °C

Secondary survey

CNS: Alert and orientated
CVS: BP 165/90 mmHg, HR 110 bpm, T 36.8 °C, cap return >2 seconds
Resp: RR 26, SaO$_2$ 96%.
GIT: Tolerating food and fluids. Bowel sounds present with a non-tender abdomen.
Renal: 50 mL/hr and no abnormalities detected.
Metabolic: BGL 5.7 mmol/L
Integumentary: Cool feet with slight oedema
BMI: 31.1
Musculoskeletal: Equal limb strength

CONCEPT MAP 4.6 Nursing assessment for Margaret

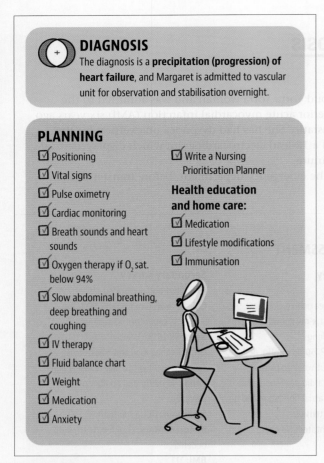

DIAGNOSIS

The diagnosis is a **precipitation (progression) of heart failure**, and Margaret is admitted to vascular unit for observation and stabilisation overnight.

PLANNING

- ☑ Positioning
- ☑ Vital signs
- ☑ Pulse oximetry
- ☑ Cardiac monitoring
- ☑ Breath sounds and heart sounds
- ☑ Oxygen therapy if O_2 sat. below 94%
- ☑ Slow abdominal breathing, deep breathing and coughing
- ☑ IV therapy
- ☑ Fluid balance chart
- ☑ Weight
- ☑ Medication
- ☑ Anxiety
- ☑ Write a Nursing Prioritisation Planner

Health education and home care:

- ☑ Medication
- ☑ Lifestyle modifications
- ☑ Immunisation

CONCEPT MAP 4.7 Diagnosis and planning for Margaret

INTERVENTIONS

1. Positioning – Fowlers
2. Vital signs 4 hourly
3. Pulse oximetry 4 hourly
4. Cardiac monitor for arrhythmia detection
5. Breath and lung sounds assessment 4 hourly
6. Oxygen therapy if O_2 sat. below 94%
7. Slow abdominal breathing, deep breathing and coughing
8. IV therapy 0.9% sodium chloride 8/24
9. Fluid balance chart hourly
10. Medication enalapril, atorvastatin, diltiazem and warfarin
11. Low fat and sodium diet
12. Relieve anxiety

Health education and home care:

- Medication – enalapril, atorvastatin, diltiazem and warfarin
- Lifestyle modification

What further assessments should be initiated?

CONCEPT MAP 4.8 Nursing interventions for Margaret

EVALUATION

The night shift handover stated that Margaret is stable. Just as the handover was completed Margaret rang the call bell for an extra blanket as her left lower leg was painful. The blanket was brought to the bed and it was observed that her left calf had a reddened appearance and was slightly oedematous. Margaret had a pain scale of 4 out of 10.

Plan:
To contact the medical team and facilitate further assessment. Advise Margaret to rest in bed until medical review. Notify RN in-charge of shift of Margaret's deterioration. Document assessment findings and nursing actions taken in Margaret's health record.

Cues

1. Why does Margaret describe her left lower leg as painful?
2. Why does the calf look reddened and slightly oedematous?
3. What has precipitated the presentation in the left calf?
4. What further assessments are required?

The medical team have been notified of Margaret's left calf and other observations remain unchanged.
While Margaret was being prepared to have an ultrasound, she complains of muscle spasms in the left calf.

5. Which blood tests should be ordered for Margaret and why?
6. Does this newly diagnosed condition relate to Margaret's reason for admission?
7. How will this newly diagnosed condition be managed and why? Consider medical and nursing management.

CONCEPT MAP 4.9 Evaluation and planning for Margaret

DISCHARGE PLANNING + COORDINATION OF CARE

How do the following areas of healthcare management **relate** to Margaret's presentation? Which members of the healthcare team are **involved** in each area of management?

Written home care instructions
Medication
INR tests
BP monitoring
Compression stockings

See GP and Practice Nurse for follow-up

Lifestyle modification:

Weight reduction, low fat and sodium diet, exercise

CONCEPT MAP 4.10 Discharge planning and coordination of care for Margaret

CONCEPT MAP SEQUENCE FOR HEART VALVE DISEASE – MITRAL REGURGITATION

Presentation

David Lee Chew is a 36-year-old chef who was brought to the emergency department by his wife. David has become fatigued over the last two months, is breathless on occasions and today has developed palpitations.

Concept maps 4.11–4.15 explore David's initial care in the emergency department.

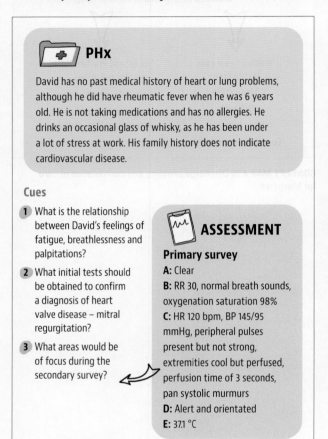

PHx

David has no past medical history of heart or lung problems, although he did have rheumatic fever when he was 6 years old. He is not taking medications and has no allergies. He drinks an occasional glass of whisky, as he has been under a lot of stress at work. His family history does not indicate cardiovascular disease.

Cues

1 What is the relationship between David's feelings of fatigue, breathlessness and palpitations?

2 What initial tests should be obtained to confirm a diagnosis of heart valve disease – mitral regurgitation?

3 What areas would be of focus during the secondary survey?

ASSESSMENT

Primary survey

A: Clear

B: RR 30, normal breath sounds, oxygenation saturation 98%

C: HR 120 bpm, BP 145/95 mmHg, peripheral pulses present but not strong, extremities cool but perfused, perfusion time of 3 seconds, pan systolic murmurs

D: Alert and orientated

E: 37.1 °C

CONCEPT MAP 4.11 Nursing assessment for David

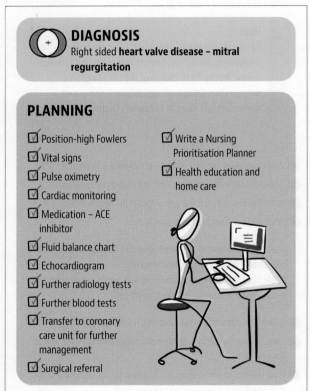

DIAGNOSIS

Right sided **heart valve disease – mitral regurgitation**

PLANNING

☑ Position-high Fowlers
☑ Vital signs
☑ Pulse oximetry
☑ Cardiac monitoring
☑ Medication – ACE inhibitor
☑ Fluid balance chart
☑ Echocardiogram
☑ Further radiology tests
☑ Further blood tests
☑ Transfer to coronary care unit for further management
☑ Surgical referral

☑ Write a Nursing Prioritisation Planner
☑ Health education and home care

CONCEPT MAP 4.12 Diagnosis and planning for David

INTERVENTIONS

1 Positioning – high Fowlers

2 Vital signs, frequency as determined by ADDS

3 Pulse oximetry and heart sounds

4 12-lead ECG

5 Medication – ACE inhibitors

6 Fluid balance chart

7 Blood tests

8 Radiology tests

9 Cardiology consultation

10 Surgical consultation

Health education and home care:

• Medication – ACE inhibitors

• Prophylactic antibiotics for surgical procedures

What further assessments should be initiated

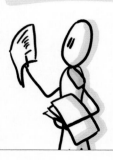

CONCEPT MAP 4.13 Nursing interventions for David

EVALUATION

David's stay in the emergency department for monitoring and further care for his heart valve disease – mitral regurgitation.

Plan:
Transfer David to the coronary care unit. Surgical team recommending a mitral valve replacement?

Cues   ① Why would a mitral valve replacement be considered as part of David's care?

CONCEPT MAP 4.14 Evaluation and planning for David

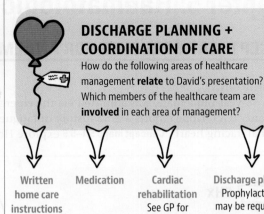

DISCHARGE PLANNING + COORDINATION OF CARE

How do the following areas of healthcare management **relate** to David's presentation? Which members of the healthcare team are **involved** in each area of management?

Written home care instructions

Medication

Cardiac rehabilitation
See GP for follow-up

Discharge planning
Prophylactic ABs may be required for some people with MV replacement who require dental work undertaken

CONCEPT MAP 4.15 Discharge planning and coordination of care for David

Chapter 5: Haematological System

CONCEPT MAP SEQUENCE FOR ANAEMIA

Presentation

Hope, a 58-year-old female, was admitted via the emergency department following referral from her general practitioner (GP). Hope reports a 2/52 history of fatigue, increased shortness of breath, headaches and an occasional 'racing heart'. **Concept maps 5.1–5.5** explore Hope's presentation in the emergency department.

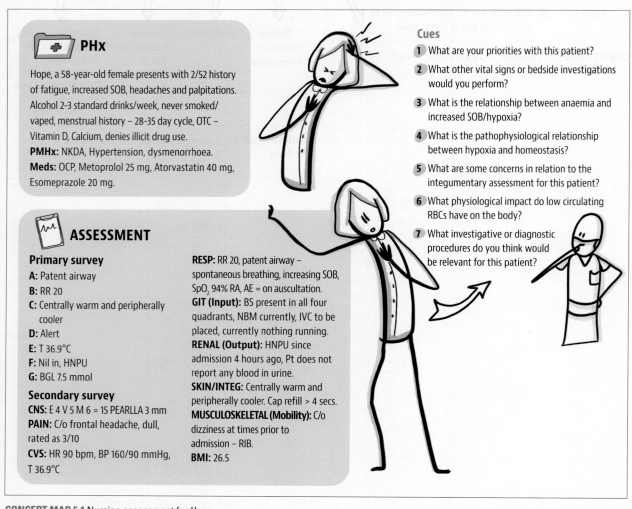

PHx

Hope, a 58-year-old female presents with 2/52 history of fatigue, increased SOB, headaches and palpitations. Alcohol 2-3 standard drinks/week, never smoked/vaped, menstrual history – 28-35 day cycle, OTC – Vitamin D, Calcium, denies illicit drug use.
PMHx: NKDA, Hypertension, dysmenorrhoea.
Meds: OCP, Metoprolol 25 mg, Atorvastatin 40 mg, Esomeprazole 20 mg.

ASSESSMENT

Primary survey
A: Patent airway
B: RR 20
C: Centrally warm and peripherally cooler
D: Alert
E: T 36.9°C
F: Nil in, HNPU
G: BGL 7.5 mmol

Secondary survey
CNS: E 4 V 5 M 6 = 15 PEARLLA 3 mm
PAIN: C/o frontal headache, dull, rated as 3/10
CVS: HR 90 bpm, BP 160/90 mmHg, T 36.9°C

RESP: RR 20, patent airway – spontaneous breathing, increasing SOB, SpO$_2$ 94% RA, AE = on auscultation.
GIT (Input): BS present in all four quadrants, NBM currently, IVC to be placed, currently nothing running.
RENAL (Output): HNPU since admission 4 hours ago, Pt does not report any blood in urine.
SKIN/INTEG: Centrally warm and peripherally cooler. Cap refill > 4 secs.
MUSCULOSKELETAL (Mobility): C/o dizziness at times prior to admission – RIB.
BMI: 26.5

Cues

1. What are your priorities with this patient?
2. What other vital signs or bedside investigations would you perform?
3. What is the relationship between anaemia and increased SOB/hypoxia?
4. What is the pathophysiological relationship between hypoxia and homeostasis?
5. What are some concerns in relation to the integumentary assessment for this patient?
6. What physiological impact do low circulating RBCs have on the body?
7. What investigative or diagnostic procedures do you think would be relevant for this patient?

CONCEPT MAP 5.1 Nursing assessment for Hope

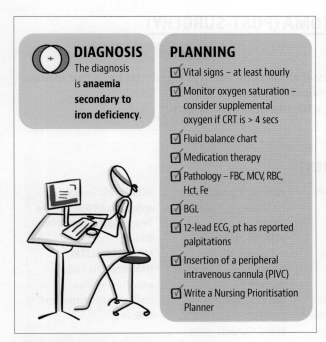

DIAGNOSIS

The diagnosis is **anaemia secondary to iron deficiency**.

PLANNING

- ☑ Vital signs – at least hourly
- ☑ Monitor oxygen saturation – consider supplemental oxygen if CRT is > 4 secs
- ☑ Fluid balance chart
- ☑ Medication therapy
- ☑ Pathology – FBC, MCV, RBC, Hct, Fe
- ☑ BGL
- ☑ 12-lead ECG, pt has reported palpitations
- ☑ Insertion of a peripheral intravenous cannula (PIVC)
- ☑ Write a Nursing Prioritisation Planner

CONCEPT MAP 5.2 Diagnosis and planning for Hope

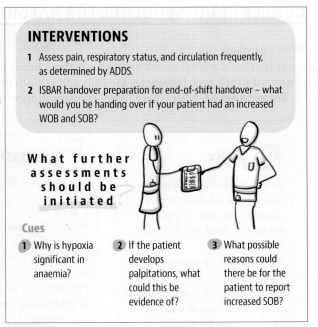

INTERVENTIONS

1 Assess pain, respiratory status, and circulation frequently, as determined by ADDS.

2 ISBAR handover preparation for end-of-shift handover – what would you be handing over if your patient had an increased WOB and SOB?

What further assessments should be initiated?

Cues

1 Why is hypoxia significant in anaemia?

2 If the patient develops palpitations, what could this be evidence of?

3 What possible reasons could there be for the patient to report increased SOB?

CONCEPT MAP 5.3 Nursing interventions for Hope

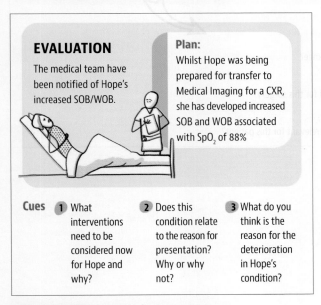

EVALUATION

The medical team have been notified of Hope's increased SOB/WOB.

Plan:
Whilst Hope was being prepared for transfer to Medical Imaging for a CXR, she has developed increased SOB and WOB associated with SpO$_2$ of 88%.

Cues

1 What interventions need to be considered now for Hope and why?

2 Does this condition relate to the reason for presentation? Why or why not?

3 What do you think is the reason for the deterioration in Hope's condition?

CONCEPT MAP 5.4 Evaluate and planning for Hope

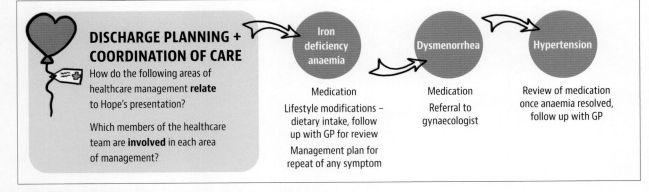

DISCHARGE PLANNING + COORDINATION OF CARE

How do the following areas of healthcare management **relate** to Hope's presentation?

Which members of the healthcare team are **involved** in each area of management?

Iron deficiency anaemia

Medication

Lifestyle modifications – dietary intake, follow up with GP for review

Management plan for repeat of any symptom

Dysmenorrhea

Medication

Referral to gynaecologist

Hypertension

Review of medication once anaemia resolved, follow up with GP

CONCEPT MAP 5.5 Discharge planning and coordination of care for Hope

CONCEPT MAP SEQUENCE FOR HAEMOTOMA (POST-SURGERY)

Presentation

Jason Jenkins is a 52-year-old male who is three hours post-femoral popliteal bypass graft. He has a past medical history of PTSD, type II diabetes mellitus and peripheral vascular disease.

Concept maps 5.6–5.10 explore Jason's presentation with a haematoma after surgery.

 PHx

Jason, a 52-year-old male, is 3 hours postoperative, following L Femoral popliteal bypass graft. (L FPBG)
PMHx: PTSD, T2DM, PVD, HTN, GORD, Hyperlipidaemia
NKDA. No alcohol or cigarettes/ illicit drugs
Meds: Escitalopram 20 mg, atorvastatin 40 mg, esomeprazole 20 mg, prazosin 2 mg, metformin 500XR

 ASSESSMENT

CNS: E4 V5 M6 = 15 PEARLA 4 mm
T: 36.4 °C
PAIN: C/o pain behind left knee. Rating as 8/10, burning, sharp, sudden onset
CVS: HR 115 bpm, regular. BP 100/65 mmHg. Centrally warm, peripherally cooler. CAP refill <3 secs, popliteal pulses DP R present, L only via Doppler, PT R present, L absent
RESP: RR 20, chest on auscultation clear throughout R = L. Nil cough. SpO$_2$ 98% RA
GIT: BS Audible in all quadrants. BGL 6.5 mmol/L
RENAL (Output): HNPU as yet

SKIN/INTEG: Surgical dressing intact with nil strike through ooze visible on the dressing
MUSCULOSKELETAL (Mobility): Strict RIB, with VTE prophylaxis - combination as documented
BMI: 24.0

Cues

1. What are your priorities with this patient?
2. What is the significance of the increase in pain and rigidity behind the knee?
3. What is the significance of VTE prophylaxis?
4. What is the pathophysiological relationship between PVD and the need for this surgery?
5. What are some concerns regarding the patient's observations?
6. What investigative or diagnostic procedures would you think would be relevant for this patient?

CONCEPT MAP 5.6 Nursing assessment for Jason

DIAGNOSIS

The diagnosis is **haematoma** post-surgery, requiring transfusion of PRBC

PLANNING

- ☑ Analgesia
- ☑ Order group and hold/ cross match if not already performed prior to surgery
- ☑ Insertion of second PIVC if not already in situ for blood transfusion
- ☑ Consent form check
- ☑ Blood product – confirm availability
- ☑ IV fluid with monitoring of fluid input and output
- ☑ Documentation – vital signs, fluid balance chart, PIVC
- ☑ VTE Prophylaxis
- ☑ Bloods and pathology
- ☑ Full physical assessment

- ☑ Write a Nursing Prioritisation Planner

Further investigations:
- ☑ 12-lead ECG
- ☑ Baseline observations prior to blood transfusion
- ☑ Surgical evacuation of haematoma?

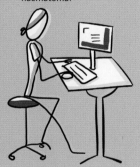

CONCEPT MAP 5.7 Diagnosis and planning for Jason

INTERVENTIONS

1 Assess pain, surgical site, blood transfusion observations, patient observations – including development of urticaria, rash, etc.

2 ISBAR handover preparation for end-of-shift handover – what would you be handing over if Jason had developed a fever during the blood transfusion?

What further assessments should be initiated?

Cues
1 What further questions or information would you like to know from Jason?

2 What is the deterioration or change in patient status here?

What is it related to pathophysiologically?

3 What clinical observations would alert you to a reaction to the PRBCs?

CONCEPT MAP 5.8 Nursing interventions for Jason

EVALUATION

The medical team have been notified of the increase in temperature to your patient during blood transfusion.

Plan:
Medical officer has requested you to hold the PRBC infusion for 30 minutes.

Cues

1 What interventions need to be considered now for your patient and why? What is your priority here?

2 If the PRBC was prescribed to be administered over four hours, and you are ceasing it for 30 mins does this impact the life of the product? What will you need to do to ensure no loss of blood product?

3 What do you think is the reasoning for increase in temperature? Is this a significant reaction and why?

CONCEPT MAP 5.9 Evaluation and planning for Jason

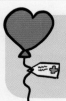

DISCHARGE PLANNING + COORDINATION OF CARE

How do the following areas of healthcare management **relate** to the patient presentation? Which members of the healthcare team are **involved** in each area of management?

Post-op bleed – reaction to PRBC	**Mobility postoperatively**	**Type 2 Diabetes**	**Wound and vascular follow–up**
Management and education to patient on delayed blood transfusion reactions.	Gait assessment – Physiotherapist	Patient education and health promotion regarding type 2 diabetes postoperatively – expectation of BGLs etc. – what to report.	Follow-up by wound care nurse in community.
Follow up with GP in one week	Management of wound site and haematoma – assessment of home surroundings for ADLs – may need OT referral also.		OPD appointment with vascular surgeon
			Review by GP for removal of staples 14 days post-op.

CONCEPT MAP 5.10 Discharge planning and coordination of care for Jason

Chapter 6: Central Nervous System

CONCEPT MAP SEQUENCE FOR AN ACUTE NEUROLOGICAL CONDITION

Presentation

Steven, an 18-year-old male, was admitted via emergency department with a base of skull fracture sustained in a high-speed MVA. He was the passenger and was wearing a seat belt. Other injuries include a fractured clavicle and closed head injury. **Concept maps 6.1–6.5** explore Steven's presentation in the emergency department.

 PHx

Steven, an **18-year-old male** was admitted via the emergency department with a **base of skull fracture** sustained in an **MVA** at high speed (>140 km/hr). He was the front seat passenger and was wearing a seat belt. He was not ejected from the vehicle. Extricated by emergency services. Other injuries include a **fractured left clavicle**, and **closed head injury**.

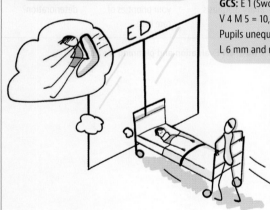

 ASSESSMENT

Primary survey
A: Patent
B: RR 14
C: Warm
D: ALOC
E: T 38.5 °C
F: IVF 166 ml/hr; IDC 50 ml/hr
G: BGL 4.6 mmol/L

Secondary survey
GCS: E 1 (Swollen shut) V 4 M 5 = 10, Pupils unequal, R 4 mm L 6 mm and non-reactive

PAIN: Responding to painful stimuli
CVS: HR 90 bpm, BP 180/95 mmHg, pedal pulses bounding. A 12-lead electrocardiogram showed a sinus rhythm with no abnormalities.
T: 38.5 °C
RESP: RR 14, patent airway – spontaneous breathing, not laborious
GIT (Input): IVF 166 mL/hr, NGT for gut decompression –

bile aspirate, strong ETOH smell, abdo soft, BS in all quadrants
RENAL (Output): IDC in situ 50 mL/hr – no sediment, straw coloured
SKIN/INTEG: Centrally and peripherally warm and well perfused.
MUSCULOSKELETAL (Mobility): Strict RIB, with chemical VTE prophylaxis
BMI: 22.4

Cues

1. What are your priorities with this patient? ABC.
2. What is the significance of the temperature in a closed head injury?
3. What is the relationship between head injury and pupillary response/s?
4. What is the pathophysiological relationship between base of skull fractures and level of consciousness?
5. What are some concerns in relation to the GCS assessment in this patient?
6. What physiological impact does a high-speed impact have on the body?
7. What investigative or diagnostic procedures do you think would be relevant for this patient?

CONCEPT MAP 6.1 Nursing assessment for Steven

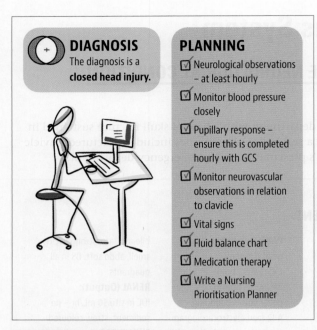

DIAGNOSIS

The diagnosis is a **closed head injury.**

PLANNING

☑ Neurological observations – at least hourly

☑ Monitor blood pressure closely

☑ Pupillary response – ensure this is completed hourly with GCS

☑ Monitor neurovascular observations in relation to clavicle

☑ Vital signs

☑ Fluid balance chart

☑ Medication therapy

☑ Write a Nursing Prioritisation Planner

CONCEPT MAP 6.2 Diagnosis and planning for Steven

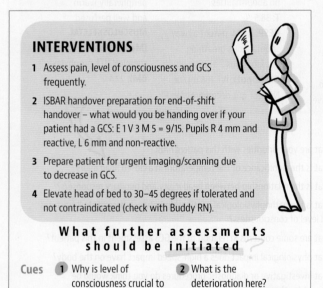

INTERVENTIONS

1 Assess pain, level of consciousness and GCS frequently.

2 ISBAR handover preparation for end-of-shift handover – what would you be handing over if your patient had a GCS: E 1 V 3 M 5 = 9/15. Pupils R 4 mm and reactive, L 6 mm and non-reactive.

3 Prepare patient for urgent imaging/scanning due to decrease in GCS.

4 Elevate head of bed to 30–45 degrees if tolerated and not contraindicated (check with Buddy RN).

What further assessments should be initiated ?

Cues

1 Why is level of consciousness crucial to observe in head injuries?

2 What is the deterioration here? What is the significance of the GCS change?

CONCEPT MAP 6.3 Nursing interventions for Steven

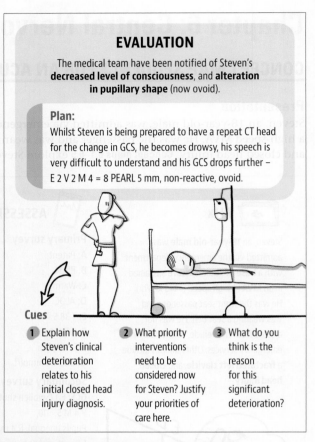

EVALUATION

The medical team have been notified of Steven's **decreased level of consciousness**, and **alteration in pupillary shape** (now ovoid).

Plan:

Whilst Steven is being prepared to have a repeat CT head for the change in GCS, he becomes drowsy, his speech is very difficult to understand and his GCS drops further – E 2 V 2 M 4 = 8 PEARL 5 mm, non-reactive, ovoid.

Cues

1 Explain how Steven's clinical deterioration relates to his initial closed head injury diagnosis.

2 What priority interventions need to be considered now for Steven? Justify your priorities of care here.

3 What do you think is the reason for this significant deterioration?

CONCEPT MAP 6.4 Evaluation and planning for Steven

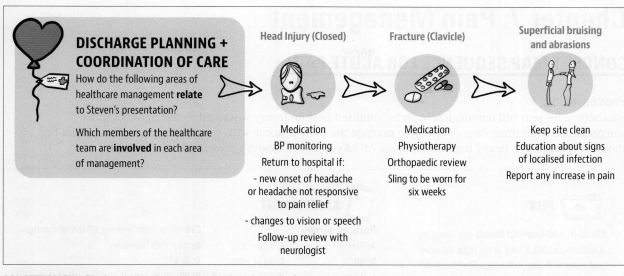

DISCHARGE PLANNING + COORDINATION OF CARE

How do the following areas of healthcare management **relate** to Steven's presentation?

Which members of the healthcare team are **involved** in each area of management?

Head Injury (Closed)

Medication
BP monitoring
Return to hospital if:
- new onset of headache or headache not responsive to pain relief
- changes to vision or speech
Follow-up review with neurologist

Fracture (Clavicle)

Medication
Physiotherapy
Orthopaedic review
Sling to be worn for six weeks

Superficial bruising and abrasions

Keep site clean
Education about signs of localised infection
Report any increase in pain

CONCEPT MAP 6.5 Discharge planning and coordination of care for Steven

Chapter 7: Pain Management

CONCEPT MAP SEQUENCE FOR ACUTE PAIN

Presentation

Elizabeth, a 39-year-old female, has been hospitalised post an injury sustained to her right shoulder. She presented after three days of trying to manage the pain at home with simple analgesia. She injured her shoulder 'dragging' a heavy bag. **Concept maps 7.1–7.5** explore Elizabeth's presentation/admission.

 PHx

Elizabeth, a **39-year-old female** was dragging a suitcase and felt a 'pop' in her right shoulder and immediate pain in the area. She continued to the hotel/destination. Ongoing pain increased over the course of the next 72 hours. Nil previous history of injury to that shoulder/arm. Elizabeth travelled from Fiji to Sydney one day ago.

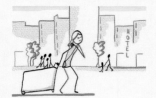

 ASSESSMENT

Primary survey

A: Patent   **E:** T 36.9 °C
B: RR 24   **F:** Nil in, HNPU
C: Warm   **G:** BGL 5.0 mmol/L
D: Alert

Secondary survey

CNS (Cognition): E 4 V 5 M 6 = 15, Pupils equal (PEARLA), 4 mm
PAIN: P – three days ago, pulling a suitcase. Q – stabbing and sharp pain. R – Pain is only in the right shoulder, with no radiation. S – at rest 7/10, movement 9/10. T – pain has been present for 3 days, getting worse. U – paracetamol, RICE, Ibuprofen with little effect.

CVS: HR 90 bpm and reg, BP 160/85 mmHg, pedal pulses bounding.
T: 36.9 °C
RESP: RR 20, patent airway – spontaneous breathing, SpO$_2$ 99% RA
GIT (Input): As tolerated.
RENAL (Output): HNPU over past 6 hours
SKIN/INTEG: Centrally and peripherally well perfused, bruising to right shoulder head, mild localised swelling to right shoulder. Otherwise grossly intact.
MUSCULOSKELETAL (Mobility): Minimal ability to mobilise due to increase in pain. Unable to dress self currently or put bra on.
BMI: 24.2

Cues

1. What are your priorities with this patient?

2. What is the significance of hypertension and tachypneoa in a patient with 9/10 pain?

3. What is your immediate course of action in regards to pain assessment? Is there any other information that you would seek?

4. What investigative or diagnostic procedures do you think would be relevant for this patient?

5. If the patient has already self-administered paracetamol and ibuprofen, could you administer this again? If so, within what time frame?

6. If you note bruising at the right shoulder head, what could this indicate?

7. Is there a risk of DVT in this patient with recent travel?

CONCEPT MAP 7.1 Nursing assessment for Elizabeth

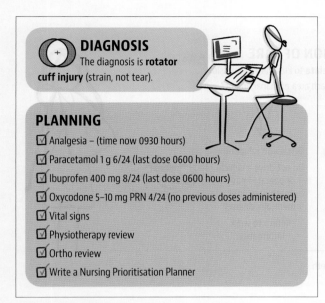

DIAGNOSIS

The diagnosis is **rotator cuff injury** (strain, not tear).

PLANNING

☑ Analgesia – (time now 0930 hours)

☑ Paracetamol 1 g 6/24 (last dose 0600 hours)

☑ Ibuprofen 400 mg 8/24 (last dose 0600 hours)

☑ Oxycodone 5–10 mg PRN 4/24 (no previous doses administered)

☑ Vital signs

☑ Physiotherapy review

☑ Ortho review

☑ Write a Nursing Prioritisation Planner

CONCEPT MAP 7.2 Diagnosis and planning for Elizabeth

INTERVENTIONS

1 Assess pain, level of consciousness, and observations.

2 ISBAR handover preparation for end-of-shift handover – what would you be handing over if your patient had a pain score of 9/10 post analgesia?

What further assessments should be initiated ?

Cues

1 What is the physiological link between vital signs and pain?

2 What possible reasons could there be for the patient to report no reduction in their pain?

CONCEPT MAP 7.3 Nursing interventions for Elizabeth

EVALUATION

The medical team have been notified of Elizabeth's pain – unchanged at 9/10.

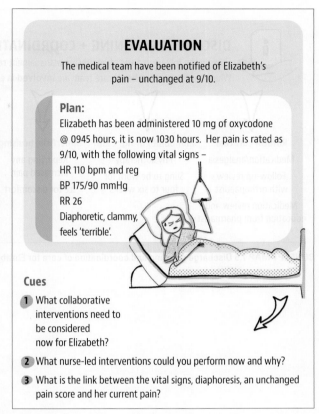

Plan:

Elizabeth has been administered 10 mg of oxycodone @ 0945 hours, it is now 1030 hours. Her pain is rated as 9/10, with the following vital signs –

HR 110 bpm and reg

BP 175/90 mmHg

RR 26

Diaphoretic, clammy, feels 'terrible'.

Cues

1 What collaborative interventions need to be considered now for Elizabeth?

2 What nurse-led interventions could you perform now and why?

3 What is the link between the vital signs, diaphoresis, an unchanged pain score and her current pain?

CONCEPT MAP 7.4 Evaluate and planning for Elizabeth

DISCHARGE PLANNING + COORDINATION OF CARE

How do the following areas of healthcare management **relate** to Elizabeth's admission?
Which members of the healthcare team are **involved** in each area of management?

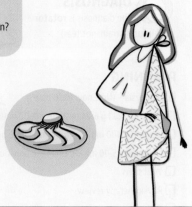

Rotator cuff tear

Medication/analgesia

Follow-up review
with orthopaedist

Medication review and
education from pharmacist

Immobility of right arm

Physiotherapy

Sling to be worn for
four to six weeks

Superficial bruising

Reporting any
increased pain

Ice for discomfort

Discharge education

Do not drive a vehicle
or operate heavy
machinery until
medically cleared

Return to work
information

CONCEPT MAP 7.5 Discharge planning and coordination of care for Elizabeth

Chapter 8: Integumentary Systems

CONCEPT MAP SEQUENCE FOR ERYTHRODERMA

Presentation

Mr James Harrison is a 35-year-old male who presented to the emergency department with generalised erythema, itchy warm skin, mildly swollen eyelids and some skin scaling. Mr Harrison also states that he feels 'shivery' at times and tired. He has not experienced generalised erythema before, and Mr Harrison thinks he may have something 'infectious'. **Concept maps 8.1–8.5** explore James' presentation/admission.

 PHx

Mr Harrison was diagnosed with **atopic dermatitis** as a child, which has been treated and controlled with topical corticosteroids. He is otherwise fit and well with no other medical or surgical history. Apart from his topical creams, Mr Harrison takes no other medications.

 ASSESSMENT

Primary survey
A: Clear
B: RR 20, SaO$_2$ 97%, nil wheeze or stridor present
C: HR 90 bpm, BP 130/80 mmHg
D: Alert and orientated complaining of severe generalised itch
E: 37.8 °C

Secondary survey
Head, face and neck: Slight eyelid swelling with mild lymphadenopathy of the neck.

Arms and hands: Generalised erythema with dry flaky skin across all surfaces and pustule-looking lesions on the elbows. Broken skin lesions on elbows and backs of hands where itch is more intense. Some oozing of lesions.
Chest, abdomen, back and buttocks: Generalised erythema across all surfaces, with lesions developing between the buttocks.
Inguinal area: Some pustules developing in skin folds including under the scrotum, with slight pungent smell noted from these lesions. No lymphadenopathy noted in the inguinal area.

Legs and feet: Generalised erythema with fine scaling present. Lesions noted across thighs, shins and in between the toes where scratching has occurred. Some discharge noted from these lesions.

(Mistry, Gupta, Alavi & Sibbald, 2015)

Cues

1. What are the general signs and symptoms at the skin level for erythroderma?
2. What are the systemic symptoms due to erthryoderma or its underlying cause?
3. What would be two important tests to assist in the diagnosis of erythroderma?
4. What other areas of the secondary survey would be documented, and are there any particular assessments that should be focused on apart from the integumentary system?

CONCEPT MAP 8.1 Nursing assessment for James

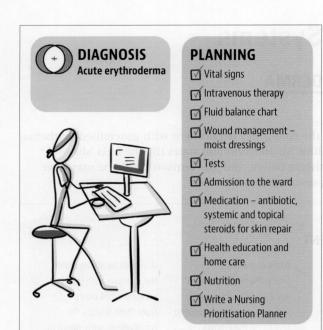

DIAGNOSIS
Acute erythroderma

PLANNING
- ☑ Vital signs
- ☑ Intravenous therapy
- ☑ Fluid balance chart
- ☑ Wound management – moist dressings
- ☑ Tests
- ☑ Admission to the ward
- ☑ Medication – antibiotic, systemic and topical steroids for skin repair
- ☑ Health education and home care
- ☑ Nutrition
- ☑ Write a Nursing Prioritisation Planner

CONCEPT MAP 8.2 Diagnosis and planning for James

INTERVENTIONS

1. Vital signs, frequency as determined by ADDS
2. Intravenous therapy
3. Fluid balance chart
4. Wound management – moist dressings
5. Tests
6. Medication – antibiotic, systemic and topical steroids for skin repair

Health education and home care:
- Wound management
- Nutrition

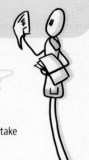

What further assessments should be initiated?

Cues
1. What other assessments should we undertake for James'?

CONCEPT MAP 8.3 Nursing interventions for James

EVALUATION

James states he feels better as the steroids and wet dressings have made his skin feel less irritated. He also noted that since taking an antibiotic his skin does not smell as much.

Plan:
James will be discharged home, with medication to assist in the repair of his skin.

Cues
1. Why is it important that James practises good wound management?
2. Which medication would James be discharged with and what are the specific roles of the medication?

CONCEPT MAP 8.4 Evaluation and planning for James

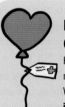

DISCHARGE PLANNING + COORDINATION OF CARE

How do the following areas of healthcare management **relate** to James' presentation? Which members of the healthcare team are **involved** in each area of management?

Skin repair
Patient education on signs and symptoms of exacerbation of erythroderma including a management plan

Follow-up appointments with the dermatologist and the GP

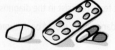

CONCEPT MAP 8.5 Discharge planning and coordination of care for James

CONCEPT MAP SEQUENCE FOR A BURN INJURY

Presentation

Mr Howard Gardener's lawn mower exploded at around 8 a.m. and his wife found him with his clothing on fire and he was rolling on the ground to stop his clothes burning. Mrs Gardener sprayed him with the hose to cool the burns and also called the ambulance service. The paramedic assessment of the burnt skin surface area was approximately 45 per cent burns to his face, arms, front and back of trunk and legs. The burns were a mixture of superficial, partial-thickness and full-thickness burns. Howard had two large bore intravenous cannulas, one in each antecubital fossa, with 0.9% sodium chloride running in each intravenous line.

Concept maps 8.6–8.10 explore Howard's initial care in the emergency department.

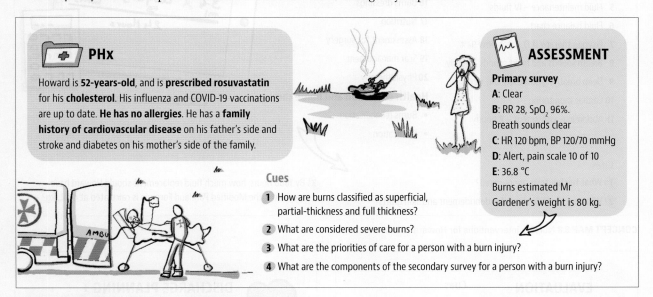

PHx

Howard is **52-years-old**, and is **prescribed rosuvastatin** for his **cholesterol**. His influenza and COVID-19 vaccinations are up to date. **He has no allergies.** He has a **family history of cardiovascular disease** on his father's side and stroke and diabetes on his mother's side of the family.

ASSESSMENT

Primary survey
A: Clear
B: RR 28, SpO$_2$ 96%.
Breath sounds clear
C: HR 120 bpm, BP 120/70 mmHg
D: Alert, pain scale 10 of 10
E: 36.8 °C
Burns estimated Mr Gardener's weight is 80 kg.

Cues

1 How are burns classified as superficial, partial-thickness and full thickness?

2 What are considered severe burns?

3 What are the priorities of care for a person with a burn injury?

4 What are the components of the secondary survey for a person with a burn injury?

CONCEPT MAP 8.6 Nursing assessment for Howard

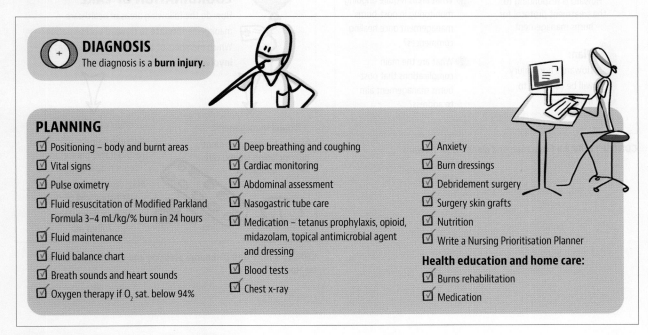

DIAGNOSIS
The diagnosis is a **burn injury**.

PLANNING

- ☑ Positioning – body and burnt areas
- ☑ Vital signs
- ☑ Pulse oximetry
- ☑ Fluid resuscitation of Modified Parkland Formula 3–4 mL/kg/% burn in 24 hours
- ☑ Fluid maintenance
- ☑ Fluid balance chart
- ☑ Breath sounds and heart sounds
- ☑ Oxygen therapy if O$_2$ sat. below 94%

- ☑ Deep breathing and coughing
- ☑ Cardiac monitoring
- ☑ Abdominal assessment
- ☑ Nasogastric tube care
- ☑ Medication – tetanus prophylaxis, opioid, midazolam, topical antimicrobial agent and dressing
- ☑ Blood tests
- ☑ Chest x-ray

- ☑ Anxiety
- ☑ Burn dressings
- ☑ Debridement surgery
- ☑ Surgery skin grafts
- ☑ Nutrition
- ☑ Write a Nursing Prioritisation Planner

Health education and home care:
- ☑ Burns rehabilitation
- ☑ Medication

CONCEPT MAP 8.7 Diagnosis and planning for Howard

INTERVENTIONS

In the burns unit:

1 Positioning – Fowlers and burns areas

2 Vital signs – hourly

3 Pulse oximetry – hourly

4 Fluid resuscitation of Modified Parkland Formula 3–4 mL/kg/% burn in 24 hours

5 Fluid maintenance – IV fluids

6 Fluid balance chart

7 Oxygen therapy if O_2 sat. below 94%

8 Breath sounds and heart sounds – hourly

9 Deep breathing and coughing – hourly

10 Cardiac monitoring

11 Abdominal assessment – 8 hourly

12 Nasogastric tube care

13 Medication – opioid infusion, midazolam infusion, topical antimicrobial agent and dressing

14 Monitor for anxiety and depression

15 Pain assessment

16 Burns dressings

17 Nutrition

18 Assessment for surgery

19 Scar management

20 Physiotherapy

Health education and home care:

• Burns rehabilitation

• Medication

What further assessments should be initiated

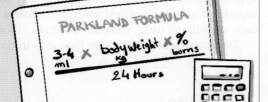

Cues

1 What further tests are required?

2 What are the indications for debridement and skin grafts?

3 By 1600 hours, how much fluid replacement should Howard have received if the Modified Parkland Formula is calculated at 4 mL/kg?

CONCEPT MAP 8.8 Nursing interventions for Howard

EVALUATION

Howard is responding to the treatment protocol for burns management.

Plan:
Howard's burn injury will be continue to monitored.

Cues

1 What areas require ongoing monitoring in post-burns management once healing commences?

2 What are the main complications that post-burns management aim to address?

CONCEPT MAP 8.9 Evaluation and planning for Howard

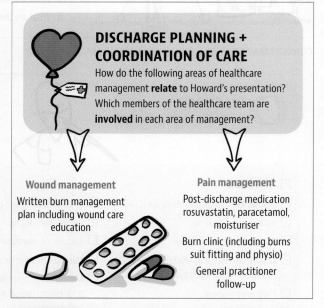

DISCHARGE PLANNING + COORDINATION OF CARE

How do the following areas of healthcare management **relate** to Howard's presentation? Which members of the healthcare team are **involved** in each area of management?

Wound management

Written burn management plan including wound care education

Pain management

Post-discharge medication rosuvastatin, paracetamol, moisturiser

Burn clinic (including burns suit fitting and physio)

General practitioner follow-up

CONCEPT MAP 8.10 Discharge planning and coordination of care for Howard

CONCEPT MAP SEQUENCE FOR A WOUND INFECTION

Presentation

Roger Kruger is a 68-year-old man who has been admitted to the intensive care unit post-cardiac surgery. His sternal surgical wound appears to be clean and dry for the first 24 hours. On the third day, the pm shift assessment of Roger's wound noted the proximal end of his sternal wound is starting to appear to be red, with increased warmth at that site. Roger's temperature is 37.3 °C and his blood glucose reading 11.9 mmol/L. Roger has a history of type 2 diabetes. It was planned to move Roger to the cardiac ward in the next 24 hours, but the infection has occurred and his blood glucose levels have been unstable postoperatively with persistent hyperglycaemia despite a short-acting insulin infusion. Because of this, the decision was made to keep Roger in the intensive care unit to stabilise his blood glucose levels and monitor the sternal wound infection.

Concept maps 8.11–8.15 explore Roger's care in the intensive care unit.

 PHx

Roger has had type 2 diabetes for the last 24 years, and the diabetes has been controlled with oral hypoglycaemics.

Cues

1 What other assessments should be made?

 ASSESSMENT

CNS: Alert and orientated
CVS: BP 135/75 mmHg, HR 80 bpm, T: 37.3 °C, peripherally perfused
Resp: Scattered fine crackles at the base of the lungs. RR 24, SaO$_2$ 96%
GIT: Bowel sounds present with a non-tender abdomen
Renal: Urine output approximate 1 mL/kg/hr

Metabolic: BGL 11.9 mmol/L
Integumentary: Warm dry skin
Wound: Length 12 cm, width 0.3 mm, depth 0.5 mm. Currently no exudate, redness to proximal end of wound, with increased warmth at that site
Musculoskeletal: Equal limb strength

CONCEPT MAP 8.11 Nursing assessment for Roger

DIAGNOSIS
Sternal wound infection post-coronary artery graft surgery

PLANNING

- ☑ Wound dressing
- ☑ Blood glucose measurement
- ☑ Sliding scale insulin
- ☑ Flucloxacillin 2 g QID IV wound infection
- ☑ Write a Nursing Prioritisation Planner

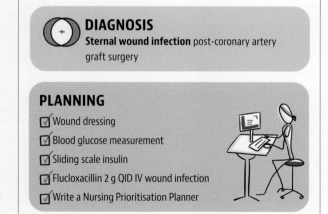

CONCEPT MAP 8.12 Diagnosis and planning for Roger

INTERVENTIONS

Postoperative care including for coronary artery graft surgery:

1 Sternal dressing daily
2 Blood glucose measurement 2 hourly
3 Sliding scale insulin
4 Flucloxacillin 2 g QID IV

Health education:

- Medication
- Cardiac rehabilitation

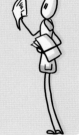

What further assessments should be initiated?

CONCEPT MAP 8.13 Nursing interventions for Roger

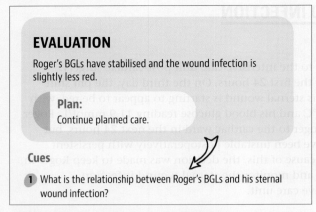

EVALUATION

Roger's BGLs have stabilised and the wound infection is slightly less red.

Plan:
Continue planned care.

Cues

1 What is the relationship between Roger's BGLs and his sternal wound infection?

CONCEPT MAP 8.14 Evaluation and planning for Roger

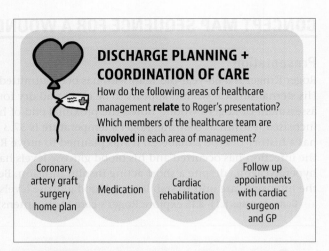

DISCHARGE PLANNING + COORDINATION OF CARE

How do the following areas of healthcare management **relate** to Roger's presentation? Which members of the healthcare team are **involved** in each area of management?

Coronary artery graft surgery home plan

Medication

Cardiac rehabilitation

Follow up appointments with cardiac surgeon and GP

CONCEPT MAP 8.15 Discharge planning and coordination of care for Roger

Chapter 9: Urinary System

CONCEPT MAP SEQUENCE FOR A PERSON WITH CHRONIC KIDNEY DISEASE (CKD)

Presentation

Maxine Broche is a 48-year-old female who was referred to the local emergency department by her general practitioner as her recent blood tests indicated abnormal renal function. Her GFR is <19. Maxine has CKD, stage four and has a past medical history of hypertension, transient ischaemic attacks, type II diabetes mellitus and is morbidly obese with a BMI of 38.

Concept maps 9.1–9.5 explore Maxine's presentation.

 PHx

Maxine is a **48-year-old female**, who has a GFR of <19. She has **CKD, stage four**, and a PMHx of HTN, TIA's, T2DM, and is **morbidly obese** with a BMI of 38.

 ASSESSMENT

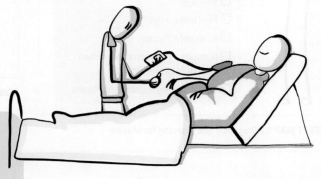

Primary survey

A: Patent

B: RR 16 bpm

C: Centrally warm

D: Alert

E: Skin coated – white crystals

F: Nil in, HNPU

G: BGL 16.2 mmol/L

Secondary survey

CNS (Cognition): E 4 V 5 M 6 = 15, Pupils equal PEARLA 4 mm

PAIN: currently denies

CVS: HR 60 bpm, BP 195/105 mmHg, pedal pulses bounding. A 12 lead electrocardiogram showed a sinus rhythm with peaked T waves.

T: 35.9 °C

RESP: RR 16, patent airway – spontaneous breathing, not laborious, metallic breath

GIT: Abdo SNT. BGL 16.2 mmol/L (2 hours post prandial)

RENAL: HNPU in >24 hours.

SKIN/INTEG: Centrally warm, peripherally cooler, 'coating' on skin.

MUSCULOSKELETAL (Mobility): Mobile.

BMI: 38

Cues

1. What are your priorities with this patient?
2. What is the significance of peaked T waves?
3. What is the relationship between renal failure and temperature regulation?
4. What is the pathophysiological relationship between blood pressure and CKD?
5. What are some concerns in relation to the skin assessment of this patient?
6. What other assessments would you consider for this patient?
7. What investigative or diagnostic procedures do you think would be relevant for this patient?

CONCEPT MAP 9.1 Nursing assessment for Maxine

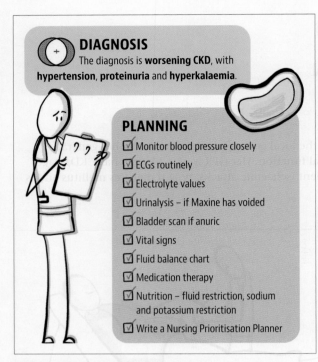

DIAGNOSIS

The diagnosis is **worsening CKD**, with **hypertension**, **proteinuria** and **hyperkalaemia**.

PLANNING

- ☑ Monitor blood pressure closely
- ☑ ECGs routinely
- ☑ Electrolyte values
- ☑ Urinalysis – if Maxine has voided
- ☑ Bladder scan if anuric
- ☑ Vital signs
- ☑ Fluid balance chart
- ☑ Medication therapy
- ☑ Nutrition – fluid restriction, sodium and potassium restriction
- ☑ Write a Nursing Prioritisation Planner

CONCEPT MAP 9.2 Diagnosis and planning for Maxine

INTERVENTIONS

1 Assess blood pressure, urine, skin and laboratory values regularly.

2 ISBAR handover preparation for end-of-shift handover – what would you be handing over if your patient had peaked T waves, arrythmias intermittently, and anuria?

What further assessments should be initiated

Cues
1 Why is blood pressure important in CKD?

2 What is the deterioration here? What is the significance of the T wave changes?

3 What possible reasons could there be for the uraemic frost on the patient's skin?

4 Does this patient need IV fluids?

CONCEPT MAP 9.3 Nursing interventions for Maxine

EVALUATION

The medical team have been notified of Maxine's increasing blood pressure to > 200 systolic, peaked T waves and irregular heart rhythm.

Plan:
Maxine's blood pressure continues to rise, and her HR is irregular, with arrythmia noted on her ECG. She is anuric, and has scaly, dry and crusted skin.

Cues
1 Undertake an A-G assessment of Maxine. What is your priority here?

2 Does this clinical deterioration relate to Maxine's CKD?

3 What do you think is the reason for this significant deterioration?

CONCEPT MAP 9.4 Evaluation and planning for Maxine

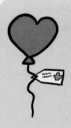

DISCHARGE PLANNING + COORDINATION OF CARE

How do the following areas of healthcare management **relate** to Maxine's presentation?

Which members of the healthcare team are **involved** in each area of management?

CKD – acute on chronic

Medication

BP monitoring

Follow-up review with nephrologist

Hypertension – exacerbation of

Medication

Diet – Na reduction, fluid restriction

Worsening CKD

Hyperkalaemia

Diet, dietitian referral

Nephrologist

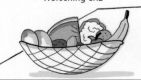
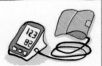

CONCEPT MAP 9.5 Discharge planning and coordination of care for Maxine

CONCEPT MAP SEQUENCE FOR A PERSON WITH FLUID OVERLOAD – HYPERVOLAEMIA

Presentation

Jessica is a 24-year-old female who is 2/7 post-laparotomy for a gangrenous appendix. She has developed hypervolaemia. She has no previous medical or surgical history.

Concept maps 9.6–9.10 explore Jessica's presentation/admission.

 PHx

Jessica is a 24-year-old female who is 2/7 post-laparotomy for a gangrenous appendix. She has no previous medical or surgical history. In the past 24 hours her fluid balance is +2785 mL, she has IVF @ 125 mL/hr and is NBM.

 ASSESSMENT

Primary survey

A: Patent

B: RR 16 bpm

C: Centrally warm

D: Alert

E: Pitting oedema

F: Nil in, IDC

G: BGL 10.2 mmol/L

Secondary survey

CNS (Cognition): E 4 V 5 M 6 = 15, Pupils equal PEARLA 4 mm

PAIN: 2/10 on movement. PCA running.

CVS: HR 120 bpm, BP 165/85 mmHg. A 12-lead electrocardiogram showed sinus arrhythmia with peaked T waves. T 37.9 °C. Bilateral pitting oedema 3+

RESP: RR 16, patent airway – spontaneous breathing, not laborious bilateral crepitus to mid/lower zones R=L

GIT: Abdo soft, tender on palpation. BS absent

RENAL: IDC in situ urine output for last four hours 42 mL. Sedimented, amber in colour

SKIN/INTEG: Centrally warm, peripherally cooler, oedema to bilateral lower limbs. Has removed ring to right index finger as it was 'tight'. TEDS in situ

MUSCULOSKELETAL (Mobility): Mobile with assistance

BMI: 24

Cues

1 What are the nurse-led priorities for this patient?

2 What are the collaborative priorities of care for Jessica?

CONCEPT MAP 9.6 Nursing assessment for Jessica

 DIAGNOSIS

The diagnosis is **hypervolaemia, hypertension, hyperkalaemia** and **hypernatraemia**

PLANNING

- ☑ Monitor blood pressure closely (consider invasive monitoring)
- ☑ ECGs routinely to monitor for T waves
- ☑ Electrolyte values
- ☑ Urinalysis
- ☑ Vital signs
- ☑ Fluid balance chart
- ☑ Medication therapy
- ☑ Remove TEDs due to oedema
- ☑ Neurovascular observations
- ☑ Write a Nursing Prioritisation Planner

CONCEPT MAP 9.7 Diagnosis and planning for Jessica

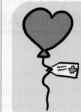

INTERVENTIONS

1 Regular ECGs due to peaked T waves.

2 Strict fluid balance chart monitoring.

3 Assess blood pressure, urine, skin and laboratory values regularly.

4 ISBAR handover preparation for end-of-shift handover – what would your clinical handover include if your patient had pitting oedema, hypertension and creps on auscultation?

What further assessments should be initiated ?

Cues

1 Why is blood pressure important in hypervolaemia?

2 What is the deterioration here? What is the significance of the urine output?

3 What possible reasons would there be for the creps on auscultation?

4 Does this patient need IV fluids?

5 What would peaked T waves indicate? What are the priorities of care in response to peaked T waves?

CONCEPT MAP 9.8 Nursing interventions for Jessica

DISCHARGE PLANNING + COORDINATION OF CARE

How do the following areas of healthcare management **relate** to Jessica's presentation? Which members of the healthcare team are **involved** in each area of management?

Hypervolaemia	Creps on auscultation	Peripheral oedema
Medication	Medication	Physiotherapist review – oedema and mobilisation
BP monitoring	Hypervolaemia – correction of electrolytes, control of BP	Occupational therapist review – if ongoing oedema
Daily weight, same scales, same time daily		
Fluid restriction management		

CONCEPT MAP 9.10 Discharge planning and coordination of care for Jessica

EVALUATION

The medical team have been notified of Jessica's developing hypertension and decrease in urine output. Noted also is her increased work of breathing (with associated creps) and arrythmias on 12-lead ECG.

Plan:
Jessica's blood pressure continues to rise, and her HR is irregular, she has worsening shortness of breath and increased work of breathing. Her urine output is 0 mL for the past hour; with 125 mL 'in'. Her fluid balance over the past 24 hours is a positive balance of 2875 mL.

Cues

1 What interventions need to be considered now for Jessica? What is your priority here?

2 Does this clinical deterioration relate to Jessica's surgery?

3 What do you think is the reason for this significant deterioration?

CONCEPT MAP 9.9 Evaluation and planning for Jessica

Chapter 10: Endocrine System

CONCEPT MAP SEQUENCE FOR A PERSON WITH AN ENDOCRINOLOGICAL CONDITION

Presentation

Wendy Mullins is a 42-year-old woman who has been hospitalised for cellulitis following an insect bite on her right forearm. Wendy initially presented to her general practitioner (GP) for review and was prescribed oral antibiotics. Since commencing these antibiotics, Wendy has developed vaginal thrush, a UTI and her cellulitis has worsened. Her BGL on her home glucometer was 22.4 mmol/L, and Wendy reports feeling 'tired, hot and sweaty, and thirsty'. **Concept maps 10.1–10.5** explore Wendy's hospitalisation.

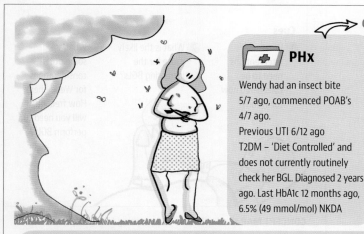

Cues

PHx

Wendy had an insect bite 5/7 ago, commenced POAB's 4/7 ago.
Previous UTI 6/12 ago
T2DM – 'Diet Controlled' and does not currently routinely check her BGL. Diagnosed 2 years ago. Last HbA1c 12 months ago, 6.5% (49 mmol/mol) NKDA

1. What are your priorities with this patient? ABC
2. What is the significance of the temperature in Wendy's current status?
3. What is the relationship between hyperglycaemia and infection?
4. What is the pathophysiological relationship between inflammation, infection and diabetes (type 2)?
5. What are some concerns in relation to CVS assessment with this patient?
6. What physiological impact does hyperglycaemia have on the patient?
7. What investigative or diagnostic procedures do you think would be relevant for this patient?

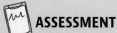

ASSESSMENT

Primary survey
A: Patent
B: RR 20
C: Warm
D: Alert
E: T 39.1 °C
F: IVF 166 mL/hr, HNPU
G: BGL 24.8 mmoL

Secondary survey
CNS (Cognition): E 4 V 5 M 6 = 15, Pupils equal, 4 mm, reactive to light (PEARLA)

PAIN: C/o pain on urination, lower abdominal pain to both R and L quadrant.
CVS: HR 105 bpm, BP 140/80 mmHg, pedal pulses bounding. A 12 lead electrocardiograph showed a sinus rhythm with no abnormalities.
T: 39.1 C
RESP: RR 20, patent airway – spontaneous breathing
GIT (Input): IVF 166 mLs/hr, BS present in all quadrants. BGL 24.8 mmol/L via glucometer.

RENAL (Output): Keytones negative. Awaiting urine sample/ward u/a. Patient denies haematuria.
SKIN/INTEG: Centrally and peripherally warm and well perfused – hot to touch.
MUSCULOSKELETAL (Mobility): Strict RIB, with VTE prophylaxis
BMI: 32.4
Wendy is in the general medical ward. She has received one dose of IV ABs; paracetamol is charted but has not yet been administered.

CONCEPT MAP 10.1 Nursing assessment for Wendy

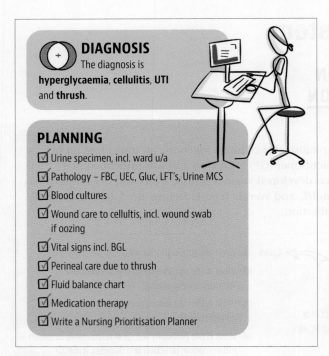

DIAGNOSIS

The diagnosis is **hyperglycaemia**, **cellulitis**, **UTI** and **thrush**.

PLANNING

- ☑ Urine specimen, incl. ward u/a
- ☑ Pathology – FBC, UEC, Gluc, LFT's, Urine MCS
- ☑ Blood cultures
- ☑ Wound care to cellultis, incl. wound swab if oozing
- ☑ Vital signs incl. BGL
- ☑ Perineal care due to thrush
- ☑ Fluid balance chart
- ☑ Medication therapy
- ☑ Write a Nursing Prioritisation Planner

CONCEPT MAP 10.2 Diagnosis and planning for Wendy

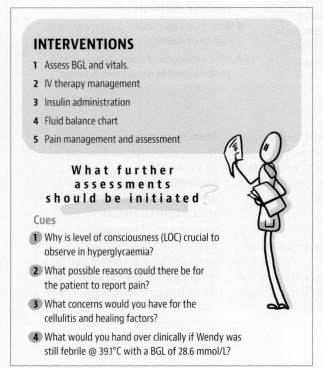

INTERVENTIONS

1. Assess BGL and vitals.
2. IV therapy management
3. Insulin administration
4. Fluid balance chart
5. Pain management and assessment

What further assessments should be initiated?

Cues

1. Why is level of consciousness (LOC) crucial to observe in hyperglycaemia?
2. What possible reasons could there be for the patient to report pain?
3. What concerns would you have for the cellulitis and healing factors?
4. What would you hand over clinically if Wendy was still febrile @ 39.1°C with a BGL of 28.6 mmol/L?

CONCEPT MAP 10.3 Nursing interventions for Wendy

EVALUATION

The medical team have been notified of Wendy's unchanged temperature and worsening hyperglycaemia (increasing BGL).

Plan:

Wendy has been prescribed an insulin infusion. Having not previously been on insulin, and weighing 94 kg, she has been prescribed insulin related to her weight. Her BGL is 28.6 mmol/L which is > 20, meaning she requires (as per the protocol outlined in the Evidence Based Practice box and Figure 10.1) 12 units of a short-acting insulin.

Cues

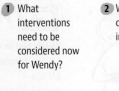

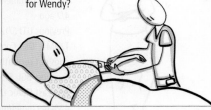

1. What interventions need to be considered now for Wendy?
2. What is the likely cause for the increasing BGLs?
3. What are some other considerations for Wendy here? How frequently will you need to perform BGLs?

CONCEPT MAP 10.4 Evaluation and planning for Wendy

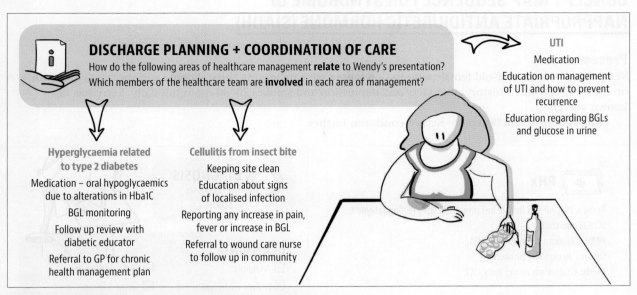

DISCHARGE PLANNING + COORDINATION OF CARE

How do the following areas of healthcare management **relate** to Wendy's presentation?
Which members of the healthcare team are **involved** in each area of management?

Hyperglycaemia related to type 2 diabetes

Medication – oral hypoglycaemics due to alterations in Hba1C

BGL monitoring

Follow up review with diabetic educator

Referral to GP for chronic health management plan

Cellulitis from insect bite

Keeping site clean

Education about signs of localised infection

Reporting any increase in pain, fever or increase in BGL

Referral to wound care nurse to follow up in community

UTI

Medication

Education on management of UTI and how to prevent recurrence

Education regarding BGLs and glucose in urine

CONCEPT MAP 10.5 Discharge planning and coordination of care for Wendy

CONCEPT MAP SEQUENCE FOR SYNDROME OF NAPPROPRIATE ANTIDIURETIC HORMONE (SIADH)

Presentation

Kerry Brouff is a 28-year-old female who has presented with increasing thirst, fatigue and shortness of breath on exertion. She has a history of anxiety and depression and smokes 20–30 cigarettes daily. Kerry has no known allergies.

Concept maps 10.6–10.10 explore Kerry's condition further.

 PHx

Kerry, a 28-year-old female has presented with feeling fatigued, SOBOE and thirst.
PMHx: Anxiety, depression. NKDA.
Smokes 20 cigs/day (tobacco)
Meds: Citalopram 20 mg daily, OCP.

 ASSESSMENT

CNS: E4 V5 M6 = 15 PEARLA 4 mm.
T: 37.4 °C
PAIN: C/o feeling exhausted. Some muscle twitching/pain but intermittent
CVS: HR 115 bpm, regular. BP 160/70 mmHg. Centrally warm, peripherally cooler. Capillary refill time < 3secs
RESP: RR 22, Increased WOB on exertion, Chest on auscultation clear throughout R=L with crepitus to lower zones bibasally. Nil cough. SpO$_2$ 98% RA.
GIT: BS audible in all quadrants. BGL 6.5 mmol/L. Nausea, reports vomiting prior to presentation
RENAL (Output): HNPU for past 4 hours
SKIN/INTEG: Poor integrity, dry skin, grossly intact. Nil skin tears. Oedema to lower limbs
MUSCULOSKELETAL (Mobility): Strict RIB, with VTE prophylaxis
BMI: 28.0

Cues

1. What are your priorities with this patient?
2. What is the significance of the increased work of breathing?
3. What is the significance of VTE prophylaxis?
4. What is the pathophysiological relationship between SIADH and presenting complaints?
5. What are some concerns in relationship to the patient's presentation?

CONCEPT MAP 10.6 Nursing assessment for Kerry

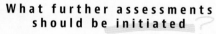 **DIAGNOSIS**
The diagnosis is **SIADH**

PLANNING

- ☑ Analgesia
- ☑ IV fluid with monitoring of fluid input and output
- ☑ BGL – sliding scale
- ☑ Documentation – vital signs, fluid balance chart, PIVC
- ☑ VTE Prophylaxis
- ☑ Bloods & Pathology
- ☑ Cease citalopram
- ☑ Serum Sodium
- ☑ Monitor for seizures
- ☑ Full physical assessment
- ☑ Write a Nursing Prioritisation Planner

Further investigations
- ☑ CXR/AXR

CONCEPT MAP 10.7 Diagnosis and planning for Kerry

INTERVENTIONS

1. Assess pain, urine output, peripheral perfusion and vital signs.
2. ISBAR handover preparation for end of shift handover – what would you be handing over if your patient had a decreasing LOC?

What further assessments should be initiated

Cues

1. What further questions or information would you like to know from the patient?
2. What is the deterioration or change in patient status here? What is it related to pathophysiologically?
3. What could be the reason for SIADH occurring?

CONCEPT MAP 10.8 Nursing interventions for Kerry

EVALUATION

The medical team have been notified of the decrease in LOC in your patient.

Plan:

Medical officer has requested further pathology (serum Na) and a repeat in vital signs, and changing IV fluids to 3% hypertonic saline.

Cues

1. What interventions need to be considered now for your patient? What is your priority here?

2. The patient has been prescribed 100 mLs of 3% NaCl. What are you nursing considerations here?

3. What do you think is the reasoning for alteration to LOC?

CONCEPT MAP 10.9 Evaluation and planning for Kerry

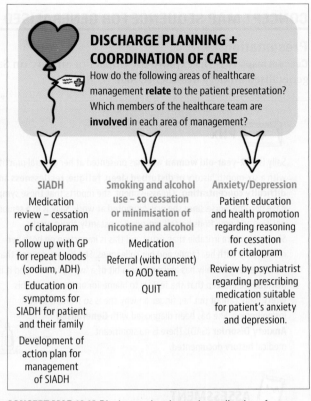

DISCHARGE PLANNING + COORDINATION OF CARE

How do the following areas of healthcare management **relate** to the patient presentation? Which members of the healthcare team are **involved** in each area of management?

SIADH

Medication review – cessation of citalopram

Follow up with GP for repeat bloods (sodium, ADH)

Education on symptoms for SIADH for patient and their family

Development of action plan for management of SIADH

Smoking and alcohol use – so cessation or minimisation of nicotine and alcohol

Medication

Referral (with consent) to AOD team.

QUIT

Anxiety/Depression

Patient education and health promotion regarding reasoning for cessation of citalopram

Review by psychiatrist regarding prescribing medication suitable for patient's anxiety and depression.

CONCEPT MAP 10.10 Discharge planning and coordination of care for Kerry

Chapter 11: Mental Health and Substance Use

CONCEPT MAP SEQUENCE FOR GENERALISED ANXIETY DISORDER (GAD)

Presentation

Concept maps 11.1–11.5 explore the impact of anxiety on Sally's life and strategies to manage the impacts of generalised anxiety disorder (GAD).

 PHx

Sally is a **32-year-old woman** who has presented at her general practitioner with a six-month history of **disturbed sleep**, **fatigue**, **restlessness** and **difficulty concentrating**. On assessment, she reports that these symptoms have become worse since she was promoted at work. Sally is in a senior position and now finds herself worrying constantly about work. She is also more irritable than usual and this is impacting on both her relationship with her family and her colleagues. She is now worried that she may lose her job. Sally has always been a bit of a 'worry bunny' and it is the disturbance in sleep that she feels is to blame for an increase in this worry. Sally cannot put her finger on why she is so worried about losing her job. She has been diagnosed with **Generalised Anxiety Disorder** (GAD). There is no significant medical history documented.

DRUG AND ALCOHOL HISTORY

Current use: Drinks a glass or two of wine while preparing dinner.
History of use: Minimal alcohol intake, usually when out with friends. No previous drug history or prescribed medication.
AUDIT score and interpretation: 8. Some simple advice on managing drinking may be offered.
Level of motivation: Does not feel motivated to change at present because Sally feels wine helps her to relax.

 ASSESSMENT

MENTAL STATUS EXAMINATION (MSE)

Behaviour: Sally appears to be quite uncomfortable during the interview, restless and sitting on the edge of her chair.
Appearance: Sally is well-dressed and well-groomed; she appears to be taking interest in her appearance.
Mood: Sally describes her mood as being fine but she is concerned about her constant worrying; affect is congruent with description of mood.
Thought form: Logical and linear, able to follow line of questioning.
Thought content: Sally appears a little distracted and brings conversation back to concerns about her job. She appears to be having difficulty focusing on anything else. There appears to be no grandiosity or disorganisation to her thought pattern.
Orientation: Sally is orientated to time, place and date.
Memory and concentration: Sally's memory appears to be intact but her

concentration appears to be affected by her anxiety and distress. Sally is finding it difficult to change focus. She describes difficulty reading and following through on work activities.
Insight and judgement: While Sally's judgement appears to be intact, her constant worry is of concern in relation to decisions she may potentially make. This in turn is having an impact upon her insight and she believes she can 'ride this through'.

FUNCTIONAL INQUIRY

Sleep: Disturbed at times, wakes up in the middle of the night with a tight chest and a light sweat; Sally cannot explain why this is happening.
Appetite: OK, but Sally sometimes skips meals as she is worried about not completing her work.
Motivation: Sally feels amotivated, which is adding to her stress and worry.
Activity and enjoyment: Sally used to enjoy swimming and walking but now

worries this is a waste of precious time.
Energy: Sally feels like she has little energy to spare as she feels exhausted all the time.

PSYCHOSOCIAL ASSESSMENT

Sally used to have regular outings with friends but feels too tired to do this now and does not want to leave the family home for fear of her husband leaving her while she is out. Sally has been married for 6 years and loves her husband but feels he is 'drifting away'. They are financially secure with both partners working and no dependants to support.

PHYSICAL ASSESSMENT

PAIN: Persistent headache
CVS: HR 76 bpm, BP 130/75 mmHg
RESP: RR 17
MUSCULOSKELETAL (Mobility): Mobile
Weight: 72 kg
Height: 165 cm
BMI: 26.45, overweight range
GASTROINTESTINAL: Occasional morning diarrhoea

Cues

1. Identify the ways anxiety can impact physical health.
2. Discuss the impact anxiety can have on family relationships.
3. Could alcohol use be contributing to Sally's increased anxiety and sleep disturbance? Why?
4. What is the relationship between anxiety and diarrhoea?
5. What is the relationship between anxiety and sleep disturbance?

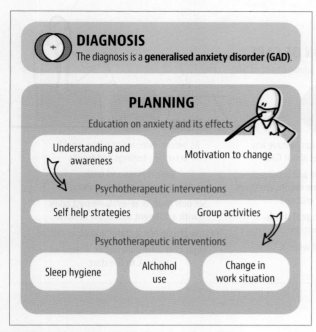

DIAGNOSIS
The diagnosis is a **generalised anxiety disorder (GAD)**.

PLANNING

Education on anxiety and its effects

Understanding and awareness

Motivation to change

Psychotherapeutic interventions

Self help strategies

Group activities

Psychotherapeutic interventions

Sleep hygiene

Alchohol use

Change in work situation

CONCEPT MAP 11.2 Diagnosis and planning for Sally

INTERVENTIONS

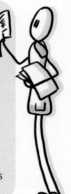

Education
1 Websites, 1:1 support
2 Family educational support
3 Education on anxiety, its impact, use of alcohol and benefits of being active
4 Substance use/abuse

Psychotherapy
1 Cognitive Behavioural Therapy (CBT)
2 Mindfulness
3 Applied relaxation techniques
4 Support groups
5 Focus on managing one aspect at a time

Lifestyle
1 Explore options to reduce workload
2 Sleep assessment and examination of routine, rumination and management of waking
3 Diet and exercise, identify achievable activities
4 Note alcohol consumption and any substance use/abuse; explore strategies to reduce this.

CONCEPT MAP 11.3 Nursing interventions for Sally

EVALUATION

Education, psychotherapeutic support and addressing lifestyle changes are all key interventions for the management of GAD. These require high commitment and may require initial intensive oversight.

Evaluation is particularly important here.

Plan:
Set a time frame with Sally (and her family) to evaluate progress sooner rather than later.

What further assessments should be initiated?

CONCEPT MAP 11.4 Evaluation and planning for Sally

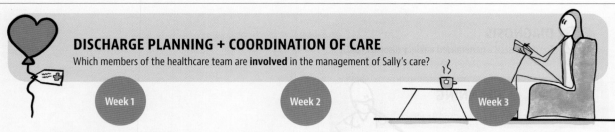

DISCHARGE PLANNING + COORDINATION OF CARE

Which members of the healthcare team are **involved** in the management of Sally's care?

Week 1

Ask Sally to keep a diary of activities and thoughts to bring to a clinical review next week

Ensure Sally has contact details, dates and appointment timesclearly recorded

Offer Sally contact details for support groups in her area or online

Ensure breathing and relaxation techniques are accessible. This could involve apps, websites or local groups

Week 2

Ask if Sally and her family have any further questions about GAD

Review of week one and progress/non-progress, explore any events, emotions, barriers and enablers

Review physiological status and observations

Set goals for week 3

Week 3

As before, evaluate previous week's activities, feelings and events

Revisit plans and goals. What is working /not working?

Set new goals or re-evaluate past goals with a different strategy if needed

Review physiological status and observations

Begin long-term planning or, if required, go back to the start.

CONCEPT MAP 11.5 Discharge planning and coordination of care for Sally

CONCEPT MAP SEQUENCE FOR DEPRESSION

Presentation

Concept maps 11.6–11.10 explore the presentation, management and planning of care for Mr Williams' depression.

 PHx

Mr Jarrah Williams is a 54-year-old Indigenous Australian male who is being assessed for poor sleep and low mood. This has been developing since Mr Williams received a diagnosis of type 2 diabetes 6 months ago. Mr Williams has been commenced on anti-depressants, but he complained that they were not working so he stopped taking them and now feels that life is not worth living any more. His family do not understand why he is not engaging in community activities any more and are concerned for his wellbeing. Mr Williams has a car but does not like to travel far from his semi-rural community and often loans it out to other community members. Mr Williams is very concerned about his diabetes as he has been instructed to eat a healthy diet and undertake more exercise, something he currently finds very challenging to achieve. Mr Williams missed his last routine diabetic follow-up appointment but has been brought to the clinic by his wife due to recently worsening mood symptoms and disengagement from friends and family. Family are concerned that Mr Williams has been saying that they are better off without him. Mr Williams has not checked his blood glucose level (BGL) for some time as he does not see the point.

 ASSESSMENT

PHYSICAL ASSESSMENT

PAIN: No pain reported

CVS: HR 82 bpm, BP 136/82 mmHg

RESP: RR 18

MUSCULOSKELETAL (Mobility): Mobile, no concerns

Weight: 88 kg

Height: 174 cm

BMI: 29.1, overweight range

Past relevant medical history

Recent diagnosis of type 2 diabetes (previous 6 months). Nil significant medical history, no previous history of mood disturbance. Has been complaining of insomnia for last 4 months, sleeping tablets prescribed with little effect. Diabetes is currently being managed with diet and exercise.

Last HbA1c result 56 mmol/mol (normal range = 48–53 mmol/mol) 5 months ago.

Functional inquiry

Sleep: disturbed at times, wakes up in the middle of the night and cannot get back to sleep.

Appetite: poor at the moment, does not feel like preparing or eating food.

Motivation: Mr Williams does not even want to get out of bed, he only gets up

to try and meet family obligations but is finding this increasingly difficult.

Activity and enjoyment: Mr Williams used to enjoy fishing and walking but now can't be bothered. He has not been to work for over 2 weeks.

Energy: Mr Williams reports having little energy to spare and feels exhausted all the time.

Cues: consider the physical impact depression has on overall health. What signs and symptoms of depression **(Figure 11.5A)** can you see here?

Mental Status Examination

Behaviour: Mr Williams appears quite morose; he is looking down and making minimal eye contact.

Appearance: Mr Williams is casually dressed but admits his wife dressed him this morning.

Mood: Mr Williams reports feeling sad and useless, he feels he is a burden to his family and community.

Thought form: logical and linear, able to follow line of questioning but responses are slow and monosyllabic.

Thought content: Mr Williams appears distracted and uninterested. Mr Williams does

not see the point of being here and feels he is just being a burden and waste of everyone's time. There appears to be no grandiosity or disorganisation to his thought pattern.

Orientation: Mr Williams is orientated to time, place and date but admits to being more forgetful lately and does not care what day it is.

Memory and concentration: Mr Williams describes difficulty reading and following through on any activities. He is concerned he is forgetting to attend important events in his community.

Insight and judgement: Mr Williams appears to have no understanding of his illness(es) or he is choosing to disengage; difficult to ascertain at the moment. This has resulted in poor judgement as he is not following his treatment routine.

Suicide assessment

As Mr Williams has indicated he feels he is a burden to everyone and they would be better off without him, it is important to ask about suicide. In order to assess this, ask about thoughts of harming or killing yourself, how often do you think of this, how you would do this, what timeframe do you have in mind and does the person have means or access and, importantly, have they

CONCEPT MAP 11.6 Nursing assessment for Mr Williams

tried suicide before (NIMH, 2022). Mr Williams denies wanting to harm or kill himself despite feeling like he is a burden. He has not made any plans and has not thought about how he would kill himself, and there have been no previous attempts reported.

Psychosocial assessment

Mr Williams lives in a small rural community to which he identifies a strong connection. Mr Williams lives with his wife, Hattie, their two children and 3 grandchildren. Mrs Williams describes this as a happy household and they have no financial stressors. Mr Williams works part time as a local mechanic and is considered an Elder in his community so he attends many ceremonial and traditional occasions. Mr Williams speaks both language (native tongue) and English.

Mr Williams used to regularly visit friends and family in his community but has not been doing this for some time.

Drug and alcohol assessment

Apart from an occasional beer at the local bar, Mr Williams drinks very little. Mr Williams has never taken illicit drugs. AUDIT score = 3

CONCEPT MAP 11.6 Nursing assessment for Mr Williams (continued)

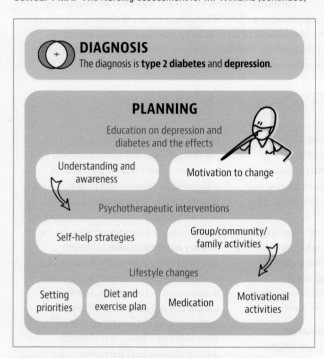

DIAGNOSIS

The diagnosis is **type 2 diabetes** and **depression**.

PLANNING

Education on depression and diabetes and the effects

Understanding and awareness

Motivation to change

Psychotherapeutic interventions

Self-help strategies

Group/community/ family activities

Lifestyle changes

Setting priorities

Diet and exercise plan

Medication

Motivational activities

CONCEPT MAP 11.7 Diagnosis and planning for Mr Williams

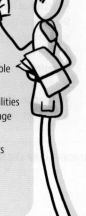

INTERVENTIONS

Education

1 Indigenous Health Worker, ACCHO, 1:1 support

2 Family educational support

3 Education on depression, its impact, use of medication and benefits of being active

4 Education on diabetes, its impact, use of food as management and benefits of being active

Medication

1 Discuss anti-depressants and how they work, timeframes for how long they take to work and potential side effects.

2 Introduce options around diabetes medication.

Psychotherapy

1 Focus on managing one aspect at a time

2 Cognitive Behavioural Therapy

3 Mindfulness

4 Community-based resources

5 Explore traditional therapies

6 Yarning

Lifestyle

1 Explore options to manage daily routines

2 Sleep assessment and examination of routine, rumination and management of waking

3 Diet and exercise; identify achievable and acceptable activities

4 Identify key community responsibilities and potential strategies to re-engage with these

5 Determine follow-up appointments around Mr Williams' usual routine

CONCEPT MAP 11.8 Nursing interventions for Mr Williams

EVALUATION

Mr Williams is going to require regular follow-up to monitor both his depression and diabetes which are of equal priority in this case.

Mr Williams really needs to take anti-depressants regularly as prescribed to gain the full effect.

Mr Williams needs to begin to re-engage in his usual activities (at his own pace) and this can be a good measure of improvement.

Education, psychotherapeutic and cultural support are all going to be key to address the long-term changes that are going to be required to manage both diabetes and depression.

Plan:
Having a clear discharge plan and future focused plan is essential and must be evaluated regularly.

Cues

1 Why is it important that any plans are developed and evaluated with Mr Williams?

2 Why is it important to connect with a local ACCHO or Indigenous Health Worker?

3 What barriers can you think of that would impede Mr Williams' engagement with healthcare services?

What further assessments could we consider following evaluation

CONCEPT MAP 11.9 Evaluation and planning for Mr Williams

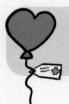

DISCHARGE PLANNING + COORDINATION OF CARE

Which members of the healthcare team are **involved** in the management of Mr Williams care?

Week 1

Ask Mr and Mrs Williams to keep a diary of meals, times and shopping budgets to bring to a clinical review next week

Ensure Mr and Mrs Williams have contact details, dates and appointment times clearly recorded

Offer Mr and Mrs Williams information on depression and diabetes

Offer Mr and Mrs Williams contact details for ACCHO or support groups in their area or online

Set a daily plan with Mr Williams with simple, achievable activities such as attending to ADLs

Ensure BGLs are being done and recorded, offer assistance as required

Week 2

Review of week 1 and progress/non-progress, explore any events, emotions, barriers and enablers

Review physiological status and observations

Align blood glucose levels with diet and exercise, illustrate the connection

Begin discussing the relationship between depression, mood and physical health

Set goals for week 3

Week 3

As before, evaluate previous week's activities, feelings and events

Revisit plans and goals, what is working what is not

Set new goals or re-evaluate past goals with a different strategy if needed

Review physiological status and observations

Begin long-term planning or, if required, go back to the start

CONCEPT MAP 11.10 Discharge planning and coordination of care for Mr Williams

CONCEPT MAP SEQUENCE FOR MANAGING ALCOHOL-INDUCED SLEEP DISTURBANCE

Presentation
Concept maps 11.11–11.15 explore the impact of Andrew's persistent insomnia.

 PHx

Andrew Jones is a 42-year-old married man who is seeking support for persistent insomnia which is affecting his day-to-day working life. Following a recent admission for day surgery for tooth extraction, Andrew has been advised to be assessed for a CPAP machine. Andrew requires a full assessment to evaluate and ascertain all possible reasons for his insomnia and disturbed sleep. Andrew's wife complains about his snoring.

DRUG & ALCOHOL HISTORY

Current use: Drinks a 'crate' of beer with friends at the weekend, has the occasional beer during the week at home. Denies any other substance use.

History of use: Since late teens, has never sought help or received treatment.

AUDIT score and interpretation: 12: indicates risky use and requires follow-up.

Level of motivation: Ambivalent, does not link alcohol to insomnia as it gets him off to sleep.

 ASSESSMENT

Functional inquiry:

Sleep: Disturbed at present, wakes up around 2–3 a.m. and struggles to get back to sleep. Feels fatigued during the day.

Appetite: Good; no changes.

Energy: Currently low, associates this with poor sleep.

Motivation: Motivated to get insomnia sorted out and go fishing but has been struggling to get up and go to work.

Concentration: Diminished, occasionally forgets things, but able to watch a movie or TV program.

Anxiety: Has been increasingly anxious about increased workload which is becoming stressful. Believes this is contributing to the insomnia.

Mood: Mood is good, just unhappy about impact insomnia is having.

NB. No requirement for an MSE on this occasion

Psychosocial assessment

Andrew has been married to Anne for 15 years. Andrew has 2 children aged 6 and 8. He works as an air traffic controller spending much of his time sitting and working shifts including night shift. Andrew is often tired after work and winds down in the evening with a couple of beers. At the weekend he watches the children playing sport then relaxes by going fishing with friends. This usually ends with 'a few bevvies' with the boys. Andrew has noticed he has become increasingly restless during the night, waking several times. He puts this down to the stress of work and the long shifts he works. He has been advised he may be suffering from sleep apnoea and may need a continuous positive airway pressure (CPAP) machine. He does not know what a CPAP machine is nor how it could help him.

Past medical history:

History of asthma since a child, currently uses Becotide OD and Ventolin PRN. Appendectomy age 12.

No significant previous history reported Last HbA1c result 52 mmol/mol (normal range = 48–53 mmol/mol) 6 months ago as part of routine medical for air traffic controllers.

Physical assessment:

PAIN: Nil

CVS: HR 76 bpm, BP 130/75 mmHg

RESP: RR 17

MUSCULOSKELETAL (Mobility): Mobile

Weight: 102 kg

Height: 171 cm

BMI: 35.3, obese range

BGL: (non-fasting) 7.4 mmol/L

Cues

① What is the relationship between disturbed sleep and alcohol use?

② What is the relationship between obesity and sleep apnoea?

③ What is the relationship between pre-diabetes and sleep disturbance?

CONCEPT MAP 11.11 Nursing assessment for Andrew

DIAGNOSIS

Sleep apnoea related to obesity and alcohol use

As evidenced by disturbed sleep and sleep/wake cycle

High alcohol consumption as evidenced by an AUDIT score of 12; risky use

PLANNING

- ☑ Write a nursing prioritisation planner in partnership with Andrew for next 2 weeks
- ☑ Brief intervention; motivation to change
- ☑ Identify and establish short term goals; i.e. lose 1 kg in weight per week/increase walking time
- ☑ Establish realistic timeframe
- ☑ Monitor blood glucose level and obtain an oral glucose tolerance test and fasting blood glucose test
- ☑ Consider assessment for introduction of a CPAP for immediate assistance

PLANNING

Education on the relationship between alcohol use and insomnia

- Understanding and awareness
- Motivation to change (brief intervention)

Psychotherapeutic interventions

- Self-help strategies
- Group/community/ family activities

Lifestyle changes

- Setting priorities
- Diet and exercise plan
- Harm minimisation
- Motivational activities

Cues

1 How might short-term use of pharmacology be useful here?

2 Can we use sleeping medication with a CPAP?

CONCEPT MAP 11.12 Diagnosis and planning for Andrew

INTERVENTIONS

Brief interventions:

1 Discuss the AUDIT

2 Complete a decisional balance chart for alcohol, food and exercise

Lifestyle planning

1 Identify behavioural patterns in relation to food and alcohol

2 Discuss daily routine

3 Identify likes/dislikes in relation to physical exercise. Planning must be realistic, achievable and affordable

4 Set small, realistic goals with Andrew

Education

1 Education on the relationship between the use of alcohol and insomnia

2 Education on the use of alcohol and weight gain

3 The benefits of being active

4 Assess motivation and areas for change

Psychotherapy

1 Brief intervention

2 Motivational interviewing

3 Support groups

4 Focus on managing one aspect at a time

5 Explore relationship with alcohol (i.e. underlying reasons for use)

Lifestyle

1 Explore options to reduce alcohol intake

2 Sleep assessment and examination of routine, and management of waking

3 Diet and exercise, identify achievable activities

4 Explore harm minimisation strategies and alternatives to alcohol use

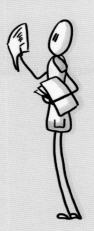

Cues

1 Why would Andrew be reluctant to consider reducing drinking at the weekends?

2 Why would all of these factors increase a sense of stress related to work?

CONCEPT MAP 11.13 Nursing interventions for Andrew

EVALUATION

Further assessment (pre-evaluation)
Andrew indicates he had not considered lifestyle factors as contributing to insomnia.

Andrew finds the decisional balance chart interesting and useful.

Cues

1 How can we use this information to plan further care?

CONCEPT MAP 11.14 Evaluation and planning for Andrew

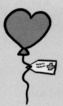

DISCHARGE PLANNING + COORDINATION OF CARE

How do the following areas of healthcare management **relate** to Andrew's presentation? Which members of the healthcare team are **involved** in each area of management?

- Diabetes
- Diet
- Snoring
- Stress management

Week 1

Engage in brief intervention and revisit the AUDIT results to explore goals

Set goals in partnership with Andrew

Ask Andrew to keep a diary of alcohol consumption and occasions

Ask Andrew to jot down sleep disturbances and effects on work, etc.

Begin to explore motivational activities

Week 2

Review of week 1 and progress/non-progress, explore any events, emotions, barriers and enablers

Review physiological status and observations

Continue discussing the relationship between alcohol use, mood and physical health

Set goals for week 3

Week 3

As before, evaluate previous week's activities, feelings and events

Revisit plans and goals; what is working, what is not

Set new goals or re-evaluate past goals with a different strategy if needed

Review physiological status and observations

Begin long-term planning or if required, go back to the start

CONCEPT MAP 11.15 Discharge planning and coordination of care for Andrew

Chapter 12: Visual and Auditory Systems

CONCEPT MAP SEQUENCE FOR OPEN-ANGLE GLAUCOMA

Presentation

Elizabeth Richardson is a 58-year-old married woman who is admitted for day surgery to reduce left eye intraocular pressure due to open-angle glaucoma. Elizabeth is scheduled for trabeculectomy filtration surgery to the left eye.

Concept maps 12.1–12.5 explore Elizabeth's initial care in the day surgery unit.

 PHx

Elizabeth, a **58-year-old female** with bilateral open-angle glaucoma (that was diagnosed 8 years ago), has now become **less responsive to antiglaucoma medication**, with increasing intraocular eye pressures, and the left eye least responsive to medication.

Elizabeth has had three changes in the types of antiglaucoma medication, due to **intraocular pressures rising to high levels**, which necessitates a change of antiglaucoma medication.

Her **older brother has also been diagnosed with bilateral glaucoma**, and has had laser surgery to control right eye pressure, and is prescribed antiglaucoma eye drops to reduce intraocular pressures.

Cues

1. What is the relationship between acute angle glaucoma and family history?

2. Why do intraocular pressures rise even though a patient is prescribed a specific antiglaucoma medication?

 ASSESSMENT

Primary survey

A: Patent
B: RR 14
C: Warm, intact
D: Alert
E: T 36.5 °C
F: Fasting, HNPU
G: BGL 4.8 mmol/L

Secondary survey

CNS (Cognition): Alert and orientated

PAIN: Nil

CVS: HR 72 bpm, BP 130/75 mmHg

RESP: RR 14

GIT (Input): Fasting since 7 a.m. for food, and for the last 2 hours for water.

MUSCULOSKELETAL (Mobility): Mobile

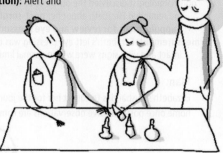

CONCEPT MAP 12.1 Nursing assessment for Elizabeth

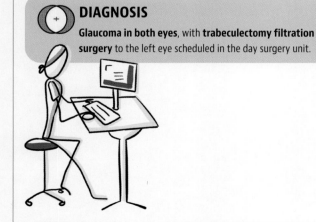 **DIAGNOSIS**

Glaucoma in both eyes, with **trabeculectomy filtration surgery** to the left eye scheduled in the day surgery unit.

PLANNING

☑ Anaesthesia, surgery and post-anaesthesia

☑ Write a Nursing Prioritisation Planner

Health education and home care:

☑ Eye dressing at night

☑ Not to touch or rub eye

☑ Pain medication – anti-inflammatory eye drops and oral paracetamol

☑ Antiglaucoma medication

☑ Avoid lifting, strenuous activity, coughing, sneezing and constipation for two weeks

☑ Avoid driving and operating heavy machinery

☑ Report eye pain, changes in vision, red eye, headache

☑ Postoperative appointment

CONCEPT MAP 12.2 Diagnosis and planning for Elizabeth

INTERVENTIONS

1 Patient health education

2 Check for valid consent

3 Accompany to anaesthetic area

4 Undertake postoperative assessments in the post-anaesthetic care unit (PACU)

5 Position with head elevated

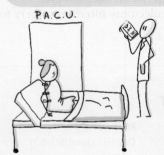

Cues

1 Why does Elizabeth state that the corner of her eye feels gritty?

What further assessments should be initiated

CONCEPT MAP 12.3 Nursing interventions for Elizabeth

EVALUATION

Whilst Elizabeth was being monitored in PACU, the ophthalmologist discussed the outcome of the surgery and reminded Elizabeth about her **post-surgical appointment for review and eye pressure measurement**. Elizabeth's left eye dressing was dry and intact and vital signs were within normal limits.

Plan:

Elizabeth's husband is to collect her for the journey home once postoperative observations are completed.

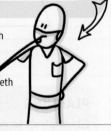

Cues **1** Why is it important that Elizabeth continues to apply antiglaucoma medication to both eyes?

2 What lifestyle changes can Elizabeth adopt to reduce the likelihood of intraocular pressures rising?

CONCEPT MAP 12.4 Evaluation and planning for Elizabeth

DISCHARGE PLANNING + COORDINATION OF CARE

How do the following areas of healthcare management **relate** to Elizabeth's presentation? Which members of the healthcare team are **involved** in each area of management?

Written postoperative instructions

Wear protective eye shield at night to protect the eye when sleeping

Postoperative medication

Anti-inflammatory eye drops and oral paracetamol

Post-surgical review

Optical prescription

Sunglasses

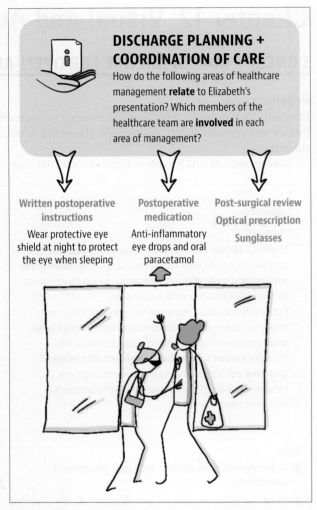

CONCEPT MAP 12.5 Discharge planning and coordination of care for Elizabeth

CONCEPT MAP SEQUENCE FOR CATARACT SURGERY

Presentation

Daphne Ferrier is an 85-year-old female who has bilateral cataracts. Daphne's visual acuity of both eyes has been decreasing, and throughout the day whatever the intensity of light is, it appears always to be glaring. At her last optometrist appointment, she was referred to an ophthalmologist for assessment. She has noticed that her dog Gemma who is white and black in colour has become shades of grey.

Concept maps 12.6–12.10 explore Daphne's initial care in the day surgery unit.

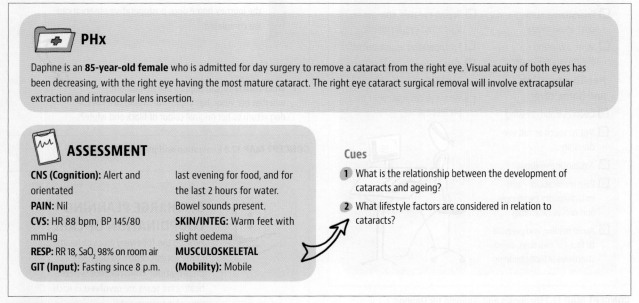

PHx

Daphne is an **85-year-old female** who is admitted for day surgery to remove a cataract from the right eye. Visual acuity of both eyes has been decreasing, with the right eye having the most mature cataract. The right eye cataract surgical removal will involve extracapsular extraction and intraocular lens insertion.

ASSESSMENT

CNS (Cognition): Alert and orientated
PAIN: Nil
CVS: HR 88 bpm, BP 145/80 mmHg
RESP: RR 18, SaO$_2$ 98% on room air
GIT (Input): Fasting since 8 p.m. last evening for food, and for the last 2 hours for water. Bowel sounds present.
SKIN/INTEG: Warm feet with slight oedema
MUSCULOSKELETAL (Mobility): Mobile

Cues

1. What is the relationship between the development of cataracts and ageing?
2. What lifestyle factors are considered in relation to cataracts?

CONCEPT MAP 12.6 Nursing assessment for Daphne

DIAGNOSIS

Bilateral cataracts, with the removal of the right eye cataract as a day surgery procedure.

PLANNING

- ☑ Preoperative medication eye drops
- ☑ Anaesthesia, surgery and post-anaesthesia
- ☑ Write a Nursing Prioritisation Planner

Health education and home care:

- ☑ Clean eye and dressing
- ☑ Not to touch or rub eye dressing
- ☑ Antibiotic eye drops
- ☑ Pain medication – anti-inflammatory eye drops and oral paracetamol
- ☑ Avoid reading and pressure to face for two days, avoid strenuous activity, bending over, lifting, coughing and sneezing for two weeks
- ☑ Report eye pain, changes in vision, red eye, headache
- ☑ Postoperative appointment
- ☑ Avoid driving or operating a vehicle
- ☑ Wear eye cover at night to protect eye

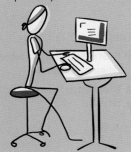

CONCEPT MAP 12.7 Diagnosis and planning for Daphne

INTERVENTIONS

1. Patient health education
2. Check for valid consent
3. Preoperative topical anaesthetic drops and mydriatic eye drops
4. Accompany to anaesthetic area
5. Undertake postoperative assessments in the post-anaesthetic care unit (PACU)

What further assessments should be initiated?

Cues **1** Why does Daphne state that her eye feels full?

CONCEPT MAP 12.8 Nursing interventions for Daphne

EVALUATION

The ophthalmologist visited Daphne in the PACU. He was happy with the surgery and will see Daphne when she has her follow-up appointment for review. Daphne's vital signs were within normal limits and the right eye dressing was dry and intact.

Plan:
Discharge Daphne in the care of a family member for the journey home once postoperative observations are completed.

1 What criteria should Daphne use to measure whether her vision has improved? Would Gemma the dog return to her original colour of black and white?

CONCEPT MAP 12.9 Evaluation and planning for Daphne

DISCHARGE PLANNING + COORDINATION OF CARE

How do the following areas of healthcare management **relate** to Daphne's presentation? Which members of the healthcare team are **involved** in each area of management?

Written postoperative instructions

Wear protective eye shield at night to protect the eye when sleeping

Postoperative medication

Antibiotic eye drops, anti-inflammatory eye drops and oral paracetamol

Post-surgical review

Optical prescription

Sunglasses

CONCEPT MAP 12.10 Discharge planning and coordination of care for Daphne

CONCEPT MAP SEQUENCE FOR OTITIS MEDIA WITH EFFUSION

Presentation

Katie Namatjira is an Aboriginal 7-year-old girl who is admitted for day surgery for bilateral myringotomy with grommets. Katie has had recurring middle ear infections for the last six months which have recurred after antibiotic treatment has been completed. Katie and her mother have come from an Aboriginal community located in far north Queensland.

Concept maps 12.11–12.15 explore Katie's initial care in the day surgery unit.

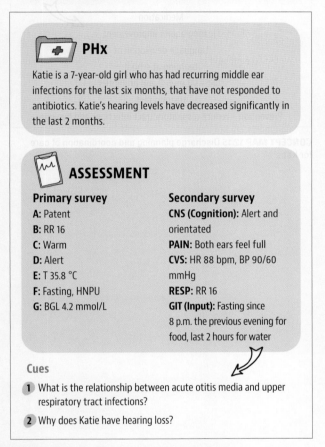

PHx

Katie is a 7-year-old girl who has had recurring middle ear infections for the last six months, that have not responded to antibiotics. Katie's hearing levels have decreased significantly in the last 2 months.

ASSESSMENT

Primary survey
A: Patent
B: RR 16
C: Warm
D: Alert
E: T 35.8 °C
F: Fasting, HNPU
G: BGL 4.2 mmol/L

Secondary survey
CNS (Cognition): Alert and orientated
PAIN: Both ears feel full
CVS: HR 88 bpm, BP 90/60 mmHg
RESP: RR 16
GIT (Input): Fasting since 8 p.m. the previous evening for food, last 2 hours for water

Cues

1 What is the relationship between acute otitis media and upper respiratory tract infections?

2 Why does Katie have hearing loss?

CONCEPT MAP 12.11 Nursing assessment for Katie

DIAGNOSIS

A 7 year old girl with **otitis media with effusion**.

PLANNING

☑ Anaesthesia, surgery and post-anaesthesia
☑ Write a Nursing Prioritisation Planner

Health education and home care:

☑ Pain medication – oral paracetamol
☑ Ear plugs for showers and swimming
☑ Report ear pain, discharge and loss of hearing
☑ Hearing regained
☑ Language development
☑ Learning at school
☑ Diet – vitamin D and probiotics

☑ Hearing test
☑ Grommets falling out within six months
☑ Prevention – reduce respiratory tract infections and hygiene
☑ Postoperative appointment

CONCEPT MAP 12.12 Diagnosis and planning for Katie

INTERVENTIONS

1 Child and mother health education
2 Check for valid consent
3 Accompany to anaesthetic area
4 Undertake postoperative assessments in the post-anaesthetic care unit (PACU)

What further assessments should be initiated

Cues 1 Katie states that everyone is very loud in PACU. What is your response?

CONCEPT MAP 12.13 Nursing interventions for Katie

EVALUATION

While Katie and her mother are in PACU, the surgeon visits and part of the discussion is to encourage attendance to the local healthcare clinic and to attend a Royal Flying Doctor Service visit that includes a review of Katie's ears.

Plan:
Discharge Katie and her mother for the journey home to far north Queensland.

Cues

1. What additional information can be provided to assist Katie's mother in providing an environment where there will be lower incidence of ear infection?

CONCEPT MAP 12.14 Evaluation and planning for Katie

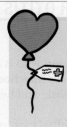

DISCHARGE PLANNING + COORDINATION OF CARE

How do the following areas of healthcare management **relate** to Katie's presentation? Which members of the healthcare team are **involved** in each area of management?

Medication
Hearing aquity improvement
Language development
Learning at school
Diet – vitamin D and probiotics
Hearing test
Prevention – reduce respiratory tract infections and hygiene

CONCEPT MAP 12.15 Discharge planning and coordination of care for Katie

CONCEPT MAP SEQUENCE FOR TINNITUS

Presentation

Francoise Cole is 37-year-old woman who is attending the general practitioner (GP) with ringing in the right ear. The ringing has been ongoing for the last three weeks, and started with a head cold but has not resolved. The ringing in the right ear has prevented the placement of her mobile telephone to the right ear.

Concept maps 12.16–12.20 explore Francoise's presentation/admission.

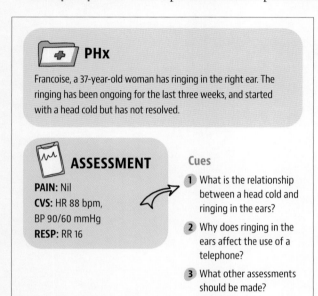

📁 PHx

Francoise, a 37-year-old woman has ringing in the right ear. The ringing has been ongoing for the last three weeks, and started with a head cold but has not resolved.

📋 ASSESSMENT

PAIN: Nil
CVS: HR 88 bpm, BP 90/60 mmHg
RESP: RR 16

Cues

1 What is the relationship between a head cold and ringing in the ears?

2 Why does ringing in the ears affect the use of a telephone?

3 What other assessments should be made?

CONCEPT MAP 12.16 Nursing assessment for Francoise

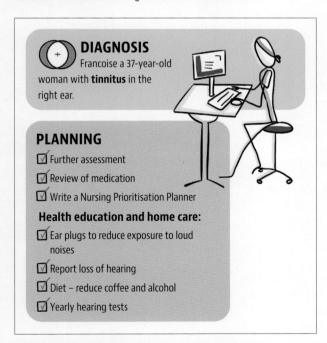

⊕ DIAGNOSIS

Francoise a 37-year-old woman with **tinnitus** in the right ear.

PLANNING

☑ Further assessment
☑ Review of medication
☑ Write a Nursing Prioritisation Planner

Health education and home care:

☑ Ear plugs to reduce exposure to loud noises
☑ Report loss of hearing
☑ Diet – reduce coffee and alcohol
☑ Yearly hearing tests

CONCEPT MAP 12.17 Diagnosis and planning for Francoise

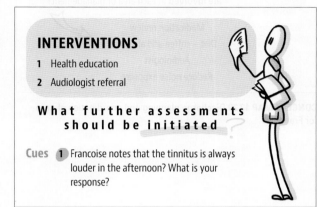

INTERVENTIONS

1 Health education
2 Audiologist referral

What further assessments should be initiated?

Cues 1 Francoise notes that the tinnitus is always louder in the afternoon? What is your response?

CONCEPT MAP 12.18 Nursing interventions for Francoise

EVALUATION

Francoise's tinnitus has evolved due to Francoise regularly attending loud rock music concerts. Francoise always likes to have headphones on while listening to loud music.

Plan:
Refer Francoise to an audiologist. Also for Francoise to limit caffeine and alcohol in her diet. Reduce exposure to loud noise.

Cues

1 How can Francoise care for hearing at work and during a rock concert?

CONCEPT MAP 12.19 Evaluation and planning for Francoise

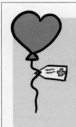

DISCHARGE PLANNING + COORDINATION OF CARE

How do the following areas of healthcare management **relate** to Francoise's presentation? Which members of the healthcare team are **involved** in each area of management?

Medication review
Diet – coffee and alcohol
Audiologist
Reduce noise exposure

CONCEPT MAP 12.20 Discharge planning and coordination of care for Francoise

Chapter 13: Gastrointestinal System

CONCEPT MAP SEQUENCE FOR DIVERTICULITIS

Presentation

Ruby is a 38-year-old woman who has been hospitalised for diverticulitis. Diverticulitis is inflammation of the diverticulum that can result in peritonitis, perforation, fistula formation or even an abscess (Craft & Gordon, 2019). **Concept maps 13.1–13.5** explore Ruby's presentation/admission.

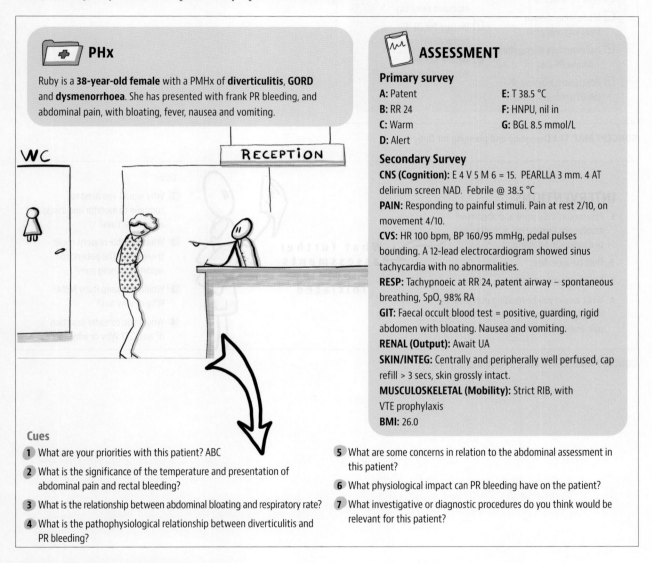

PHx

Ruby is a **38-year-old female** with a PMHx of **diverticulitis**, **GORD** and **dysmenorrhoea**. She has presented with frank PR bleeding, and abdominal pain, with bloating, fever, nausea and vomiting.

WC

RECEPTION

ASSESSMENT

Primary survey

A: Patent

B: RR 24

C: Warm

D: Alert

E: T 38.5 °C

F: HNPU, nil in

G: BGL 8.5 mmol/L

Secondary Survey

CNS (Cognition): E 4 V 5 M 6 = 15. PEARLLA 3 mm. 4 AT delirium screen NAD. Febrile @ 38.5 °C

PAIN: Responding to painful stimuli. Pain at rest 2/10, on movement 4/10.

CVS: HR 100 bpm, BP 160/95 mmHg, pedal pulses bounding. A 12-lead electrocardiogram showed sinus tachycardia with no abnormalities.

RESP: Tachypnoeic at RR 24, patent airway – spontaneous breathing, SpO$_2$ 98% RA

GIT: Faecal occult blood test = positive, guarding, rigid abdomen with bloating. Nausea and vomiting.

RENAL (Output): Await UA

SKIN/INTEG: Centrally and peripherally well perfused, cap refill > 3 secs, skin grossly intact.

MUSCULOSKELETAL (Mobility): Strict RIB, with VTE prophylaxis

BMI: 26.0

Cues

1. What are your priorities with this patient? ABC

2. What is the significance of the temperature and presentation of abdominal pain and rectal bleeding?

3. What is the relationship between abdominal bloating and respiratory rate?

4. What is the pathophysiological relationship between diverticulitis and PR bleeding?

5. What are some concerns in relation to the abdominal assessment in this patient?

6. What physiological impact can PR bleeding have on the patient?

7. What investigative or diagnostic procedures do you think would be relevant for this patient?

CONCEPT MAP 13.1 Nursing assessment for Ruby

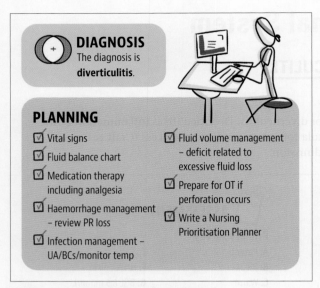

DIAGNOSIS
The diagnosis is **diverticulitis**.

PLANNING

☑ Vital signs

☑ Fluid balance chart

☑ Medication therapy including analgesia

☑ Haemorrhage management – review PR loss

☑ Infection management – UA/BCs/monitor temp

☑ Fluid volume management – deficit related to excessive fluid loss

☑ Prepare for OT if perforation occurs

☑ Write a Nursing Prioritisation Planner

CONCEPT MAP 13.2 Diagnosis and planning for Ruby

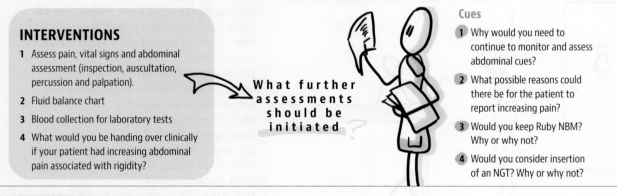

INTERVENTIONS

1 Assess pain, vital signs and abdominal assessment (inspection, auscultation, percussion and palpation).

2 Fluid balance chart

3 Blood collection for laboratory tests

4 What would you be handing over clinically if your patient had increasing abdominal pain associated with rigidity?

What further assessments should be initiated?

Cues

1 Why would you need to continue to monitor and assess abdominal cues?

2 What possible reasons could there be for the patient to report increasing pain?

3 Would you keep Ruby NBM? Why or why not?

4 Would you consider insertion of an NGT? Why or why not?

CONCEPT MAP 13.3 Nursing interventions for Ruby

EVALUATION

The medical team have been notified of Ruby's increasing abdominal pain (despite analgesia) and increased rigidity.

Plan:

Whilst Ruby was being prepared to have a repeat CT abdomen for the alterations in condition, she becomes hypotensive and tachycardic.

Cues

1 What interventions need to be considered now for Ruby? Prioritise these interventions in order of urgency.

2 Does this deterioration in her condition relate to the reason for presentation?

3 What do the deteriorations in vital signs indicate pathophysiologically?

CONCEPT MAP 13.4 Evaluation and planning for Ruby

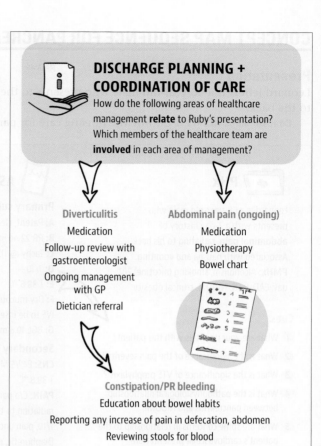

DISCHARGE PLANNING + COORDINATION OF CARE

How do the following areas of healthcare management **relate** to Ruby's presentation? Which members of the healthcare team are **involved** in each area of management?

Diverticulitis

Medication

Follow-up review with gastroenterologist

Ongoing management with GP

Dietician referral

Abdominal pain (ongoing)

Medication

Physiotherapy

Bowel chart

Constipation/PR bleeding

Education about bowel habits

Reporting any increase of pain in defecation, abdomen

Reviewing stools for blood

CONCEPT MAP 13.5 Discharge planning and coordination of care for Ruby

CONCEPT MAP SEQUENCE FOR PANCREATITIS

Presentation

Leonard Jeffers is a 66-year-old male who presents to the emergency department with abdominal pain radiating to the back.

Concept maps 13.6–13.10 outline the nursing care for pancreatitis for Leonard.

 PHx

Leonard is a 68-year-old male who presents with a 2-day history of **abdominal pain**, radiating to his back. Associated with nausea and vomiting.
PMHx: Alcoholism, smoking (nicotine) 20/day, CAD, HTN, NIDDM, truncal obesity.

Cues

1. What are your priorities with this patient?
2. What is the significance of the pain severity?
3. What is the significance of VTE prophylaxis?
4. What is the pathophysiological relationship between pancreatitis and NIDDM?
5. What are some concerns in relationship to the patient's cardiovascular presentation?
6. What investigative or diagnostic procedures would you think would be relevant for this patient?

 ASSESSMENT

Primary survey
A: Patent, clear
B: RR 22 no increased WOB
C: Tachy @ 115, regular
D: 7/10
E: T 38.6 °C
F: Dry mucous membranes, IVF to be inserted
G: BGL 10.6 mmol/L

Secondary survey
CNS: E4 V5 M6 = 15 PEARLA 4 mm. T 38.8 °C
PAIN: C/o pain to abdomen, and radiating to the back – rated as 7/10, pain unchanged on movement. Diaphoretic, generalised.
CVS: HR 115 bpm, regular. BP 110/70 mmHg. Centrally warm, peripherally cooler. cap refill <3 secs

RESP: RR 22, no increased WOB, related to pain? Chest on auscultation clear throughout R = L with decreased AE bibasally. Nil cough. SpO$_2$ 98% RA. Clubbing.
GIT: BS Audible in all quadrants. Pain to RUQ/epigastric region, radiating to back. BGL 12.5 mmol/L. Nausea, reports vomiting prior to presentation.
RENAL (output): HNPU for past 6 hours.
SKIN/INTEG: Poor integrity, dry skin, grossly intact. Nil skin tears.
MUSCULOSKELETAL (mobility): Strict RIB, with VTE prophylaxis. Tremor present.
BMI: 28.0

CONCEPT MAP 13.6 Nursing assessment for Leonard

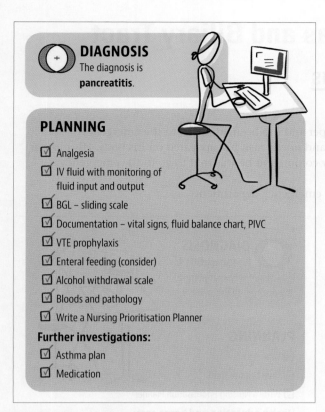

DIAGNOSIS

The diagnosis is **pancreatitis**.

PLANNING

- ☑ Analgesia
- ☑ IV fluid with monitoring of fluid input and output
- ☑ BGL – sliding scale
- ☑ Documentation – vital signs, fluid balance chart, PIVC
- ☑ VTE prophylaxis
- ☑ Enteral feeding (consider)
- ☑ Alcohol withdrawal scale
- ☑ Bloods and pathology
- ☑ Write a Nursing Prioritisation Planner

Further investigations:

- ☑ Asthma plan
- ☑ Medication

CONCEPT MAP 13.7 Diagnosis and planning for Leonard

INTERVENTIONS

1. Assess pain, BGLs and vital signs.
2. Assess alcohol withdrawal scale hourly or more frequently if required.
3. ISBAR handover preparation for end-of-shift handover – what would you be handing over if your patient has increasing pain?

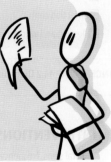

What further assessments should be initiated?

Cues
1. What further questions or information would you like to know from the patient?
2. What is the deterioration or change in patient status here?
3. What could be the pathophysiological reason for the increase in pain?

CONCEPT MAP 13.8 Nursing interventions for Leonard

EVALUATION

The medical team have been notified of the increase in your patient's pain. It is now rated as 9/10.

Plan:
Medical officer has requested further analgesia, and a repeat in vital signs, including BGL.

Cues
1. What interventions need to be considered now for your patient? What is your priority here?
2. The patient has been prescribed 5 mg subcutaneous morphine. What are the considerations for administration of this medication?
3. What do you think is the reason for the increase in pain?

CONCEPT MAP 13.9 Evaluation and planning for Leonard

DISCHARGE PLANNING + COORDINATION OF CARE

How do the following areas of healthcare management **relate** to Leonard's presentation? Which members of the healthcare team are **involved** in each area of management?

Pancreatitis
Medication
Diet review
Pain management plan
Follow-up with GP for repeat lipase and other indices

Smoking and alcohol use – cessation or minimisation of nicotine and alcohol
Medication
Referral (with consent) to AOD team
QUIT

NIDDM
Patient education and health promotion on BGL management
Diet review
Alcohol and impact on NIDDM – follow up with Diabetic Educator

CONCEPT MAP 13.10 Discharge planning and coordination of care for Leonard

Chapter 14: Liver, Pancreas and Biliary Tract

CONCEPT MAP SEQUENCE FOR HEPATITIS

Presentation

Ngoc Bui is a 28-year-old information technology developer and has been admitted to the emergency department with nausea and vomiting for the last week, and now a rash has appeared on his body. His mother noted that the white part of his eyes has a tinge of yellow colour, and he was told to go to the emergency department straight away.

Concept maps 14.1–14.5 explore Ngoc's initial care in the emergency department.

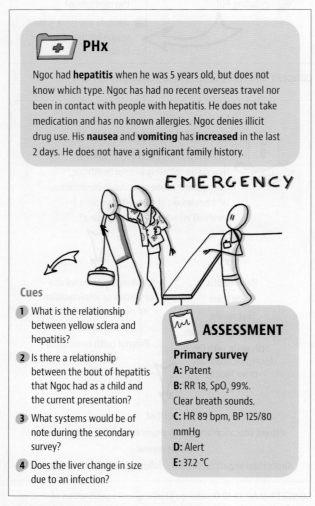

PHx

Ngoc had **hepatitis** when he was 5 years old, but does not know which type. Ngoc has had no recent overseas travel nor been in contact with people with hepatitis. He does not take medication and has no known allergies. Ngoc denies illicit drug use. His **nausea** and **vomiting** has **increased** in the last 2 days. He does not have a significant family history.

EMERGENCY

Cues

1. What is the relationship between yellow sclera and hepatitis?

2. Is there a relationship between the bout of hepatitis that Ngoc had as a child and the current presentation?

3. What systems would be of note during the secondary survey?

4. Does the liver change in size due to an infection?

ASSESSMENT

Primary survey
A: Patent
B: RR 18, SpO$_2$ 99%. Clear breath sounds.
C: HR 89 bpm, BP 125/80 mmHg
D: Alert
E: 37.2 °C

CONCEPT MAP 14.1 Nursing assessment for Ngoc

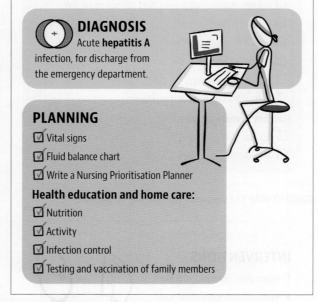

DIAGNOSIS

Acute **hepatitis A** infection, for discharge from the emergency department.

PLANNING

☑ Vital signs

☑ Fluid balance chart

☑ Write a Nursing Prioritisation Planner

Health education and home care:

☑ Nutrition

☑ Activity

☑ Infection control

☑ Testing and vaccination of family members

CONCEPT MAP 14.2 Diagnosis and planning for Ngoc

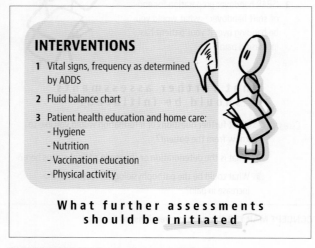

INTERVENTIONS

1. Vital signs, frequency as determined by ADDS

2. Fluid balance chart

3. Patient health education and home care:
   - Hygiene
   - Nutrition
   - Vaccination education
   - Physical activity

What further assessments should be initiated

CONCEPT MAP 14.3 Nursing interventions for Ngoc

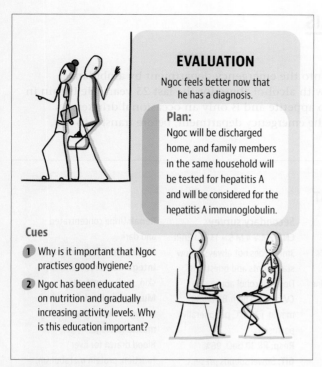

EVALUATION

Ngoc feels better now that he has a diagnosis.

Plan:
Ngoc will be discharged home, and family members in the same household will be tested for hepatitis A and will be considered for the hepatitis A immunoglobulin.

Cues

1. Why is it important that Ngoc practises good hygiene?
2. Ngoc has been educated on nutrition and gradually increasing activity levels. Why is this education important?

CONCEPT MAP 14.4 Evaluation and planning for Ngoc

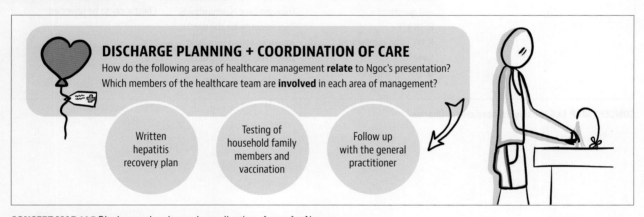

DISCHARGE PLANNING + COORDINATION OF CARE

How do the following areas of healthcare management **relate** to Ngoc's presentation? Which members of the healthcare team are **involved** in each area of management?

- Written hepatitis recovery plan
- Testing of household family members and vaccination
- Follow up with the general practitioner

CONCEPT MAP 14.5 Discharge planning and coordination of care for Ngoc

CONCEPT MAP SEQUENCE FOR CIRRHOSIS

Presentation

Charles Wilson is a 62-year-old man who was brought into the emergency department by ambulance. Charles' wife states that he has had ongoing problems with alcohol abuse for the last 25 years. He is thin in build and has a florid face. Charles states that he has no appetite and is only an occasional drinker.

Concept maps 14.6–14.10 explore Charles' initial care in the emergency department, before transfer to the medical ward for further care.

 PHx

Charles had a **bleeding gastric ulcer** 3 years ago, which was treated. He now has had significant weight loss, and nausea and vomiting for the last 3 weeks. Charles states that he does not have an alcohol problem, and the gastric ulcer was not caused by alcohol.

 ASSESSMENT

Primary survey
A: Clear
B: RR 28, pulse oximetry 96% on room air, breath sounds reveal lower lobe bilateral fine crackles on auscultation.
C: HR 102 bpm, BP 150/90 mmHg, spider angiomas on cheeks and nose
D: Orientated but does not always follow statements and questions
E: 38.3 °C
F: IVF to be commenced, urine dark
G: BGL 7.2 mmol/L

Secondary survey
CNS: E 4 V 4 M 5 = 13/15 PEARL 3mm. Does not always follow statements and questions. Denies alcohol abuse.
CVS: HR 104 bpm, BP 155/90 mmHg, T 38.6 °C, peripherally perfused
Resp: RR 30, SaO$_2$ 96%
GIT: Bowel sounds present. Left upper quadrant tender. Enlarged liver. Haemorrhoids. Poor appetite for the last 3 weeks, so eating very little. So has regular constipation.

Renal: Urine concentrated and dark
Metabolic: BGL 7.2 mmol/L
Integumentary: Warm dry skin, spider angiomas.
Musculoskeletal: Equal limb strength with limbs showing muscle wastage.
Blood drawn for liver function, protein metabolism, and lipid metabolism.
Chest x-ray to be reviewed.

CONCEPT MAP 14.6 Nursing assessment for Charles

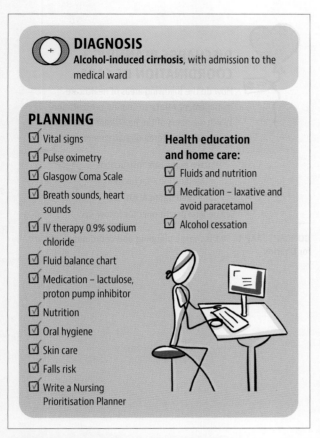

DIAGNOSIS

Alcohol-induced cirrhosis, with admission to the medical ward

PLANNING

- ☑ Vital signs
- ☑ Pulse oximetry
- ☑ Glasgow Coma Scale
- ☑ Breath sounds, heart sounds
- ☑ IV therapy 0.9% sodium chloride
- ☑ Fluid balance chart
- ☑ Medication – lactulose, proton pump inhibitor
- ☑ Nutrition
- ☑ Oral hygiene
- ☑ Skin care
- ☑ Falls risk
- ☑ Write a Nursing Prioritisation Planner

Health education and home care:

- ☑ Fluids and nutrition
- ☑ Medication – laxative and avoid paracetamol
- ☑ Alcohol cessation

CONCEPT MAP 14.7 Diagnosis and planning for Charles

INTERVENTIONS

1. Vital signs 4 hourly
2. Pulse oximetry 4 hourly
3. Glasgow Coma Scale 4 hourly
4. Breath sounds and heart sounds daily
5. Hourly alcohol withdrawal scale
6. IV therapy 0.9% sodium chloride 8/24
7. Fluid balance chart
8. Lactulose 6 hourly, Esomeprazole daily
9. High protein diet
10. Oral care after meals and snacks
11. Skin care 2 hourly
12. Falls risk 8 hourly

Health education and home care:

- Nutrition – small regular meals and increased fluid intake
- Medication – lactulose, esomeprazole
- Alcohol cessation program

What further assessments should be initiated?

CONCEPT MAP 14.8 Nursing interventions for Charles

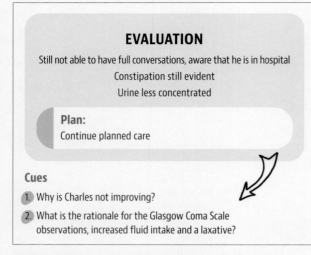

EVALUATION

Still not able to have full conversations, aware that he is in hospital

Constipation still evident

Urine less concentrated

Plan:

Continue planned care

Cues

1. Why is Charles not improving?

2. What is the rationale for the Glasgow Coma Scale observations, increased fluid intake and a laxative?

CONCEPT MAP 14.9 Evaluation and planning for Charles

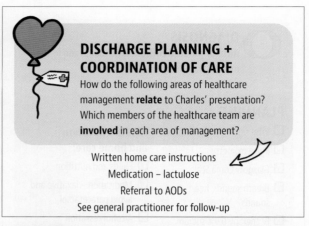

DISCHARGE PLANNING + COORDINATION OF CARE

How do the following areas of healthcare management **relate** to Charles' presentation? Which members of the healthcare team are **involved** in each area of management?

Written home care instructions

Medication – lactulose

Referral to AODs

See general practitioner for follow-up

CONCEPT MAP 14.10 Discharge planning and coordination of care for Charles

CONCEPT MAP SEQUENCE FOR GALLSTONES (CHOLELITHIASIS)

Presentation

Rosa Futura is a 56-year-old woman who was brought to the emergency department by her husband. Rosa was making pasta sauce for dinner, when suddenly she felt excruciating pain on her upper right side and bent over with pain. Rosa's face is quite sweaty.

Concept maps 14.11–14.15 explore Rosa's presentation/admission.

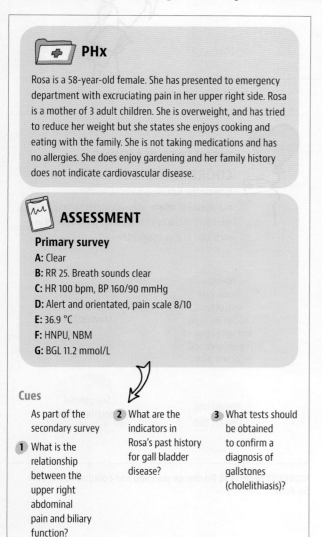

PHx

Rosa is a 58-year-old female. She has presented to emergency department with excruciating pain in her upper right side. Rosa is a mother of 3 adult children. She is overweight, and has tried to reduce her weight but she states she enjoys cooking and eating with the family. She is not taking medications and has no allergies. She does enjoy gardening and her family history does not indicate cardiovascular disease.

ASSESSMENT

Primary survey

A: Clear
B: RR 25. Breath sounds clear
C: HR 100 bpm, BP 160/90 mmHg
D: Alert and orientated, pain scale 8/10
E: 36.9 °C
F: HNPU, NBM
G: BGL 11.2 mmol/L

Cues

As part of the secondary survey

1 What is the relationship between the upper right abdominal pain and biliary function?

2 What are the indicators in Rosa's past history for gall bladder disease?

3 What tests should be obtained to confirm a diagnosis of gallstones (cholelithiasis)?

CONCEPT MAP 14.11 Nursing assessment for Rosa

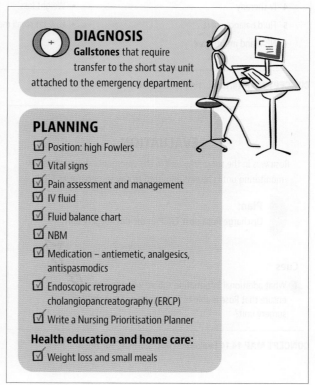

DIAGNOSIS

Gallstones that require transfer to the short stay unit attached to the emergency department.

PLANNING

☑ Position: high Fowlers
☑ Vital signs
☑ Pain assessment and management
☑ IV fluid
☑ Fluid balance chart
☑ NBM
☑ Medication – antiemetic, analgesics, antispasmodics
☑ Endoscopic retrograde cholangiopancreatography (ERCP)
☑ Write a Nursing Prioritisation Planner

Health education and home care:

☑ Weight loss and small meals

CONCEPT MAP 14.12 Diagnosis and planning for Rosa

INTERVENTIONS

1. Positioning – high Fowlers
2. Vital signs – every 2 hours, then 4 hourly overnight
3. Pain scale hourly
4. IV therapy
5. Fluid balance chart
6. NBM and mouth care
7. Medication – ondansetron, morphine and atropine
8. Prepare for ERCP next day.

Health education and home care:
- Weight loss
- Low fat small meals

What further assessments should be initiated

CONCEPT MAP 14.13 Nursing interventions for Rosa

EVALUATION

Rosa was in the short stay unit in the emergency department for monitoring until she was admitted to day surgery for an ERCP.

Plan:
Discharge Rosa post-ERCP in the day surgery unit.

Cues

 1. What additional information should we obtain to ensure that Rosa is able to be discharged from the day surgery unit?

CONCEPT MAP 14.14 Evaluation and planning for Rosa

DISCHARGE PLANNING + COORDINATION OF CARE

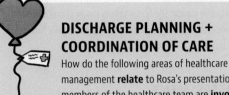 How do the following areas of healthcare management **relate** to Rosa's presentation? Which members of the healthcare team are **involved** in each area of management?

- Written home care instructions, including signs and symptoms of recurrence and action plan
- Medication
- Weight loss Low fat diet
- See general practitioner for follow-up

CONCEPT MAP 14.15 Discharge planning and coordination of care for Rosa

Chapter 15: Musculoskeletal System

CONCEPT MAP SEQUENCE FOR A FRACTURE

Presentation

Michael, a 15-year-old male, was admitted to the surgical short stay unit after a fall from an electric scooter at approx. 20 km/hr. Michael sustained a FOOSH (fall on outstretched hand) resulting in a distal radial fracture to his right arm. He has been hospitalised overnight for monitoring post-sedation to a closed reduction. Post-sedation, Michael will have a POP cast put in place.

Concept maps 15.1–15.5 explore Michael's admission.

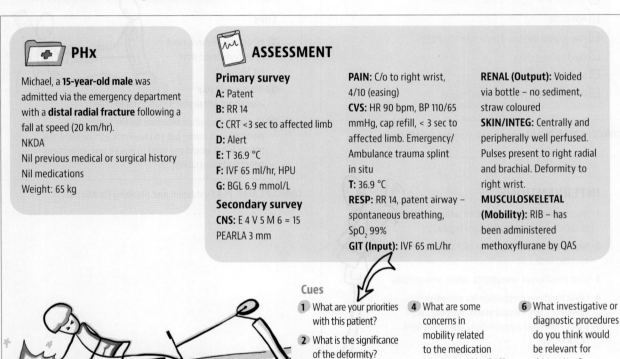

PHx

Michael, a **15-year-old male** was admitted via the emergency department with a **distal radial fracture** following a fall at speed (20 km/hr).
NKDA
Nil previous medical or surgical history
Nil medications
Weight: 65 kg

ASSESSMENT

Primary survey
A: Patent
B: RR 14
C: CRT <3 sec to affected limb
D: Alert
E: T 36.9 °C
F: IVF 65 ml/hr, HPU
G: BGL 6.9 mmol/L

Secondary survey
CNS: E 4 V 5 M 6 = 15
PEARLA 3 mm

PAIN (Output): C/o to right wrist, 4/10 (easing)
CVS: HR 90 bpm, BP 110/65 mmHg, cap refill, < 3 sec to affected limb. Emergency/Ambulance trauma splint in situ
T: 36.9 °C
RESP: RR 14, patent airway – spontaneous breathing, SpO_2 99%
GIT (Input): IVF 65 mL/hr

RENAL (Output): Voided via bottle – no sediment, straw coloured
SKIN/INTEG: Centrally and peripherally well perfused. Pulses present to right radial and brachial. Deformity to right wrist.
MUSCULOSKELETAL (Mobility): RIB – has been administered methoxyflurane by QAS

Cues

1 What are your priorities with this patient?

2 What is the significance of the deformity?

3 What is the relationship between the FOOSH and the distal fracture?

4 What are some concerns in mobility related to the medication administered by QAS?

5 How frequently would you assess pain levels?

6 What investigative or diagnostic procedures do you think would be relevant for this patient?

CONCEPT MAP 15.1 Nursing assessment for Michael

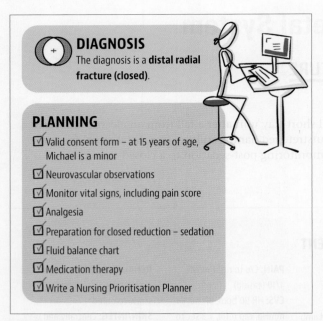

DIAGNOSIS

The diagnosis is a **distal radial fracture (closed)**.

PLANNING

- ☑ Valid consent form – at 15 years of age, Michael is a minor
- ☑ Neurovascular observations
- ☑ Monitor vital signs, including pain score
- ☑ Analgesia
- ☑ Preparation for closed reduction – sedation
- ☑ Fluid balance chart
- ☑ Medication therapy
- ☑ Write a Nursing Prioritisation Planner

CONCEPT MAP 15.2 Diagnosis and planning for Michael

INTERVENTIONS

1. Assess pain, neurovascular observations, level of consciousness and vital signs regularly
2. Neurovascular assessment of POP cast and affected limb
3. Limb elevation as tolerated to reduce limb oedema
4. ISBAR handover preparation for end-of-shift handover – what would you be handing over if your patient had a diminished pulse to his right radial artery?

What further assessments should be initiated?

Cues

1. Why are neurovascular observations crucial to fractures?
2. What possible reasons could there be for the patient to report pain?
3. What has likely occurred for Michael's pulse to be diminished in the right radial artery?

CONCEPT MAP 15.3 Nursing interventions for Michael

EVALUATION

The medical team have been notified of Michael's **decreased sensation** and **increased pain** to his right wrist.

Plan:

Michael is to have a closed reduction, under sedation, and then a plaster of paris (POP) applied in the ED. He will be admitted to the short stay surgical unit overnight due to age and sedation.

Cues

1. What interventions need to be considered now for Michael?
2. What would your assessment entail post sedation for Michael?
3. Michael is prescribed ketamine for the sedation (one medication of many) but you have not administered this before. What would you need to ensure and understand prior to administration?

CONCEPT MAP 15.4 Evaluation and planning for Michael

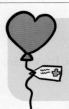
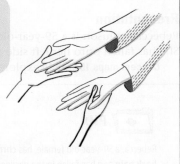

DISCHARGE PLANNING + COORDINATION OF CARE

How do the following areas of healthcare management **relate** to Michael's presentation? Which members of the healthcare team are **involved** in each area of management?

Fractured distal radius

Medication/analgesia

Follow-up review with fracture clinic (appointment made prior to discharge)

Education handout for fractures

Report any increase in pain

Report any decrease in sensation to affected limb

Occupational therapist referral for aids for dominant hand

Post sedation observation

Instructions to parents/ care giver for any side effects (ketamine-induced nightmares)

Superficial bruising and abrasions

Keeping site clean

Education about signs of localised infection

Reporting any increase in pain

CONCEPT MAP 15.5 Discharge planning and coordination of care for Michael

CONCEPT MAP SEQUENCE FOR BACK PAIN

Presentation

Rebecca Ferguson is a 59-year-old-female who has presented post a fall, with a background of chronic back pain. She has fallen onto her left side and is complaining of pain in her lower back and shoulder.

Concept maps 15.6–15.10 explore Rebecca's admission.

 PHx

Rebecca, a 59-year-old female, has **chronic back pain** and has fallen in the garden today on a slippery tile. She has fallen onto her left side and is complaining of pain to her lower back, and shoulder. Her 'normal' back pain is in her cervical and thoracic region from a motor vehicle accident 25 years ago.

PMHx, #T9-11 – MVA 25 years ago.

Meds – amitriptyline 25 mg, targin 40/10 BD, telmisarten 40 mg, aspirin 100 mg. NKDA.

Smokes 15 cigs/day

ETOH – 2 wines/day

 ASSESSMENT

Primary survey

A: Patent
B: RR 20
C: Warm
D: Alert
E: T 36.2 °C
F: HNPU nil in
G: BGL 6.5 mmol/L

Secondary survey

CNS: E 4 V 5 M 6 = 15 PEARL 4 mm
PAIN: C/o pain to mid lower back, centralised, pain also in her right shoulder from fall. Rating pain as 7/10.

Has taken her a.m. dose of targin (it is now 1400 hours)

CVS: HR 82 bpm, regular. BP 140/65 mmHg. Centrally and peripherally warm, cap refill <3 sec. T 36.2 °C

RESP: RR 20, chest on auscultation clear throughout R=L. Nil cough. SpO$_2$ 98% RA

GIT: BS audible in all quadrants. BGL 6.5 mmol/L

RENAL (output): HNPU as yet

SKIN/INTEG: Abrasions to right shoulder, nil other breaks in integument

MUSCULOSKELETAL (mobility): Await physio review due to pain

Cues

1 What are your priorities with this patient?

2 What is the concern regarding analgesia here?

3 What does targin do? Will it be safe to administer this patient further analgesia?

4 What are the concerns for this patient with acute on chronic pain?

5 How could you assess her right shoulder for pain? Would you also perform neurovascular observations?

6 What investigative or diagnostic procedures do you think would be relevant for this patient?

CONCEPT MAP 15.6 Nursing assessment for Rebecca

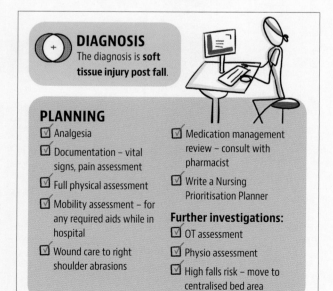

DIAGNOSIS
The diagnosis is **soft tissue injury post fall**.

PLANNING

☑ Analgesia

☑ Documentation – vital signs, pain assessment

☑ Full physical assessment

☑ Mobility assessment – for any required aids while in hospital

☑ Wound care to right shoulder abrasions

☑ Medication management review – consult with pharmacist

☑ Write a Nursing Prioritisation Planner

Further investigations:

☑ OT assessment

☑ Physio assessment

☑ High falls risk – move to centralised bed area

CONCEPT MAP 15.7 Diagnosis and planning for Rebecca

INTERVENTIONS

1 Assess pain, abrasions and neurovascular observations to affected limb. Assess for falls risk in hospital.

2 Referral to pain specialist

3 Establish acute on chronic pain management in collaboration with healthcare team

4 ISBAR handover preparation for end-of-shift handover – what would you be handing over if your patient was a high falls risk?

What further assessments should be initiated

Cues **1** What further questions or information would you like to know from the patient?

2 What is the potential impact on the patient's mobility if she already has chronic back pain in her upper back, and now has pain in her lower back?

3 What frequency would you assess her pain?

CONCEPT MAP 15.8 Nursing interventions for Rebecca

EVALUATION

The medical team have been notified of the increase in pain to your patient's shoulder and lower back.

Plan:
Medical officer has requested you to administer 10 mg oxycodone PO.

Cues

1 What interventions need to be considered now for your patient? What is your priority here?

2 If your patient has already had targin 40/10 is it safe to administer 10 mg oxycodone? What are the nursing considerations here?

3 What do you think is the reason for increase in pain? Is this a deterioration or an expected occurence?

CONCEPT MAP 15.9 Evaluation and planning for Rebecca

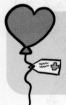

DISCHARGE PLANNING + COORDINATION OF CARE

How do the following areas of healthcare management **relate** to the patient presentation? Which members of the healthcare team are **involved** in each area of management?

Soft tissue injury – right shoulder and lumbar spine

Management and education to patient on non-pharmaceutical analgesia such as change of position, movement, etc.

Ongoing review of chronic pain management with current pain medication

Follow up with GP in one week

Mobility post-fall and wound care

Gait assessment – physiotherapist

Management of wound – keep abrasions clean and dry, for review by GP in one week

Pain management

Patient education and health promotion regarding pain management and activity

Review by chronic pain team to establish analgesia for old injury

Review by physiotherapist for ongoing management of acute pain

CONCEPT MAP 15.10 Discharge planning and coordination of care for Rebecca

Chapter 16: Female Reproductive System

CONCEPT MAP SEQUENCE FOR ENDOMETRIOSIS

Presentation

Lee Jones is a 28-year-old receptionist who has attended the general practice clinic to work out why she has painful periods. The painful periods started when she was 17 years old, and the period pain has recently become so debilitating that she now needs to take time off from work.

Concept maps 16.1–16.5 explore Lee's initial care with the general practice nurse.

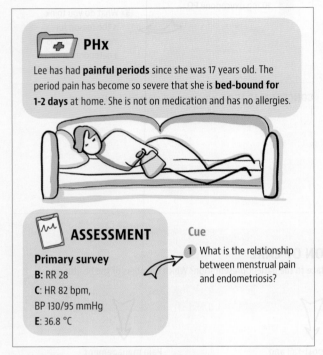

PHx

Lee has had **painful periods** since she was 17 years old. The period pain has become so severe that she is **bed-bound for 1-2 days** at home. She is not on medication and has no allergies.

ASSESSMENT

Primary survey
B: RR 28
C: HR 82 bpm, BP 130/95 mmHg
E: 36.8 °C

Cue

1. What is the relationship between menstrual pain and endometriosis?

CONCEPT MAP 16.1 Nursing assessment for Lee

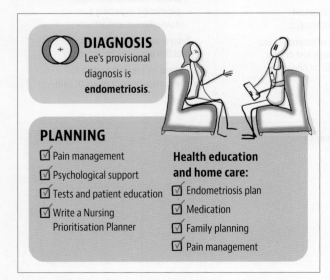

DIAGNOSIS
Lee's provisional diagnosis is **endometriosis**.

PLANNING

☑ Pain management
☑ Psychological support
☑ Tests and patient education
☑ Write a Nursing Prioritisation Planner

Health education and home care:

☑ Endometriosis plan
☑ Medication
☑ Family planning
☑ Pain management

CONCEPT MAP 16.2 Diagnosis and planning for Lee

INTERVENTIONS

Health education and home care:
Endometriosis plan – NSAIDs

What further assessments should be initiated

CONCEPT MAP 16.3 Nursing interventions for Lee

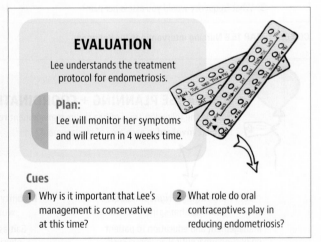

EVALUATION

Lee understands the treatment protocol for endometriosis.

Plan:
Lee will monitor her symptoms and will return in 4 weeks time.

Cues

1. Why is it important that Lee's management is conservative at this time?

2. What role do oral contraceptives play in reducing endometriosis?

CONCEPT MAP 16.4 Evaluation and planning for Lee

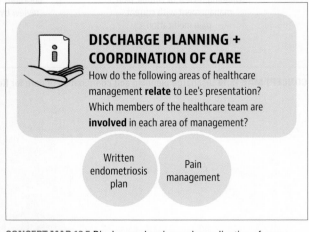

DISCHARGE PLANNING + COORDINATION OF CARE
How do the following areas of healthcare management **relate** to Lee's presentation? Which members of the healthcare team are **involved** in each area of management?

Written endometriosis plan

Pain management

CONCEPT MAP 16.5 Discharge planning and coordination of care for Lee

CONCEPT MAP SEQUENCE FOR POLYCYSTIC OVARY SYNDROME

Presentation

Justine Rebeiro is a 32-year-old woman who has presented to her general practice for an appointment with the practice nurse who is also a midwife. The practice nurse notes Justine is experiencing difficulty in becoming pregnant. Justine has irregular periods and has tried to eat a healthy diet as she acknowledges she is overweight.

Concept maps 16.6–16.10 explore Justine's care in the practice nurse's office.

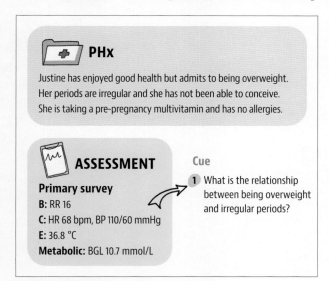

PHx

Justine has enjoyed good health but admits to being overweight. Her periods are irregular and she has not been able to conceive. She is taking a pre-pregnancy multivitamin and has no allergies.

ASSESSMENT

Primary survey
B: RR 16
C: HR 68 bpm, BP 110/60 mmHg
E: 36.8 °C
Metabolic: BGL 10.7 mmol/L

Cue
1 What is the relationship between being overweight and irregular periods?

CONCEPT MAP 16.6 Nursing assessment for Justine

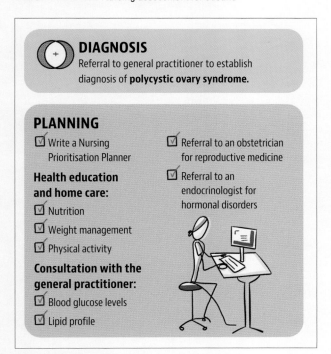

DIAGNOSIS
Referral to general practitioner to establish diagnosis of **polycystic ovary syndrome.**

PLANNING
☑ Write a Nursing Prioritisation Planner

Health education and home care:
☑ Nutrition
☑ Weight management
☑ Physical activity

Consultation with the general practitioner:
☑ Blood glucose levels
☑ Lipid profile

☑ Referral to an obstetrician for reproductive medicine
☑ Referral to an endocrinologist for hormonal disorders

CONCEPT MAP 16.7 Diagnosis and planning for Justine

INTERVENTIONS

1 Referred to general practitioner for follow up:
- blood glucose level
- lipid profile
- referrals to obstetrician and endocrinologist as needed

Health education and home care:
- Nutrition – moderate carbohydrate and fat intake
- Physical activity
- Weight measurement

What further assessments should be initiated

CONCEPT MAP 16.8 Nursing interventions for Justine

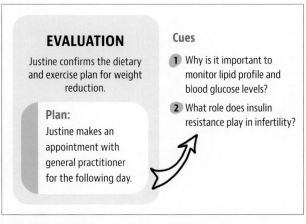

EVALUATION

Justine confirms the dietary and exercise plan for weight reduction.

Plan:
Justine makes an appointment with general practitioner for the following day.

Cues
1 Why is it important to monitor lipid profile and blood glucose levels?
2 What role does insulin resistance play in infertility?

CONCEPT MAP 16.9 Evaluation and planning for Justine

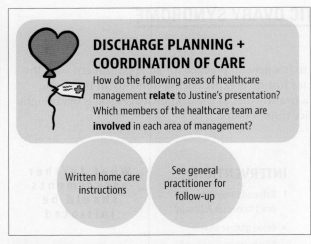

DISCHARGE PLANNING + COORDINATION OF CARE

How do the following areas of healthcare management **relate** to Justine's presentation? Which members of the healthcare team are **involved** in each area of management?

Written home care instructions

See general practitioner for follow-up

CONCEPT MAP 16.10 Discharge planning and coordination of care for Justine

CONCEPT MAP SEQUENCE FOR CHLAMYDIA

Presentation

Vera Voroski is a 22-year-old university student who has experienced painful urination for the last three days. She has made an appointment with the practice nurse at her general practitioner's office.

Concept maps 16.11–16.15 explore Vera's care in the practice nurse's office.

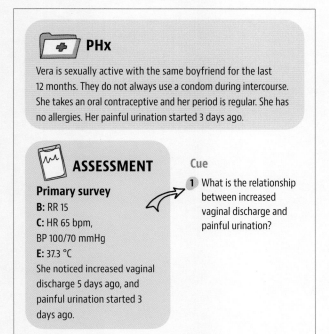

PHx

Vera is sexually active with the same boyfriend for the last 12 months. They do not always use a condom during intercourse. She takes an oral contraceptive and her period is regular. She has no allergies. Her painful urination started 3 days ago.

ASSESSMENT

Primary survey
B: RR 15
C: HR 65 bpm,
BP 100/70 mmHg
E: 37.3 °C
She noticed increased vaginal discharge 5 days ago, and painful urination started 3 days ago.

Cue
1 What is the relationship between increased vaginal discharge and painful urination?

CONCEPT MAP 16.11 Nursing assessment for Vera

INTERVENTIONS

1 Urine test

2 Referral to general practitioner for examination; Doxycycline for Vera and her partner, antibiotic for both chlamydia and gonorrhoea

Health education and home care:

- Abstain from sex while on antibiotic
- Always use a condom
- Follow up in 3 months

What further assessments should be initiated

CONCEPT MAP 16.13 Nursing interventions for Vera

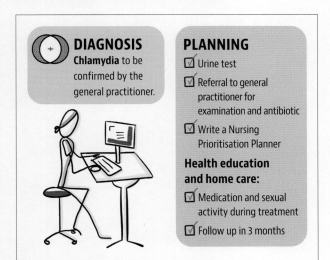

DIAGNOSIS
Chlamydia to be confirmed by the general practitioner.

PLANNING
☑ Urine test
☑ Referral to general practitioner for examination and antibiotic
☑ Write a Nursing Prioritisation Planner

Health education and home care:
☑ Medication and sexual activity during treatment
☑ Follow up in 3 months

CONCEPT MAP 16.12 Diagnosis and planning for Vera

EVALUATION

Vera was able to explain what was required to ensure treatment was followed while her chlamydia infection was being resolved.

Plan:
Vera was able to see the general practitioner immediately after the consultation with the practice nurse.

Cue
1 What additional information would the general practitioner require to be able to differentiate chlamydia and gonorrhoea infections?

CONCEPT MAP 16.14 Evaluation and planning for Vera

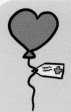

DISCHARGE PLANNING + COORDINATION OF CARE

How do the following areas of healthcare management **relate** to Vera's presentation? Which members of the healthcare team are **involved** in each area of management?

| Written home care instructions | Return in 3 months for follow-up | Antimicrobial stewardship |

CONCEPT MAP 16.15 Discharge planning and coordination of care for Vera

Chapter 17: Male Reproductive System

CONCEPT MAP SEQUENCE FOR A URINARY TRACT INFECTION (UTI)

Presentation

Peter Carrington is a 58-year-old male who presented two days prior with an upper respiratory tract infection. He has developed urinary symptoms during his hospitalisation.

Concept maps 17.1–17.5 explore Peter's presentation/admission.

 PHx

Peter, a **58-year-old male**, day 2 on medical ward. Presented initially with upper respiratory tract infection, now complaining of difficulty in urinating, and an increase in urgency and frequency in urination.
PMHx – NKDA, Hypertension, COVID-19 May 2022, Asthma.
Meds – Telmisartan 20 mg, Atorvastatin 40 mg, Esomeprazole 20 mg, Salbutamol 2 puffs daily.

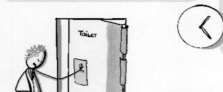

 ASSESSMENT

Primary survey
A: Patent
B: RR 16 bpm
C: Warm and well perfused
D: Alert
E: Nil concerns
F: Difficulty urinating
G: BGL 6.2 mmol/L

Secondary survey
CNS: E 4 V 5 M 6 = 15 PEARLA 3 mm
PAIN: C/o pain on urination 4/10
CVS: HR 90 bpm, BP 160/90 mmHg, T: 37.7 °C

RESP: RR 16 bpm, patent airway – spontaneous breathing, SpO$_2$ 98% RA, AE = on auscultation
GIT (Input): IVC to be placed, currently nothing running
RENAL (Output): C/o frequency, pain on urination, Pt reports blood passed on urination
SKIN/INTEG: Centrally warm and peripherally cooler. Cap refill time < 3 sec.
MUSCULOSKELETAL (Mobility): Steady gait, SOBOE prior to admission – RIB
BMI: 28.5

Cues
1 What are your priorities with this patient?
2 What other vital signs or bedside investigations would you perform?
3 What is the relationship between dysuria, frequency and urgency?
4 What is the pathophysiological relationship of UTI and frequency, dysuria and urgency?
5 What investigative or diagnostic procedures do you think would be relevant for this patient?

CONCEPT MAP 17.1 Nursing assessment for Peter

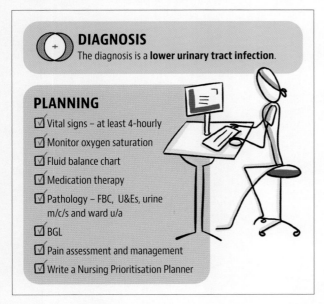 **DIAGNOSIS**
The diagnosis is a **lower urinary tract infection**.

PLANNING
☑ Vital signs – at least 4-hourly
☑ Monitor oxygen saturation
☑ Fluid balance chart
☑ Medication therapy
☑ Pathology – FBC, U&Es, urine m/c/s and ward u/a
☑ BGL
☑ Pain assessment and management
☑ Write a Nursing Prioritisation Planner

CONCEPT MAP 17.2 Diagnosis and planning for Peter

INTERVENTIONS

1 Assess urinary symptoms with each void.

2 Fluid intake and output – fluid balance chart

3 Nutrition status

4 Vital signs

5 Pain assessment and management

6 ISBAR handover preparation for end-of-shift handover – what would you be handing over regarding your patient's condition?

What further assessments should be initiated

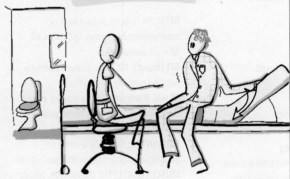

Cues

1 What are the symptoms relevant to a UTI here?

2 What patient education could you provide to Peter?

3 If the patient develops tachycardia and becomes more febrile what could this be evidence of?

CONCEPT MAP 17.3 Nursing interventions for Peter

EVALUATION

The medical team have been notified of Peter's increasing temperature (now 38.1 °C) and HR 105 bpm and regular.

Plan:
Commence IVABs, collect urine m/c/s, administer paracetamol.

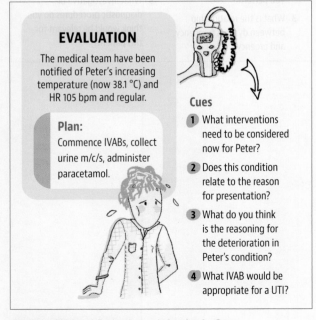

Cues

1 What interventions need to be considered now for Peter?

2 Does this condition relate to the reason for presentation?

3 What do you think is the reasoning for the deterioration in Peter's condition?

4 What IVAB would be appropriate for a UTI?

CONCEPT MAP 17.4 Evaluation and planning for Peter

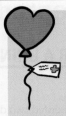

DISCHARGE PLANNING + COORDINATION OF CARE

How do the following areas of healthcare management **relate** to Peter's presentation? Which members of the healthcare team are **involved** in each area of management?

UTI

Medication

Lifestyle modifications – dietary intake, follow-up with GP for review.

Management plan for a repeat of any symptoms

Hypertension, asthma and URTI follow-up

Review of blood pressure and any unresolved symptoms from hospitalisation, follow-up with GP

CONCEPT MAP 17.5 Discharge planning and coordination of care for Peter

Chapter 21: Complex Care

CONCEPT MAP SEQUENCE FOR A PERSON WITH COVID-19

Presentation

Caitlyn-Rose is a 28-year-old female who has presented to the emergency department via ambulance for increased shortness of breath, fever and coughing. **Concept maps 21.1–21.5** explore Caitlyn-Rose's initial care in the emergency department.

 PHx

Caitlyn-Rose, a 28-year-old female with a 2/7 history of shortness of breath, non-productive cough, subjective fevers, fatigue, and headache. Works in retail.
No medical or surgical history.
Presents via ambulance, who were called to her workplace due to increased SOB and coughing.

 ASSESSMENT

Primary survey
A: Patent
B: RR 24
C: Warm
D: ALOC GCS 14
E: T 38.2°C
F: IVF @ 166 ml/hr voided
G: BGL 6.5 mmol/L

Secondary survey
CNS (Cognition): E 4 V4 (disorientated to time/person/place) M 6 = 14 PEARL 4 mm
PAIN: c/o headache, not rating pain
CVS: HR 90 bpm and reg, BP 100/65 mmHg, pedal pulses bounding. A 12-lead electrocardiogram showed sinus rhythm

with no abnormalities. T 38.2 °C (has had paracetamol 1 g 60 mins ago)
RESP: RR 24, SpO$_2$ 94%, patent airway – spontaneous breathing, increased work of breathing, spontaneous cough, non-productive. AE decreased BB
GIT (input): IVF 166 mL/hr. Abdo soft, non-tender, BS audible in all quadrants
RENAL (output): voided via pan, 240 mL – some sediment, amber coloured
SKIN/INTEG: Centrally warm and peripherally cooler
MUSCULOSKELETAL (mobility): RIB currently due to confusion
BMI: 23.0

Cues

1. What are your priorities with this patient?

2. What is the significance of her temperature?

3. What is the relationship between work of breathing and respiratory rate?

4. What is the pathophysiological relationship between a viral infection, such as COVID-19, and multi-organ dysfunction?

5. What are some concerns in relationship to the GCS assessment in this patient?

6. What physiological impact can a prolonged fever cause?

7. What investigative or diagnostic procedures would you think would be relevant for this patient?

CONCEPT MAP 21.1 Nursing assessment for Caitlyn-Rose

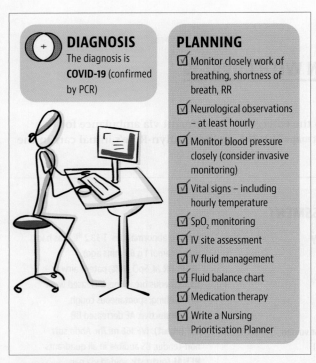

DIAGNOSIS

The diagnosis is **COVID-19** (confirmed by PCR)

PLANNING

☑ Monitor closely work of breathing, shortness of breath, RR

☑ Neurological observations – at least hourly

☑ Monitor blood pressure closely (consider invasive monitoring)

☑ Vital signs – including hourly temperature

☑ SpO$_2$ monitoring

☑ IV site assessment

☑ IV fluid management

☑ Fluid balance chart

☑ Medication therapy

☑ Write a Nursing Prioritisation Planner

CONCEPT MAP 21.2 Diagnosis and planning for Caitlyn-Rose

INTERVENTIONS

1 Assess RR, WOB and SpO$_2$, level of consciousness and GCS frequently

2 Position the patient into semi-Fowlers or high-Fowlers postion if they can tolerate it

3 Isolation procedures

4 Respiratory precautions

5 ISBAR handover preparation for end-of-shift handover – what would you be handing over if your patient had a GCS of E4 V4 M5, PEARL 4 mm+, was febrile and had an increased RR?

What further assessments should be initiated

Cues ① Why is chest auscultation and work of breathing crucial in this patient?

② What possible reasons would there be for the patient to be experiencing SOB?

③ What has precipitated the change in GCS? How has this occurred?

CONCEPT MAP 21.3 Nursing interventions for Caitlyn-Rose

EVALUATION

The medical team have been notified of Caitlyn's altered SpO$_2$ (95%) associated with increase in RR and WOB.

Plan:
Supplementary oxygen support – high flow nasal prongs, 35 L, FiO$_2$ 0.3
Position in high Fowlers as tolerated
NBM

Cues ① What interventions need to be considered now for Caitlyn?

② What is the significance of NBM?

③ How does HFNP assist patients' airways? What does it 'do'?

CONCEPT MAP 21.4 Evaluation and planning for Caitlyn-Rose

DISCHARGE PLANNING + COORDINATION OF CARE

How do the following areas of healthcare management **relate** to Caitlyn-Rose's presentation? Which members of the healthcare team are **involved** in each area of management?

Respiratory – increased work of breathing, shortness of breath, hypoxia

Medication

Spirometry

Follow-up review with physiotherapist

Deep breathing and cough exercises

Worksheet for patient

Physiotherapy

Infection control measures

Contact tracing

Advice on presentation for testing if symptomatic

Vaccination information for when well again

Follow-up with GP

CONCEPT MAP 21.5 Discharge planning and coordination of care for Caitlyn-Rose

CONCEPT MAP SEQUENCE FOR CORONARY ARTERY BYPASS GRAFT SURGERY

Presentation

John Kennedy is a 78-year-old man that has been admitted to the emergency department (ED) with chest pain and breathlessness for the last two hours. He is pale and sweaty and is admitted to the monitored area of the ED.

Concept maps 21.6–21.10 explore John's presentation/admission.

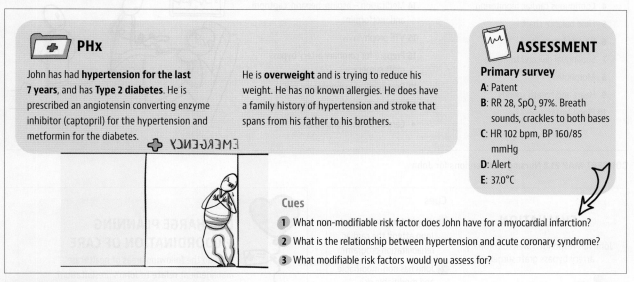

PHx

John has had **hypertension for the last 7 years**, and has **Type 2 diabetes**. He is prescribed an angiotensin converting enzyme inhibitor (captopril) for the hypertension and metformin for the diabetes.

He is **overweight** and is trying to reduce his weight. He has no known allergies. He does have a family history of hypertension and stroke that spans from his father to his brothers.

ASSESSMENT

Primary survey

A: Patent

B: RR 28, SpO$_2$ 97%. Breath sounds, crackles to both bases

C: HR 102 bpm, BP 160/85 mmHg

D: Alert

E: 37.0°C

Cues

1. What non-modifiable risk factor does John have for a myocardial infarction?
2. What is the relationship between hypertension and acute coronary syndrome?
3. What modifiable risk factors would you assess for?

CONCEPT MAP 21.6 Nursing assessment for John

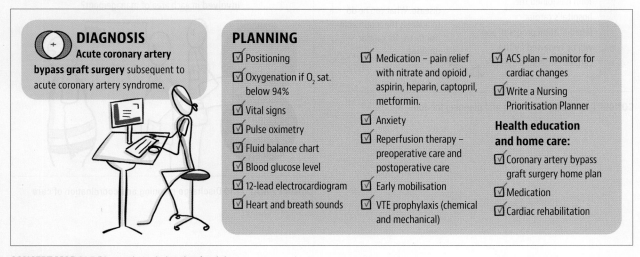

DIAGNOSIS

Acute coronary artery bypass graft surgery subsequent to acute coronary artery syndrome.

PLANNING

- ☑ Positioning
- ☑ Oxygenation if O$_2$ sat. below 94%
- ☑ Vital signs
- ☑ Pulse oximetry
- ☑ Fluid balance chart
- ☑ Blood glucose level
- ☑ 12-lead electrocardiogram
- ☑ Heart and breath sounds
- ☑ Medication – pain relief with nitrate and opioid , aspirin, heparin, captopril, metformin.
- ☑ Anxiety
- ☑ Reperfusion therapy – preoperative care and postoperative care
- ☑ Early mobilisation
- ☑ VTE prophylaxis (chemical and mechanical)
- ☑ ACS plan – monitor for cardiac changes
- ☑ Write a Nursing Prioritisation Planner

Health education and home care:

- ☑ Coronary artery bypass graft surgery home plan
- ☑ Medication
- ☑ Cardiac rehabilitation

CONCEPT MAP 21.7 Diagnosis and planning for John

INTERVENTIONS

1   Position upright
2   Oxygen if O$_2$ sat. below 94%
3   Vital signs and pulse oximetry
4   Continuous cardiac monitoring
5   Fluid balance chart
6   Blood glucose level
7   Sublingual glyceryl trinitrate
8   Morphine
9   Heart and breath sounds
10 Blood tests

11 12-lead ECG
12 Monitor for stress and anxiety
13 Psychosocial support
14 Medication – aspirin, heparin, captopril and metformin
15 VTE prophylaxis
16 Prepare for coronary artery bypass graft surgery
17 Post surgical management in ICU

Health education and home care:

• Cardiac rehabilitation plan

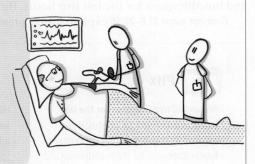

What further assessments should be initiated

CONCEPT MAP 21.8 Nursing interventions for John

EVALUATION

John has responded well to coronary artery bypass graft surgery.

Plan:
John has joined the hospital's cardiac rehabilitation program, and will be reviewed by the cardiac surgeon in 3 weeks.

Cues

1   Why is it important that John attend the cardiac rehabilitation program?

2   John has non-modifiable and modifiable risk factors for cardiac disease. What can he do to address the modifiable risk factor for cardiac disease?

CONCEPT MAP 21.9 Evaluation and planning for John

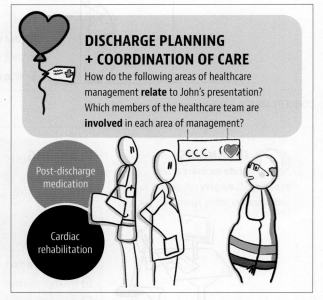

DISCHARGE PLANNING + COORDINATION OF CARE

How do the following areas of healthcare management **relate** to John's presentation? Which members of the healthcare team are **involved** in each area of management?

Post-discharge medication

Cardiac rehabilitation

CONCEPT MAP 21.10 Discharge planning and coordination of care for John

CONCEPT MAP SEQUENCE FOR SHOCK AND DISSEMINATED INTRAVASCULAR COAGULATION

Presentation

Subra Manorama is a 55-year-old man who was brought into the ED by ambulance. Subra fell off a ladder while pruning an apple tree. He landed on his left side and the blade of the open secateurs pierced his upper left thigh. His daughter, who has a first aid certificate, applied a compression bandage to the bleeding wound. When paramedics arrived to assess Subra, considerable blood seepage was occurring around the bandage and there was a pool of blood on the ground. Paramedics applied a further compression pad before transporting Subra to the ED.

Concept maps 21.11–21.15 explore Subra's initial care in the ED, before transfer to the operating theatre and the surgical ward for further care.

 PHx

Subra has enjoyed good health which he attributes to being a gardener and walker. He takes ginger for a healthy immune system and cardiac strength aspirin for his heart. He has no allergies. He takes aspirin as his family has a history of heart disease.

 ASSESSMENT

Primary Survey
A: Patent
B: RR 22, pulse oximetry 97% on room air, breath sounds normal
C: HR 118 bpm, BP 130/80 mmHg, skin pale. Wound on left thigh oozing blood through compression bandage
D: Alert and orientated
E: 36.7°C

F: IV to be commenced, wound ooze
G: BGL 5.7 mmol/L

Secondary Survey
CNS: Alert and orientated. GCS E 4 V 5 M 6 = 15.
CVS: BP 130/80 mmHg, HR 118 bpm, T 36.8°C, centrally and peripherally cool
Resp: RR 20, SpO$_2$ 96%

GIT: Bowel sounds present with a non-tender abdomen.
Renal: Urine concentrated but no abnormalities detected
Metabolic: BGL 5.7 mmol/L
Integumentary: Cool dry skin
Musculoskeletal: equal limb strength with pain at the wound site.
Left thigh x-ray and chest x-ray to be reviewed.

CONCEPT MAP 21.11 Nursing assessment for Subra

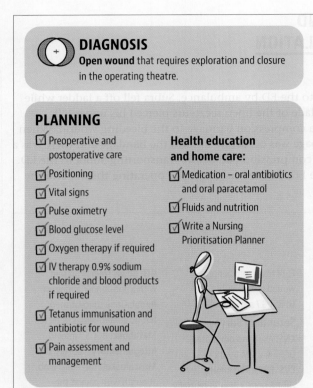

DIAGNOSIS

Open wound that requires exploration and closure in the operating theatre.

PLANNING

- ☑ Preoperative and postoperative care
- ☑ Positioning
- ☑ Vital signs
- ☑ Pulse oximetry
- ☑ Blood glucose level
- ☑ Oxygen therapy if required
- ☑ IV therapy 0.9% sodium chloride and blood products if required
- ☑ Tetanus immunisation and antibiotic for wound
- ☑ Pain assessment and management

Health education and home care:

- ☑ Medication – oral antibiotics and oral paracetamol
- ☑ Fluids and nutrition
- ☑ Write a Nursing Prioritisation Planner

CONCEPT MAP 21.12 Diagnosis and planning for Subra

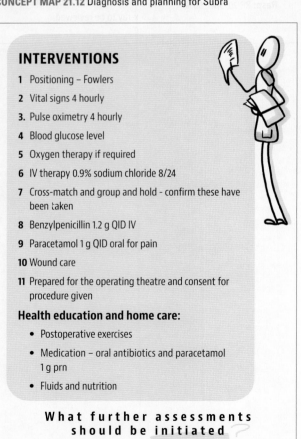

INTERVENTIONS

1. Positioning – Fowlers
2. Vital signs 4 hourly
3. Pulse oximetry 4 hourly
4. Blood glucose level
5. Oxygen therapy if required
6. IV therapy 0.9% sodium chloride 8/24
7. Cross-match and group and hold - confirm these have been taken
8. Benzylpenicillin 1.2 g QID IV
9. Paracetamol 1 g QID oral for pain
10. Wound care
11. Prepared for the operating theatre and consent for procedure given

Health education and home care:

- Postoperative exercises
- Medication – oral antibiotics and paracetamol 1 g prn
- Fluids and nutrition

What further assessments should be initiated?

CONCEPT MAP 21.13 Nursing interventions for Subra

EVALUATION

During the cleansing and closing of the wound in theatre, the wound would not stop oozing. Subra was transferred to the ICU for monitoring, fluid maintenance and wound management. Subra's wound is still oozing and his vital signs show tachypnoea, tachycardia and borderline hypotension. Subra states he is feeling anxious, and wonders if he will ever see his garden again.

Plan:

To take blood sample for full blood count and clotting profile.

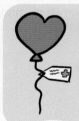

Cues

1. Why is Subra deteriorating?
2. What is the medical management for disseminated coagulopathy?
3. What nursing interventions would you instigate for Subra?

CONCEPT MAP 21.14 Evaluation and planning for Subra

DISCHARGE PLANNING + COORDINATION OF CARE

How do the following areas of healthcare management **relate** to Subra's presentation? Which members of the healthcare team are **involved** in each area of management?

- Written home care instructions for wound care, antibiotic therapy and pain management
- Medication – review self-prescribed ginger and aspirin dosage in view of bleeding disorder
- Outpatient clinic appointment

CONCEPT MAP 21.15 Discharge planning and coordination of care for Subra

CONCEPT MAP SEQUENCE FOR ACUTE RESPIRATORY DISTRESS SYNDROME

Presentation

Juan Montoya is a 36-year-old plumber who went to the general practitioner with an infected cut on his right calf. Juan was prescribed antibiotics for the infected wound and has been taking them for the last two days. This morning he woke up flushed and sweaty, and feels very nauseated. His mother brought him to the ED. Juan has noticed that his breathing has quickened.

Concept maps 21.16–21.20 explore Juan's initial care in the ED.

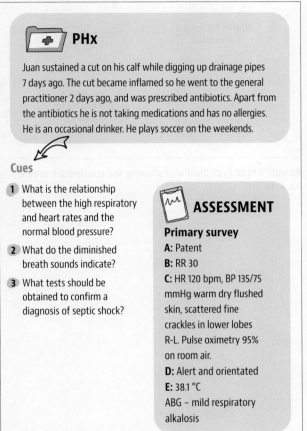

PHx

Juan sustained a cut on his calf while digging up drainage pipes 7 days ago. The cut became inflamed so he went to the general practitioner 2 days ago, and was prescribed antibiotics. Apart from the antibiotics he is not taking medications and has no allergies. He is an occasional drinker. He plays soccer on the weekends.

Cues

1 What is the relationship between the high respiratory and heart rates and the normal blood pressure?

2 What do the diminished breath sounds indicate?

3 What tests should be obtained to confirm a diagnosis of septic shock?

ASSESSMENT

Primary survey

A: Patent

B: RR 30

C: HR 120 bpm, BP 135/75 mmHg warm dry flushed skin, scattered fine crackles in lower lobes R–L. Pulse oximetry 95% on room air.

D: Alert and orientated

E: 38.1 °C

ABG – mild respiratory alkalosis

CONCEPT MAP 21.16 Nursing assessment for Juan

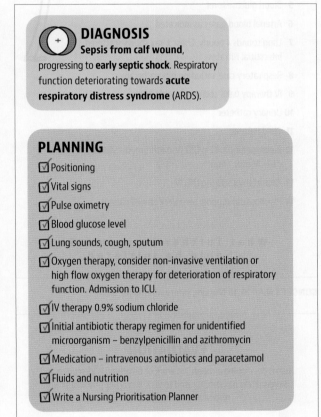

DIAGNOSIS

Sepsis from calf wound, progressing to **early septic shock**. Respiratory function deteriorating towards **acute respiratory distress syndrome** (ARDS).

PLANNING

☑ Positioning

☑ Vital signs

☑ Pulse oximetry

☑ Blood glucose level

☑ Lung sounds, cough, sputum

☑ Oxygen therapy, consider non-invasive ventilation or high flow oxygen therapy for deterioration of respiratory function. Admission to ICU.

☑ IV therapy 0.9% sodium chloride

☑ Initial antibiotic therapy regimen for unidentified microorganism – benzylpenicillin and azithromycin

☑ Medication – intravenous antibiotics and paracetamol

☑ Fluids and nutrition

☑ Write a Nursing Prioritisation Planner

CONCEPT MAP 21.17 Diagnosis and planning for Juan

INTERVENTIONS

1   Positioning – high Fowlers

2   Oxygen via mask to keep oxygen saturation above 94%

3   Vital signs hourly

4   Pulse oximetry hourly

5   Blood glucose level

6   Arterial blood gases as indicated

7   Lung sounds 4 hourly. Chest x-ray shows scattered interstitial filtrates.

8   Respiratory care, including physiotherapy

9   IV therapy 0.9% sodium chloride 8/24

10 Urinary catheter

11 Fluid balance

12 Benzylpenicillin 1.2 g QID IV; azithromycin 500 mg daily IV over 1 hour

13 Paracetamol 500 mg QID IV

14 Psychosocial support for a very unwell patient

What further assessments should be initiated?

CONCEPT MAP 21.18 Nursing interventions for Juan

EVALUATION

Juan is developing a cough, his work of breathing is increasing and oxygenation has deteriorated to 90% and is not physiologically responding to the increased FiO_2.

Plan:
For endotracheal intubation and mechanical ventilation to address deteriorating oxygen levels.

Cues

1   What additional information should we obtain about Juan's respiratory status?

CONCEPT MAP 21.19 Evaluation and planning for Juan

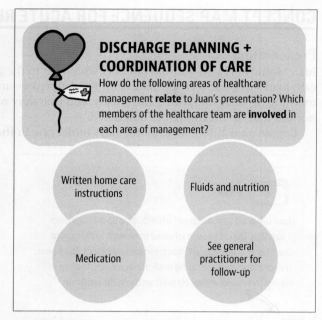

DISCHARGE PLANNING + COORDINATION OF CARE

How do the following areas of healthcare management **relate** to Juan's presentation? Which members of the healthcare team are **involved** in each area of management?

Written home care instructions

Fluids and nutrition

Medication

See general practitioner for follow-up

CONCEPT MAP 21.20 Discharge planning and coordination of care for Juan

Chapter 22: Cancer Care

CONCEPT MAP SEQUENCE FOR COLORECTAL CANCER (CRC)

Presentation

The patient presenting with CRC is Darby Fuller, a 78-year-old male. **Concept maps 22.1–22.5** explore Darby's presentation/admission.

PHx

Darby is a 78-year-old male who is presenting post a rectal bleed this a.m. Darby describes the bleed as 'bright red and a lot'. He reports infrequent defecation, with associated lower abdominal pain. He has a history of COPD, HTN and obesity.

Cues

1. What are your priorities with this patient?.
2. What is the significance of tachycardia post rectal bleeding?
3. What is the relationship between bleeding and anaemia?
4. What is the pathophysiological relationship between CRC and anaemia?
5. What are some concerns in relationship to the GIT assessment in this patient?
6. What physiological impact does tachypnoea, tachycardia and temperature have on the patient?
7. What investigative or diagnostic procedures do you think would be relevant for this patient?

ASSESSMENT

Primary survey
A: Patent
B: RR 24
C: Warm centrally
D: Alert
E: T 38 °C
F: IVT to commence, dark urine
G: BGL 6.2 mmol/L

Secondary survey
CNS: (E4 V5 M6 = 15, PEARLA 3 mm). Febrile @ 38 °C
PAIN: Abdo pain LLQ 6/10. Headaches infrequently.
CVS: HR 105 bpm, irregular and thready, NIBP 100/80 mmHg, ECG – sinus arrythmia

RESP: RR 24, patent airway – spontaneous breathing, SpO_2 90%
GIT: Nausea and vomiting, abdo tender in LLQ, BS on auscultation hypoactive. Faecal odour on breath. Blood in faeces reported.
RENAL (output): Pt reports no changes to habits. Dark, urine, await ward UA
SKIN/INTEG: Centrally warm, peripherally cooler. Skin intact, however, fragile
MUSCULOSKELETAL (mobility): strict RIB, with VTE prophylaxis
BMI: 31.0

CONCEPT MAP 22.1 Nursing assessment for Darby

DIAGNOSIS
CRC – likely in descending colon.

PLANNING

☑ Diagnostic tests – x-ray abdo, CT scan

☑ For theatre – for bowel resection +/- -ostomy

☑ Conservative treatment if the cancer has spread and is inoperable

☑ Write a Nursing Prioritisation Planner

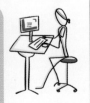

CONCEPT MAP 22.2 Diagnosis and planning for Darby

INTERVENTIONS

1. Assess bowel function

2. Assess pain, fluid balance and cardiovascular function regularly

3. ISBAR handover preparation for end-of-shift handover – what would you be handing over if your patient was due for theatre in 30 mins?

What further assessments should be initiated

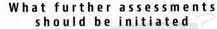

Cues
1. What specific preoperative requirements does Darby have?

2. What possible reasons would there be for the patient to report pain?

3. What has the bleeding been caused by?

CONCEPT MAP 22.3 Nursing interventions for Darby

EVALUATION

The medical team have been notified of Darby's decreasing blood pressure (90 mmHg systolic) and increasing HR – 120 bpm, irregular and weak.

Plan:

While Darby is being prepared for OT for a bowel resection, his vital signs deteriorate. He is yet to have the nasogastric tube (NGT) that was ordered inserted.

Cues

1. What interventions need to be considered now for Darby?

2. Does this deterioration relate to his presentation?

3. Why do you think an NGT is required?

4. If there was a delay in inserting the NGT, what impact do you think this could have had on Darby's pain?

CONCEPT MAP 22.4 Evaluation and planning for Darby

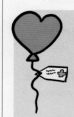

DISCHARGE PLANNING + COORDINATION OF CARE

How do the following areas of healthcare management **relate** to Darby's presentation?

Which members of the healthcare team are **involved** in each area of management?

Colorectal cancer (CRC)

Medication

BP monitoring

Follow-up review with oncologist and surgical team (general surgeon)

+/- ostomy formation

Keeping site clean – and assessing perfusion

Education about signs of localised infection

Reporting any increase in pain

Monitoring discharge – consistency, frequency, etc.

Cardiovascular compromise

Medication

Physiotherapy

Post-op ECG and follow up in community for BP measurement

CONCEPT MAP 22.5 Discharge planning and coordination of care for Darby

CONCEPT MAP SEQUENCE FOR LUNG CANCER

Presentation

Janice is a 55-year-old female who has had a cough lasting longer than three weeks and associated fatigue. She has a family history of lung cancer (father) and has been a passive smoker for 30 years. She has also worked in a diesel fitters' business for the past 25 years as the office manager. Janice has a diagnosis of COPD (asthma and emphysema) which was confirmed seven years ago.

Concept maps 22.6–22.10 explore Janice's admission.

 PHx

Janice, a 55-year-old female presents with increasing shortness of breath, associated with cough (different to normal COPD cough) for past month. Fatigue ++
Presents to medical centre.
PMHx – COPD, non-smoker, osteoporosis, TAH 10 years ago.

Cues

1. What are your priorities with this patient?
2. What is the significance of cap refill?
3. What is the relationship between chest pain, cough and hypoxia?
4. What is the pathophysiological relationship between COPD and lung cancer?
5. What are some concerns in relation to respiratory presentation of this patient?
6. What is the relevance of the warmth to one calf?
7. What investigative or diagnostic procedures would you think would be relevant for this patient?

 ASSESSMENT

Primary survey
A: Spontaneous, inc. WOB
B: RR 26
C: Poor perfusion
D: Alert
E: T 37.9 °C
F: HNPU
G: BGL 4.7 mmol/L

Secondary survey
CNS: E4 V5 M6 = 15 PEARLA 4 mm. T 37.9 °C
PAIN: c/o pain to chest 'tight' and shoulder pain – rated as 7/10, worse on deep inspiration
CVS: HR 110 bpm, regular. BP 150/90 mmHg. Centrally warm, centrally cyanotic and poorly perfused. cap refill >4 sec
RESP: RR 26 SpO$_2$ 88% RA, increased WOB, use of accessory muscles, pursed lip breathing, tripoding. Chest on auscultation, minimal air entry to bases, R=L, creps throughout midzones. Pt reports green sputum when able to expectorate.
GIT: SNT BS audible in all quadrants. BNO >3 days. BGL 4.7 mmol/L
RENAL (output): HNPU as yet
SKIN/INTEG: Poor integrity, poor peripheral perfusion. Nil skin tears. Clubbing. Left calf warmer than right.
MUSCULOSKELETAL (mobility): Strict RIB, with VTE prophylaxis – sit upright @ 45 degrees minimum
BMI: 22.4

CONCEPT MAP 22.6 Nursing assessment for Janice

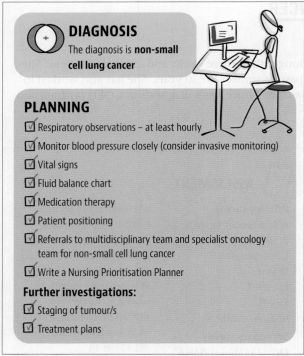

DIAGNOSIS

The diagnosis is **non-small cell lung cancer**

PLANNING

- ☑ Respiratory observations – at least hourly
- ☑ Monitor blood pressure closely (consider invasive monitoring)
- ☑ Vital signs
- ☑ Fluid balance chart
- ☑ Medication therapy
- ☑ Patient positioning
- ☑ Referrals to multidisciplinary team and specialist oncology team for non-small cell lung cancer
- ☑ Write a Nursing Prioritisation Planner

Further investigations:

- ☑ Staging of tumour/s
- ☑ Treatment plans

CONCEPT MAP 22.7 Diagnosis and planning for Janice

INTERVENTIONS

1 Assess pain, respiratory function, patient condition including psychosocial support.

2 ISBAR handover preparation for end-of-shift handover – what would you be handing over if your patient had increasing WOB and SOB? With SpO$_2$ <87%?

What further assessments should be initiated

Cues

1 What further questions or information would you like to know from Janice?

2 What is the deterioration here? How has the lung cancer been 'missed' for so long?

3 What possible reasons would there be for the patient to report pain in her chest and shoulder?

4 What could be the pathophysiological reason for pain and swelling to left calf?

CONCEPT MAP 22.8 Nursing interventions for Janice

EVALUATION

The medical team have been notified of Janice's increased WOB and SOB with associated hypoxia @ 86% SpO$_2$

Plan:

Medical officer has requested an arterial blood gas (ABG) analysis. While organising this test (it is not within RN scope at all facilities), Janice becomes anxious regarding her breathing, she is 'panicking' as she 'cannot breathe' and is worried 'that this will be my last few breaths'. She is only able to speak in words, not sentences.

Cues

1 What interventions need to be considered now for Janice? What is your priority here?

2 Does this newly diagnosed condition relate to the reason for presentation?

3 What do you think is the reason for this significant deterioration?

CONCEPT MAP 22.9 Evaluation and planning for Janice

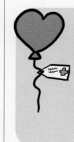

DISCHARGE PLANNING + COORDINATION OF CARE

How do the following areas of healthcare management **relate** to Janice's presentation? Which members of the healthcare team are **involved** in each area of management?

Non-small cell carcinoma/cancer

Medication

Oncology review and planning of care

Follow-up review with thoracic specialist or nurse practitioner – respiratory

Palliative care team if care is not curative

COPD

Medication

Physiotherapy

Occupational therapist to review home setting

Anxiety

Referral to psychologist and potentially psychiatrist, dependent upon patient's response

Patient education and 'coping' techniques

Breathing education and exercises

CONCEPT MAP 22.10 Discharge planning and coordination of care for Janice

Chapter 23: Chronic Disease Management

CONCEPT MAP SEQUENCE FOR HEART FAILURE AND PORTAL HYPERTENSION

Presentation

George Bouzounis is a 71-year-old retired builder that has been admitted to the emergency department (ED) with breathlessness for the last two hours. George has an audible wheeze and is producing frothy sputum. He has a history of hypertension, acute myocardial infarction, worsening heart failure and fatty liver disease.

Concept maps 23.1–23.5 explore George's presentation and admission.

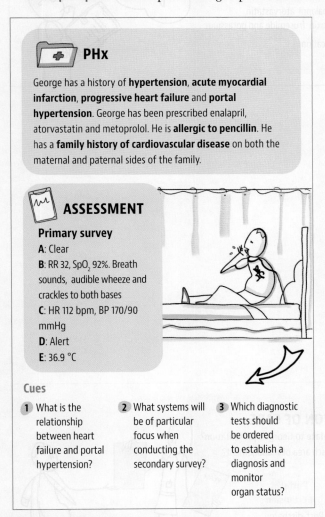

PHx

George has a history of **hypertension**, **acute myocardial infarction**, **progressive heart failure** and **portal hypertension**. George has been prescribed enalapril, atorvastatin and metoprolol. He is **allergic to pencillin**. He has a **family history of cardiovascular disease** on both the maternal and paternal sides of the family.

ASSESSMENT

Primary survey

A: Clear

B: RR 32, SpO₂ 92%. Breath sounds, audible wheeze and crackles to both bases

C: HR 112 bpm, BP 170/90 mmHg

D: Alert

E: 36.9 °C

Cues

1. What is the relationship between heart failure and portal hypertension?

2. What systems will be of particular focus when conducting the secondary survey?

3. Which diagnostic tests should be ordered to establish a diagnosis and monitor organ status?

CONCEPT MAP 23.1 Nursing assessment for George

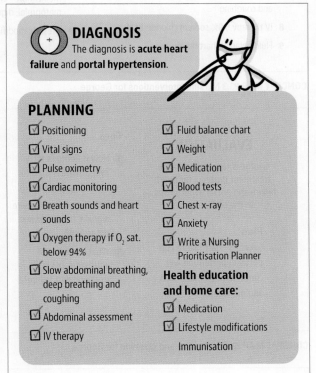

DIAGNOSIS

The diagnosis is **acute heart failure** and **portal hypertension**.

PLANNING

- ☑ Positioning
- ☑ Vital signs
- ☑ Pulse oximetry
- ☑ Cardiac monitoring
- ☑ Breath sounds and heart sounds
- ☑ Oxygen therapy if O₂ sat. below 94%
- ☑ Slow abdominal breathing, deep breathing and coughing
- ☑ Abdominal assessment
- ☑ IV therapy
- ☑ Fluid balance chart
- ☑ Weight
- ☑ Medication
- ☑ Blood tests
- ☑ Chest x-ray
- ☑ Anxiety
- ☑ Write a Nursing Prioritisation Planner

Health education and home care:

- ☑ Medication
- ☑ Lifestyle modifications

Immunisation

CONCEPT MAP 23.2 Diagnosis and planning for George

INTERVENTIONS

1 Positioning – Fowlers
2 Vital signs 4-hourly
3 Pulse oximetry 4-hourly
4 Cardiac monitor for arrhythmia detection
5 Breath and lung sounds assessment 4-hourly
6 Oxygen therapy if O$_2$ sat. below 94%
7 Slow abdominal breathing, deep breathing and coughing
8 IV therapy 0.9% sodium chloride 8/24
9 Fluid balance chart hourly

10 Medication enalapril, atorvastatin, metoprolol, digoxin, frusemide and potassium
11 Low fat and sodium diet
12 Relieve anxiety
13 Abdominal assessment

Health education and home care:

- Medication – enalapril, atorvastatin, metoprolol, digoxin, frusemide and potassium
- Lifestyle modification

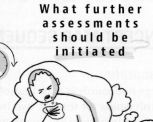

What further assessments should be initiated

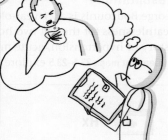

CONCEPT MAP 23.3 Nursing interventions for George

EVALUATION

George is responding to the treatment protocol for heart failure and portal hypertension in the cardiac ward.

Plan:

George's heart failure and portal hypertension will continue to be monitored and managed.

Cues

1 How is George's fatty liver disease related to portal hypertension?
2 Why does George require digoxin, frusemide and potassium?
3 What is the role of anticoagulants in treating heart failure?

CONCEPT MAP 23.4 Evaluation and planning for George

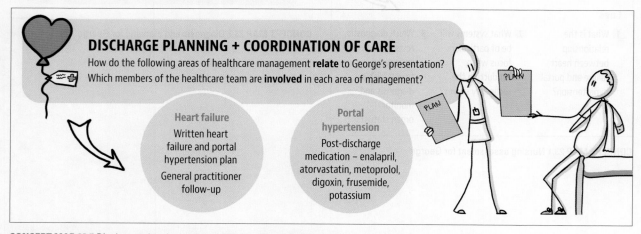

DISCHARGE PLANNING + COORDINATION OF CARE

How do the following areas of healthcare management **relate** to George's presentation? Which members of the healthcare team are **involved** in each area of management?

Heart failure
Written heart failure and portal hypertension plan
General practitioner follow-up

Portal hypertension
Post-discharge medication – enalapril, atorvastatin, metoprolol, digoxin, frusemide, potassium

CONCEPT MAP 23.5 Discharge planning and coordination of care for George

CONCEPT MAP SEQUENCE FOR CANCER OF THE LARYNX

Presentation

Chun Wong is a 49-year-old man who has been admitted to the respiratory ward for a laryngectomy and modified neck dissection. He has been a smoker for 25 years and developed hoarseness in the last three months. He has been diagnosed with cancer of the larynx and the cancer lesions are advanced so a total laryngectomy is required, but with a modified neck dissection. After Chun recovers from surgery, he will commence chemotherapy. Chun's wife is with him while you conduct his admission to the ward.

Concept maps 23.6–23.10 explore Chun's care in the respiratory ward.

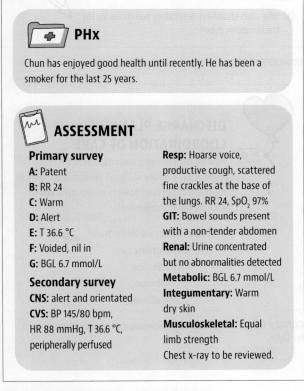

PHx

Chun has enjoyed good health until recently. He has been a smoker for the last 25 years.

ASSESSMENT

Primary survey

A: Patent
B: RR 24
C: Warm
D: Alert
E: T 36.6 °C
F: Voided, nil in
G: BGL 6.7 mmol/L

Secondary survey

CNS: alert and orientated
CVS: BP 145/80 bpm, HR 88 mmHg, T 36.6 °C, peripherally perfused

Resp: Hoarse voice, productive cough, scattered fine crackles at the base of the lungs. RR 24, SpO_2 97%
GIT: Bowel sounds present with a non-tender abdomen
Renal: Urine concentrated but no abnormalities detected
Metabolic: BGL 6.7 mmol/L
Integumentary: Warm dry skin
Musculoskeletal: Equal limb strength
Chest x-ray to be reviewed.

CONCEPT MAP 23.6 Nursing assessment for Chun

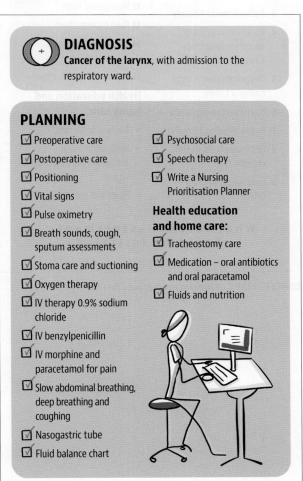

DIAGNOSIS

Cancer of the larynx, with admission to the respiratory ward.

PLANNING

- ☑ Preoperative care
- ☑ Postoperative care
- ☑ Positioning
- ☑ Vital signs
- ☑ Pulse oximetry
- ☑ Breath sounds, cough, sputum assessments
- ☑ Stoma care and suctioning
- ☑ Oxygen therapy
- ☑ IV therapy 0.9% sodium chloride
- ☑ IV benzylpenicillin
- ☑ IV morphine and paracetamol for pain
- ☑ Slow abdominal breathing, deep breathing and coughing
- ☑ Nasogastric tube
- ☑ Fluid balance chart
- ☑ Psychosocial care
- ☑ Speech therapy
- ☑ Write a Nursing Prioritisation Planner

Health education and home care:

- ☑ Tracheostomy care
- ☑ Medication – oral antibiotics and oral paracetamol
- ☑ Fluids and nutrition

CONCEPT MAP 23.7 Diagnosis and planning for Chun

INTERVENTIONS

Preoperative and postoperative care including:

1 Positioning – Fowlers

2 Vital signs – postoperative and then 4 hourly

3 Pulse oximetry 4 hourly

4 Breath sounds, cough, sputum assessments 4 hourly

5 Oxygen therapy – nasal prongs 4 L/min

6 Stoma suctioning hourly

7 Stoma dressing 4 hourly

8 IV therapy 0.9% sodium chloride 8/24

9 Benzylpenicillin 1.2 g QID IV

10 Morphine 1 mg/hr via PCA and paracetamol 1 g QID IV oral for pain

11 Slow abdominal breathing, deep breathing and coughing hourly while awake

12 Nasogastric tube

13 Fluid balance chart

14 Monitor for anxiety and depression

15 Liaise with speech therapy

Health education and home care:

- Tracheostomy care

- Medication – oral antibiotics and paracetamol 1 g prn

- Fluids and nutrition

What further assessments should be initiated

CONCEPT MAP 23.8 Nursing interventions for Chun

EVALUATION

Chun had a disturbed sleep as the stoma required frequent suctioning during the night.

Plan:
Consult with the respiratory surgeon today.

Cue

1 Why does Chun have respiratory secretions via the tracheostomy tube?

CONCEPT MAP 23.9 Evaluation and planning for Chun

DISCHARGE PLANNING + COORDINATION OF CARE

How do the following areas of healthcare management **relate** to Chun's presentation? Which members of the healthcare team are **involved** in each area of management?

Written home care instructions

Tracheostomy care

Medication

Nutrition

Chemotherapy

CONCEPT MAP 23.10 Discharge planning and coordination of care for Chun

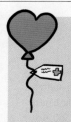

CONCEPT MAP SEQUENCE FOR CHRONIC OBSTRUCTIVE PULMONARY DISEASE (COPD)

Presentation

Victor Kostenko, a 71-year-old man, arrives via ambulance to the ED. His wife called for an ambulance as he became short of breath and restless. He has a barrel-shaped chest. He states that his sputum is green and the salbutamol has stopped working.

Concept maps 23.11–23.15 explore Victor's care in hospital.

 PHx

Victor, a 71-year-old male, is a long-term smoker. He has smoked cigarettes for the last 52 years, and is only smoking occasionally now as he finds it hard to completely give up smoking. Recently he has noticed that he has a cough mainly in the morning. While working in his shed he sometimes has to sit down and catch his breath. He has noticed that he has lost weight especially around his waistline. His GP diagnosed emphysema 12 months ago, and prescribed salbutamol.

 ASSESSMENT

Primary survey
A: Clear
B: RR 28, accessory muscle use, breath sounds diminished with widespread crackles, percussion hyper-resonant
C: HR 118 bpm, BP 162/88 mmHg. Breath sounds diminished, O_2 sat 92%
D: Alert and orientated
E: 37.9 °C

Secondary survey significant findings:
Chest x-ray reveals flat low diaphragm with lung hyperinflation

Pulmonary function tests show decreased tidal volume and vital capacity
Increased total lung capacity
Prolonged forced expiratory volume
Arterial blood gas reveals compensated chronic respiratory alkalosis – pH 7.26, PaO_2 79, $PaCO_2$ 57, HCO_3 – 27, O_2 sat 90%
Increased RBC and WBC count

CONCEPT MAP 23.11 Nursing assessment for Victor

 DIAGNOSIS

Emphysema. In short stay unit attached to the emergency department until respiratory ward bed available.

PLANNING

- ☑ Positioning
- ☑ Oxygen
- ☑ Vital signs
- ☑ Pulse oximetry
- ☑ Salbutamol 5 mg nebulised
- ☑ Prednisolone 40 mg oral daily
- ☑ Ceftriaxone 1 g daily IV
- ☑ Roxithromycin 300 mg daily oral
- ☑ Huffing
- ☑ Percussion and postural drainage every 8 hours
- ☑ Pursed lip breathing and abdominal breathing hourly
- ☑ Breath sounds
- ☑ Tests – Arterial blood gases and sputum
- ☑ Fluid balance chart
- ☑ Weigh daily
- ☑ Increasing mobility
- ☑ Family coping
- ☑ Write a Nursing Prioritisation Planner

CONCEPT MAP 23.12 Diagnosis and planning for Victor

INTERVENTIONS

1. Positioning: high Fowlers
2. Oxygen 2 L/min nasal prongs
3. Vital signs hourly
4. Pulse oximetry hourly
5. 5 mg salbutamol nebulised, reassessed at 20 minutes then hourly
6. Prednisolone 40 mg daily oral for 5 days
7. Ceftriaxone 1 g daily IV for 7 days
8. Roxithromycin 300 mg daily oral for 10 days
9. Huffing
10. Percussion and postural drainage every 8 hours
11. Pursed lip breathing and abdominal breathing hourly while awake
12. Breath sounds 8 hourly
13. Tests – arterial blood gases and sputum as needed
14. Fluid balance chart
15. Weigh daily
16. Increasing mobility
17. Family coping

What further assessments should be initiated

CONCEPT MAP 23.13 Nursing interventions for Victor

EVALUATION

Victor's response to therapy was noted by decreased breathlessness, decreased work of breathing and improved oxygen saturation.

Plan:

Transfer to the respiratory ward when a bed becomes available.

Cue

 What additional information can be given to Victor and his wife to provide health education while in the short stay unit to prepare them for transfer to the respiratory ward and then discharge to the home environment?

CONCEPT MAP 23.14 Evaluation and planning for Victor

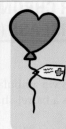

DISCHARGE PLANNING + COORDINATION OF CARE

How do the following areas of healthcare management **relate** to Victor's presentation? Which members of the healthcare team are **involved** in each area of management?

Medication – salbutamol puffer

Nutrition and hydration

Prevention – reduce respiratory tract infections, activity strengthening and respiratory hygiene

CONCEPT MAP 23.15 Discharge planning and coordination of care for Victor

GLOSSARY

A

abdominal aortic aneurysm

An enlargement of the aorta, the main blood vessel that delivers blood to the body, at the level of the abdomen.

acute myocardial infarction

An ischaemic event within a coronary artery that produces necrosis of myocardial cells.

addiction

Addiction is marked by a change in behaviour caused by the biochemical changes in the brain after continued substance abuse. Substance use becomes the main priority of the addict, regardless of the harm they may cause to themselves or others. An addiction causes people to act irrationally when they don't have the substance they are addicted to in their system.

altered mental health

A disruption in how the brain works that causes a change in behaviour.

anaemia

A condition in which the number of red blood cells or the haemoglobin concentration within them is lower than normal, and therefore a lowered ability of the blood to carry oxygen.

asthma

The inflammation of the airways, which results in bronchoconstriction, hyper-responsive airways and oedema.

atrial fibrillation

Disorganised atrial electrical activity which produces ineffective atrial contraction.

B

balanitis

An inflammation of the head of the penis and the foreskin. It can be caused by infection, irritation or an allergic reaction. Symptoms include redness, itching and soreness of the affected area. Hygiene is a big cause – more typical in younger boys.

benign prostatic hyperplasia (BPH)

A non-cancerous enlargement of the prostate gland that can cause difficulty urinating, frequent urination and weak urine flow. Common cause of UTI in older males.

best practice

Agreed approaches or procedures that are most effective and will provide best possible outcomes for those in your care.

bronchiolitis

A viral infection of the lungs, with inflammation of the airways and subsequent mucus build-up.

burn

Injury to skin and body tissue due to exposure to heat, radiation, chemicals, friction, cold exposure or electrical current.

C

cancer of the larynx

Malignant cells formation in the tissues of the larynx.

cataract

An opacity within the lens of the eye.

chlamydia

A sexually transmitted infection of the reproductive organs.

chronic kidney disease (CKD)

CKD is defined (as per Kidney Health Australia) as a 'Glomerular Filtration Rate of <60 mL/min/1.73 m2 that is present for >/= 3 months with or without evidence of kidney damage; or evidence of kidney damage without decreased GFR that is present for >/= 3 months as evidenced by any of the following: microalbuminuria, proteinuria, glomerular haematuria, pathological abnormalities (e.g. abnormal renal biopsy) or anatomical abnormalities (e.g. scarring on imaging or polycystic kidneys).

chronic obstructive pulmonary disease (COPD)

A chronic inflammatory lung disease that produces obstructed airflow in the airways of the lung.

cirrhosis

Fibrosis of the liver.

clinical decision making

The deliberate collection of information which is analysed and informs decisions in performing subsequent actions.

clinical judgement

Produces conclusions that provide direction for choosing specific actions.

clinical pathways

Standardised management plans that are evidence-based and are applicable to the multidisciplinary healthcare team.

closed head injury

A type of traumatic brain injury in which the skull and dura mater remain intact.

co-morbidities

The presence of one or more diseases; so if a patient has diabetes and hypertension, for example, these are co-morbidities when they present with chest pain.

complex

Complicated and intricate – in health care it relates to patients who have multiple conditions or diseases that impact upon the presenting condition.

concept maps

A graphic presentation of the linkage (relationships) of concepts (information) within a presentation (situation).

critical thinking

A cognitive process of analysing information to facilitate clinical judgement and clinical decision making.

cultural determinants of health

These centre on an Indigenous definition of health, concentrating on social and emotional wellbeing from which individuals, families and communities can draw strength, resilience and empowerment (World Health Organization).

D

deep vein thrombosis

Thrombus formation and inflammation within a deep vein in the lower extremities.

dependence

Usually refers to a physical dependence on a substance. Dependence is characterised by the symptoms of tolerance and withdrawal.

diagnostic overshadowing

The failure, when assessing an individual with multiple disabilities, to discern the presence of one disability because its features are attributed to another, primary disability (APA, https://dictionary.apa.org/diagnostic-overshadowing).

diverticulitis

Inflammation of the diverticulum that can result in peritonitis, perforation, fistula formation or even an abscess.

E

endometriosis

Deposits of endometrial-like tissue that develop within the pelvic cavity.

epididymitis

An inflammation of the epididymis, a small organ located at the back of the testicles that stores and carries sperm. It can be caused by an infection, injury or other underlying condition. Symptoms include pain and swelling in the testicles and fever. Typically caused by sexually transmitted infections (STIs).

erythroderma

Generalised inflammatory skin disease, usually associated with atopic dermatitis.

evidence-based practice

Approaches and procedures that have been validated by research findings.

F

fluid balance chart (FBC)

A chart used for calculating and recording the amount of fluid entering the body and comparing it to the amount of fluid leaving the body.

G

gallstones (cholelithiasis)

Calculi that are developed in the gallbladder and biliary duct.

glaucoma

The increased intraocular pressure within the eye, with or without symptoms, and produces optic nerve atrophy and reduction in the peripheral visual field.

H

haematoma

A collection (or pooling) of blood outside of blood vessels, usually due to trauma or injury.

heart failure

The heart is unable to pump an adequate flow of blood to meet the metabolic demands of cells within the body.

heart valve disease

A valve within the heart does not open or close effectively.

hepatitis

Inflammation of the liver.

hyperglycaemia

When the level of sugar in the blood is too high.

hysterectomy

The surgical removal of the uterus.

I

intoxication

The condition of having physical or mental control markedly diminished by the effects of alcohol or drugs.

intraoperative phase

It begins when the patient is transferred to the operating room and ends when the patient is transported to the recovery room for immediate postanaesthetic care.

M

Meniere's disease

An inner ear disease which is characterised by sudden episodic vertigo, tinnitus and fluctuating hearing loss.

mental health

Mental health includes our emotional, psychological, and social wellbeing. It affects how we think, feel, and act. It also helps determine how we handle stress, relate to others, and make choices.

mitral regurgitation

Where the mitral valve incompletely closes during systole and blood flows backward from the left ventricle to the left atrium.

N

neoplasm

An abnormal tissue mass that forms when cells divide or grow in abnormal ways.

nursing process

A systematic problem-solving tool for providing nursing care.

O

objective data

Measurable data that is not influenced by feelings or opinions. Objective data includes vital signs, laboratory findings and BGL.

otitis media with effusion

An infection of the middle ear with retained fluid and exudate.

P

PACU

Postanaesthetic care unit

pancreatitis

Inflammation of the pancreas.

person-centred care

Age-appropriate care that is underpinned by ethical and legal principles, and is negotiated with the person and their significant others in equal partnership with the nurse.

phimosis

A condition where the foreskin becomes trapped behind the head of the penis and cannot be returned to its original position. It can cause pain, swelling and difficulty with urination. Will require circumcision; it can be a surgical emergency due to the swelling of the glans.

pneumonia

The infection of lung bronchioles and alveoli, which produces exudate in the alveoli and reduces gas exchange and impacts on ventilation.

pneumothorax

The pleural space is breached and air enters the pleural space and lung inflation is decreased.

polycystic ovary syndrome

A hormonal disorder where there is an increased level of insulin and androgens.

portal hypertension

Increased blood pressure in the portal venous system.

postoperative phase

It begins when the patient is transferred to the ward and ends when the patient is safely discharged home.

preoperative phase

The patient is prepared for surgery.

pressure injury

Ischaemia of the skin and associated tissue due to external pressure that impedes circulation to the area.

priapism

A condition characterised by a prolonged and painful erection of the penis, lasting for several hours without sexual stimulation. It can be caused by various factors, including blood disorders, certain medications and injury to the penis. Management of priapism depends on the underlying cause and the duration of the erection. In cases of ischaemic priapism (low-flow priapism), which is caused by a buildup of blood in the penis that is not flowing out, the primary goal is to reduce the blood flow to the penis and alleviate the pain.

primary health care

The first step in a patient's care and is focused on health promotion, illness prevention, care of the sick, advocacy and community development.

problem solving

Involves identification of a problem by collecting data and identifying the cause, and then producing a solution to the problem.

prostate cancer

The most common cancer in men, it occurs when cells in the prostate gland begin to grow uncontrollably. Symptoms include difficulty urinating, blood in the urine, and pain in the lower back or pelvis.

R

RPAO

Routine postanaesthetic observation

S

sentinel event

An adverse patient safety event that was wholly preventable and results in serious harm to, or death of, a patient. They are the most serious incidents reported through state and territory incident reporting systems.

sinusitis

Involves one or more of the sinuses and is the inflammation of the mucous membranes within the sinus.

social determinants of health

The non-medical factors that influence health outcomes. They are the conditions in which people are born, grow, work, live and age, and the wider set of forces and systems shaping the conditions of daily life.

subjective data

Data obtained from a patient that is based on their feelings, views and experiences. Subjective data cannot be verified (e.g. pain rated as 9/10 cannot be 'checked').

substance use disorder

Disorders involving using too much alcohol, tobacco or other drugs; also known as substance abuse, substance dependence or addictions.

T

testicular cancer

A type of cancer that develops in the testicles (the male reproductive organs that produce sperm). Symptoms include a lump or swelling in the testicles, pain or discomfort and changes in the testicle shape or size. Usually occurs in younger males.

testicular torsion

A medical emergency that occurs when the spermatic cord, which provides blood flow to the testicle, becomes twisted. This can cause severe pain and swelling in the affected testicle, and if not treated quickly can lead to the loss of the testicle. Needs to be reversed within four hours.

tinnitus

The sensation of the person hearing a sound such as ringing, chirping, buzzing or roaring, and it is a sound that no other person can hear externally.

V

varicocele

A condition where the veins in the testicles become enlarged, causing discomfort and reducing fertility. Swelling is typically unilateral.

W

wound infection

An injury to external skin structure and/or body tissue which has become infected with a micro-organism.

INDEX